OXFORD MEDICAL PUBLICATIONS

Stroke Medicine

Published and forthcoming Oxford Specialist Handbooks

General Oxford Specialist Handbooks
Cardiopulmonary Transplantation and
    Mechanical Circulatory Support
Infection in the Immunocompromised Host
Pharmaceutical Medicine
Postoperative Complications, 2e
Prison Medicine and Health
Retrieval Medicine

**Oxford Specialist Handbooks in
    Anaesthesia**
Anaesthesia for Emergency Care
Global Anaesthesia
Obstetric Anaesthesia
Paediatric Anaesthesia
Regional Anaesthesia, Stimulation, and
    Ultrasound Techniques
Thoracic Anaesthesia
Vascular Anaesthesia

**Oxford Specialist Handbooks in
    Cardiology**
Adult Congenital Heart Disease
Cardiac Catheterization and Coronary
    Intervention
Cardiovascular Computed Tomography
Cardiovascular Imaging
Cardiovascular Magnetic Resonance
Echocardiography, 3e
Fetal Cardiology, 2e
Heart Disease in Pregnancy
Inherited Cardiac Disease, 2e
Nuclear Cardiology, 2e
Pacemakers and ICDs, 2e
Paediatric Cardiology
Pulmonary Hypertension
Valvular Heart Disease

**Oxford Specialist Handbooks in End
    of Life Care**
End of Life Care in Dementia
End of Life Care in Heart Failure
End of Life Care in Kidney Disease
End of Life Care in Respiratory Disease

**Oxford Specialist Handbooks in
    Neurology**
Parkinson's Disease and Other Movement
    Disorders, 2e
Stroke Medicine, 3e

**Oxford Specialist Handbooks in
    Obstetrics and Gynaecology**
Fetal Medicine

Obstetric Medicine
Urogynaecology

**Oxford Specialist Handbooks in
    Oncology**
Myeloproliferative Neoplasms
Practical Management of Complex Cancer
    Pain, 2e
Radiotherapy Planning

**Oxford Specialist Handbooks in
    Paediatrics**
Management of Childhood Infections:
    The Blue Book, 4e
Neurodisability and Community Child Health
Paediatric Dermatology, 2e
Paediatric Endocrinology and Diabetes, 2e
Paediatric Gastroenterology, Hepatology, and
    Nutrition, 2e
Paediatric Haematology and Oncology, 2e
Paediatric Intensive Care
Paediatric Nephrology, 3e
Paediatric Palliative Medicine, 2e
Paediatric Respiratory Medicine, 2e
Paediatric Rheumatology, 2e

**Oxford Specialist Handbooks in
    Psychiatry**
Eating Disorders
Forensic Psychiatry
Medical Psychotherapy

**Oxford Specialist Handbooks in
    Radiology**
Head and Neck Imaging
Interventional Radiology
Musculoskeletal Imaging
Thoracic Imaging

**Oxford Specialist Handbooks in
    Surgery**
Burns
Cardiothoracic Surgery, 2e
Colorectal Surgery, 2e
Current Surgical Guidelines, 2e
Gastric and Oesophageal Surgery
Hand Surgery
Oral and Maxillofacial Surgery, 3e
Otolaryngology and Head and Neck Surgery
Paediatric Surgery, 2e
Plastic and Reconstructive Surgery, 2e
Urological Surgery, 2e
Vascular Surgery, 2e

Oxford Specialist Handbooks in Neurology

Stroke Medicine

THIRD EDITION

Hugh Markus
Professor of Stroke Medicine
University of Cambridge, and Consultant Neurologist
Addenbrooke's Hospital, Cambridge, UK

Anthony Pereira
Consultant Neurologist
Department of Neurology
St George's Hospital, London, UK

Geoffrey Cloud
Professor of Stroke Medicine
Monash University, and
Consultant Stroke Physician
Alfred Hospital, Melbourne, Australia

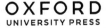

OXFORD
UNIVERSITY PRESS

OXFORD
UNIVERSITY PRESS

Great Clarendon Street, Oxford, OX2 6DP,
United Kingdom

Oxford University Press is a department of the University of Oxford.
It furthers the University's objective of excellence in research, scholarship,
and education by publishing worldwide. Oxford is a registered trade mark of
Oxford University Press in the UK and in certain other countries.

Published in the United States of America by Oxford University Press
198 Madison Avenue, New York, NY 10016, United States of America.

British Library Cataloguing in Publication Data
Data available

Library of Congress Control Number: 2025933832

ISBN 978–0–19–890626–1

DOI: 10.1093/med/9780198906261.001.0001

Printed and bound by
CPI Group (UK) Ltd., Croydon, CR0 4YY.

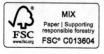

The manufacturer's authorized representative in the EU for product safety is Oxford
University Press España S.A., Parque Empresarial San Fernando de Henares, Avenida
de Castilla, 2 – 28830 Madrid (www.oup.es/en or product.safety@oup.com). OUP
España S.A. also acts as importer into Spain of products made by the manufacturer.

Preface to the Third Edition

Stroke has advanced rapidly since our last edition was published in 2017. It is an exciting time to be working in the field. Thrombectomy is now routine in stroke care. Advances are beginning to transform care for patients with intracerebral haemorrhage. The COVID-19 pandemic had an enormous impact on stroke care worldwide, not only because COVID-19 increases stroke risk, but also because of its impact on delivery of care. One positive consequence has been the increasing use of telemedicine to deliver care.

In this third edition we have completely revised and updated the text to take into account these, and many other, advances. We hope it will continue to provide a useful and easily accessible portable reference for both stroke trainees and specialists in their daily clinical practice.

Hugh Markus
Anthony Pereira
Geoffrey Cloud

Preface to the Second Edition

There have been major advances in the management of stroke since the last edition in 2010. These culminated in a series of trials, led by the MR CLEAN trial, showing that patients who had occlusion of the large cerebral vessels had a better outcome if treated with thrombectomy compared with intravenous thrombolysis. The past five years have also provided more data showing how the organization of stroke care can have a major impact on outcome. For example, centralizing care within London into eight hyperacute stroke units with direct ambulance transfer to these units resulted in an approximately 30% reduction in mortality. These are exciting times for stroke.

In this Second Edition we have completely revised and updated the text to take into account these and many other advances.

The First Edition received excellent feedback and we are grateful for all the helpful comments we received. We are grateful to Hannah Cock for contributing to the section on post-stroke epilepsy in this edition.

Hugh Markus
Anthony Pereira
Geoffrey Cloud

Preface to the First Edition

Recent years have seen a revolution in the profile of stroke. Often thought of as an untreatable disease we now realize that, not only can many strokes be prevented, but acute treatment can have a major impact on outcome. Organized care within stroke units markedly reduces mortality. Thrombolysis is transforming the way in which acute stroke services are organized. It is encouraging both the medical profession and the general public to think of stroke as a potentially treatable 'brain attack' requiring urgent diagnosis, transfer to hospital, and treatment. Recent data has shown that minor stroke and TIA are followed by a high risk of early recurrent stroke, much higher than previously appreciated. Preventing this early recurrence prevents major challenges in how we reconfigure services, and determine which early secondary prevention strategies are most effective.

These advances in stroke present many challenges in delivering services. In many countries stroke has been a 'Cinderella' specialty, and there have been few senior doctors specifically trained in stroke care. Specialists from geriatric medicine, neurology, and other disciplines are having to train themselves in hyperacute stroke management, and familiarize themselves with the many other advances in management which are required to deliver comprehensive stroke care. We will need many more stroke specialists in the future and this has led to the establishment of dedicated stroke training programmes, such as the UK Stroke Specialty training programme, and similar schemes in other countries.

Clinicians looking after stroke patients need rapid access to up-to-date practical information on how to look after stroke patients. We hope this textbook of stroke medicine will provide such a source. It is written by two neurologists and a stroke physician, who together run a busy district and regional stroke service. It is aimed to provide a ready source of information for both stroke trainees and consultants. It is written to cover the syllabus of the UK stroke specialist training programme and other similar programmes worldwide.

Hugh Markus
Anthony Pereira
Geoffrey Cloud

Preface to the First Edition

Hugh MacKenzie
Anthony Pereira
Geoffrey Cloud

Contents

Contents

Symbols and abbreviations

ACA	Anterior cerebral artery	DSA	Digital subtraction angiography
ADC	Apparent diffusion coefficient	DVLA	Driver Vehicle Licensing Authority
AF	Atrial fibrillation	DWI	Diffusion-weighted imaging
AHA	American Heart Association	DWP	Department of Work and Pensions
AI	Artificial intelligence	EDV	End-diastolic velocity
ANH	Artificial nutrition and hydration	EPA	Enduring Power of Attorney
ASL	Arterial spin labelling	ESR	Erythrocyte sedimentation rate
ASPECTS	Alberta Stroke Programme Early CT score	ESUS	Embolic stroke of undetermined source
AVM	Arteriovenous malformation	FES	Functional electrical stimulation
BMA	British Medical Association		
BMET	Brief Memory and Executive Test	FLAIR	Fluid-attenuated inversion recovery
BMI	Body mass index	GAS	Goal attainment scaling
BMT	Best Medical Treatment	GCS	Glasgow Coma Score
BP	Blood pressure	GDB	Goal-directed behaviour
CAA	Cerebral amyloid angiopathy	GDP	Gross domestic product
CADASIL	Cerebral autosomal dominant arteriopathy with subcortical infarcts and leucoencephalopathy	GDS	Geriatric Depression Scale
		GE	Gradient echo
		GOM	Granular osmiophilic material
		GWAS	Genome-wide association scan
CART	Combination anti-retroviral therapies	HADS	Hospital Anxiety and Depression Scale
CBF	Cerebral blood flow	HDL	High-density lipoprotein
CBV	Cerebral blood volume	HRT	Hormone replacement therapy
CCD	Cognitive communication disorder		
		HSP	Hemiplegic shoulder pain
CCM	Cerebral cavernous malformations	ICA	Internal Carotid artery
		ILAE	International League Against Epilepsy
CDU	Carotid duplex ultrasound		
CNS	Central nervous system	ILR	Implantable loop recorder
COC	Combined oral contraceptive	IMCA	Independent Mental Capacity Advocate
CPSP	Central post-stroke pain		
CSF	Cerebral spinal fluid	INR	International normalized ratio
CT	Computed tomography	IPC	Intermittent pneumatic compression
CTA	Computed tomography angiography		
		KCT	Kaolin cephalin time
CTIMP	Clinical trials of investigational medicinal products	LA	Lenticulostriate artery
		LACI	Lacunar infarct
CVT	Cerebral venous thrombosis	LDL	Low-density lipoprotein
DALY	Disability-adjusted life-years	LMIC	Low- and middle-income countries
DOAC	Direct-acting oral anticoagulants		
		LMWH	Low-molecular-weight heparin
DoLS	Deprivation of Liberty Safeguards		

LOC	Level of Consciousness	PFO	Patent foramen ovale
LPA	Lasting Power of Attorney	PICA	Posterior interior cerebral artery
LVO	Large vessel occlusion	PSD	Post-stroke depression
MCA	Mental Capacity Act	PSF	Post-stroke fatigue
MCA	Middle cerebral artery	PSV	Peak systolic velocity
MCS	Minimally conscious state	PVR	Post-voiding residual
MELAS	Mitochondrial encephalopathy with lactic acidosis and stroke-like	RCT	Randomized controlled trial
		RCVS	Reversible cerebral vasoconstriction syndrome
MoCA	Montreal Cognitive Assessment	RF	Radio frequency
MR	Magnetic resonance	RIG	Radiologically Inserted Gastrostomy
MRA	Magnetic resonance angiography	RoPE	Risk of Parodoxical Embolism
MRI	Magnetic resonance imaging	SLT	Speech and language therapy
MRS	Magnetic resonance spectroscopy	SNP	Single nucleotide polymorphism
MRV	MR venography	STICH	Supratentorial lobar intracerebral haematomas
MTT	Mean transit time	SVD	Small-vessel disease
NHANES	National Health and Nutrition Examination survey	SWI	Susceptibility-weighted imaging
NIHSS	NIH Stroke Scale	TACI	Total anterior circulation infarct
NINDS	National Institute for Neurological Disorders and Stroke	TENS	Transcutaneous electrical nerve stimulation
		TFNE	Transient focal neurological episodes
NMDA	N-methyl-D-aspartate	TIA	Transient ischaemic attack
NSF	Nephrogenic systemic fibrosis	TXA	Tranexamic acid
OR	Odds ratio	VA	Vertebral artery
OSA	Obstructive sleep apnoea	VASES	Visual Analogue Self-esteem Scale
OT	Occupational therapy	VCI	Vascular cognitive impairment
PAN	Polyarteritis nodosa	VOR	Vestibulo-Ocular Reflex
PDOC	Prolonged disorders of consciousness	VS	Vegetative state
PEG	Percutaneous endoscopic gastrostomy	WBC	White blood cell count
		WHO	World Health Organization
PEJ	Percutaneous endoscopic jejunostomy	WMH	White matter hyperintensities
PET	Positron emission tomography		

Chapter 1

Epidemiology and stroke risk factors

Introduction

- Stroke is common. Someone suffers a stroke every 5 minutes in the UK, every 40 seconds in the USA, and every 3 seconds worldwide.
- Every year over 12.2 million people throughout the world suffer a stroke and 5 million are left significantly disabled with an estimated 100 million people globally living with the effects of stroke.
- The most recent Global Burden of Disease (GBD) 2019 stroke burden estimates showed that stroke remains the second leading cause of death and the third leading cause of death and disability combined.
- The estimated global cost of stroke is over US$891 billion (1.12% of the global GDP).
- From 1990 to 2019, the burden (in terms of the absolute number of cases) increased substantially (70.0% increase in incident strokes, 43.0% deaths from stroke, 102.0% prevalent strokes) with the bulk of the global stroke burden (86.0% of deaths) residing in lower-income and lower-middle-income countries (LMICs).
- The lifetime risk of stroke has also increased over the last 20 years by 50%—and is now one in four people.
- One-quarter of strokes are recurrent events.
- Because stroke is such a common disease, preventative interventions which have only a small benefit to individual patients can have a large population benefit.
- Approximately 8 of 10 strokes are avoidable through a combination of stopping smoking, increasing exercise, reducing obesity, reducing blood pressure (BP), and improving diet.

Definitions for epidemiological studies

Stroke

- A standardized definition of stroke is vital for epidemiological studies.
- The World Health Organization (WHO) definition of stroke dates from 1970 and has been used for most studies and defines stroke as:
  'Rapidly developing clinical signs of focal (or global) disturbance of cerebral function, with symptoms lasting 24 hours or longer, or leading to death, with no apparent cause other than of vascular origin'.
- This definition *includes* ischaemic stroke, intracerebral haemorrhage, and subarachnoid haemorrhage. It *excludes* transient ischaemic attack (TIA), subdural haematoma, and haemorrhage or infarction secondary to tumour or infection.
- More recently the ICD 11 has incorporated the results of imaging in the definition—so that evidence on brain imaging of acute infarction or haemorrhage, even if symptoms last less than 24 hours is diagnosed as stroke (see Box 1.1).

Transient ischaemic attack

- Stroke symptoms which last less than 24 hours are termed TIA.
- In the new ICD 11 definition if there is an infarct or haemorrhage on brain imaging then it would be diagnosed as stroke and not TIA.
- One should not think of TIA as an independent entity but rather a very short-lived stroke—that does not leave a 'footprint' of acute ischaemia or haemorrhage on acute brain imaging.

About 15% of strokes are preceded by a TIA

Box 1.1 Cerebrovascular disease categories and definitions (selected) in the ICD-11

Stroke

Cerebral ischaemic stroke

Definition: acute focal neurological dysfunction caused by focal infarction at single or multiple sites of the brain or retina. Evidence of acute infarction may either come from
a) symptom duration lasting more than 24 hours
b) neuroimaging or other technique in the clinically relevant area of the brain

Intracerebral haemorrhage

Definition: acute neurological dysfunction caused by haemorrhage within the brain parenchyma or in the ventricular system

Subarachnoid haemorrhage

Definition: acute neurological dysfunction caused by subarachnoid haemorrhage

Stroke not known if ischaemic or haemorrhagic

Definition: acute focal neurological dysfunction lasting more than 24 hours (or lead to death in less than 24 hours), but subtype of stroke (ischaemic or haemorrhagic) has not been determined by neuroimaging or other techniques

Transient ischaemic attack*

Definition: a transient episode of focal neurological dysfunction caused by focal brain or retinal ischaemia without acute infarction in the clinically relevant area of the brain or retina. Symptoms should resolve completely within 24 hours

Cerebrovascular disease with no acute cerebral symptom*

- Silent cerebral infarct (defined as an infarct demonstrated on neuroimaging or at autopsy that has not caused cute dysfunction of the brain)
- Silent cerebral microbleed
- Silent white matter abnormalities associated with vascular disease (defined as abnormalities in the cerebral white matter of proven or assumed vascular origin)

* Categories not classified as 'stroke'

Stroke subtyping

- The definition of stroke does not differentiate between haemorrhagic and ischaemic stroke or between subtypes of ischaemic stroke
- Brain imaging is required to differentiate between haemorrhagic and ischaemic stroke
- Ischaemic stroke subtyping has been attempted using the following classifications.

Clinical classifications

These rely on clinical features and were introduced before the widespread availability of brain and cerebral vascular imaging. The most used is the Oxfordshire Community Stroke Project Classification (OCSP, Table 1.1). The OCSP:

- is simple and easy to apply
- relates to prognosis and is useful to look at case mix between populations
- does not differentiate pathophysiological subtypes well, for example, the OCSP stroke syndrome may not match the identified infarct (e.g. a lacunar infarct (LACI) frequently turns out to be caused by a non-lacunar infarct, such as a small cortical infarct or a striatocapsular infarct)
- is less suited to look at the pathological process causing the stroke, and the risk factor profiles for different stroke subtypes.

Pathophysiological classifications

Here the results of additional investigations are taken into account before identifying a pathophysiological subtype of stroke. For example, brain imaging may show a cortical infarct, the Doppler may show 80% stenosis due to atherosclerotic plaque, and the echocardiogram (echo) and electrocardiogram (ECG) may be normal. This stroke is then classified as a large-artery atherosclerotic infarct.

Table 1.1 Oxfordshire community stroke project classification

Stroke type	Symptoms/presentation
LACI (lacunar infarct) Outcome = sometimes good	Pure motor or pure sensory stroke or a combination of motor and sensory (sensorimotor) or ataxic hemiparesis
TACI (total anterior circulation infarct) Outcome = usually poor	Motor and/or sensory deficits which affect the arm, leg and face in at least two areas and hemianopia (visual problems) and higher cerebral dysfunction such as dysphasia
PACI (partial anterior circulation infarct) Outcome = varied	Any two components of a TACI or isolated cerebral dysfunction, which are more restrictive than in a LACI classification
POCI (posterior circulation infarct) Outcome = varied	Symptoms of brainstem dysfunction or hemianopia (isolated)

Reproduced from *Lancet*, 337(8756), Bamford J, Sandercock P, *et al.*, Classification and natural history of clinically identifiable subtypes of cerebral infarction, p. 1521, Copyright (1991), with permission from Elsevier.

Pathophysiological classifications:
- are aimed at identifying the causes of individual subtypes
- need intensive investigation (e.g. extracranial and ideally intracranial cerebral artery imaging, echo, etc. if they are to provide useful data)
- may not identify a mechanism even if the patient is fully investigated (approximately 25% of strokes remain of unknown cause).

The most used is the Trial of Org 10172 in Acute Stroke Treatment (TOAST) study, which was a 7-year, randomized, double-blind, placebo-controlled, multicentre study of 1281 acute stroke patients in 36 centres across the USA, sponsored by the National Institute of Neurological Disorders and Stroke (NINDS).

Trial of Org 10172 in Acute Stroke Treatment (TOAST) classification

The TOAST classification denotes five subtypes of ischaemic stroke:
1. Large-artery atherosclerosis
2. Cardioembolism
3. Small-vessel occlusion
4. Stroke of other determined aetiology
5. Stroke of undetermined aetiology
6. Stroke caused by more than one potential cause

The original TOAST classification:
- Divided most causes into probable and possible. However, many clinicians use only one category for both probable and possible when using it clinically or for research
- Used risk factors in the definition of subtype, e.g. hypertension for lacunar stroke. This is often not applied, particularly in studies looking at risk factor profiles, as it will, of course, exaggerate the role of hypertension as a risk factor for lacunar stroke.

Incidence and prevalence

Incidence is the number of new cases of stroke per annum in a population.

Prevalence is the total number of patients who have had a stroke at any time within a population.

Very useful reference figures on global stroke incidence and prevalence can be obtained from the World Stroke Organization: Global Fact Sheet 2025. ℘ https://doi.org/10.1177/17474930241308142

Stroke incidence

Stroke incidence is probably under-reported for several reasons:
- Owing to the limitations of epidemiological studies using the WHO clinical definition alone.
- The fact that not all stroke patients go to hospital.
- Stroke diagnosis may not be recorded in those individuals who die shortly after stroke onset (brain imaging is required to confirm a diagnosis of stroke).
- There are few reliable estimates of incidence in developing countries.

Globally there are 2.2 million new stroke per year, and one in four people over 25 will have a stroke in their lifetime.

There are large geographical differences in age-standardized stroke incidence (6-fold), mortality (15-fold), and prevalence (4-fold), with the highest rates in LMICs (particularly in Eastern Europe, Asia, and Sub-Saharan Africa).

In most high-income countries, the incidence of stroke overall has been reducing over the last two decades, although the risk in young individuals (<55 years) has not shown the same decrease. For example, over 20 years or more of prospective study in Oxford (UK), incorporating both OCSP and OXVASC, incidence seems to have fallen by about a third (other estimates have UK stroke incidence falling by 19% from 1990 to 2010). This is thought to be due principally to a reduction in levels of hypertension and smoking within the population, and the introduction of statin and antiplatelet therapy for primary prevention of those with vascular risk factors. In LMICs this decrease is not being seen, and in many stroke incidence is increasing.

The Global Burden of Disease Study 2021 identified studies published between 1990 and 2019. It concluded that although age-standardized rates of stroke mortality have decreased worldwide in the past two decades, the absolute number of people who have a stroke every year, stroke survivors, related deaths, and the overall global burden of stroke (disability-adjusted life-years (DALYs) lost) are great and increasing.

Stroke prevalence

- In the UK, there are over 1 million stroke survivors and over half are dependent on others for everyday activities, with 300 000 living with significant disability from their stroke
- In the USA, there are over 7.8 million survivors (approximately 3.1% of the total population).

- A global increase in stroke prevalence is now being seen driven by LMICs, with 89% of global death and disability combined occurring in LMICs.
- Stroke affects people of all ages but is age related. Prevalence under 55 years in the US and Australia is 1% compared with 12–16% in those aged over 80 years. Generally, stroke is more common in men than women.
- The latest Global Burden of Disease Study on stroke, published in 2021, reported that between 1990 and 2019 there was an 85% rise in prevalence of stroke survivors, 70% increase in all strokes, and a 43% increase in the number of deaths due to stroke.

Stroke mortality

- Estimates of stroke mortality are more robust than those of incidence as minor (almost always non-fatal) strokes are more easily missed than major ones
- Within Europe, there is a fivefold gradient of increased stroke mortality, from France and Switzerland with the lowest mortality rates to Russia and the former Soviet bloc with the highest. This difference is mainly determined by **socioeconomic factors**. About 66% of the variance can be ascribed to the amount of gross domestic product (GDP) countries spend on stroke care. GDP is not the whole story, however, as countries such as Norway with high GDP spent on stroke care still have relatively increased stroke mortality rates in comparison to other countries such as France
- Overall, rates of stroke mortality are:
  - decreasing in Western Europe
  - increasing in Eastern Europe
  - seem to have 'bottomed out' in both the USA and Japan
- Stroke mortality is falling in the UK (30-day mortality has fallen from approximately 1 in 4 to 1 in 8), but still 25% of people die within a year of stroke—with case fatality twice as high in patients aged over 85 as those below 65 years
- Early stroke mortality is frequently reported at 30 days and should always be adjusted for case mix, especially age, stroke severity (e.g. NIHSS) and stroke sub-type (e.g. haemorrhagic vs. ischaemic). Atrial fibrillation-related stroke is also associated with increased 30-day mortality

The economic cost of stroke care

- Acute stroke care in England is responsible for 6% of all NHS expenditure
- More recent estimates of the total aggregated annual cost of UK care published in 2020 (incorporating post-acute care costs) show the total has risen to £26 billion (NHS £3.4 billion, 13%; Personal Social Services £5.2 billion, 20%; unpaid care £15.8 billion, 61%; lost productivity £1.6 billion, 6%) (Table 1.2)
- The cost of stroke in the USA was estimated in 2020 to be $78 billion and is expected to rise to $208 billion by 2030 (Fig. 1.1)
- Over one-quarter of strokes occur in people of working age (18-65yrs)
- Cerebrovascular disease is also the second commonest cause of dementia, is the commonest cause of late-onset epilepsy, and a major cause of depression, compounding the healthcare economic burden of stroke
- In an ageing population, the incidence, prevalence, and cost are all set to rise

Table 1.2 Aggregate cost (£ million) of incident and prevalent stroke in the UK: base, high, and low case estimates

	Mean aggregate cost base case estimates[‡]	Mean aggregate cost, high estimates	Mean aggregate cost, high estimates[‡]
Incident and prevalent stroke cost			
NHS	3404	3298	3510
Formal social care	5181	4695	5668
Unpaid care	15 828	12 811	18 845
Lost productivity	1555	913	2196
NHS & PSS perspective	8586	8066	9105
Societal perspective	25 970	21 792	30 148

[‡]Low- and high-cost estimates based on range of mean cost.

Adapted from Patel et al. (2020) Age Ageing 49: 270–276.

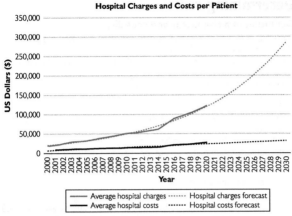

Fig. 1.1. Mean hospital charges and costs per stroke patient in the USA from 2000 to 2020 with trend forecasts to 2030

Reproduced from Alexis Iorio, Carlos Garcia-Rodriguez, Ali Seifi; Two Decades of Stroke in the United States: A Healthcare Economic Perspective. Neuroepidemiology 2 April 2024; 58 (2): 143–150. https://doi.org/10.1159/000536011. Copyright © 2024, Silverchair publisher.

Determining risk

Definition of a risk factor and causality

A risk factor for stroke is a characteristic which, when possessed by an individual, increases their liability to suffer a stroke.

Such an association does not necessarily imply causality. Causality depends upon a number of factors, including:

- biological and epidemiological plausibility
- a temporal sequence between risk factor and stroke
- the strength of the association
- the reproducibility and consistency of the association in different studies and populations
- independence from confounding factors
- the demonstration that reduction or treatment of that risk factor reduces stroke risk.

Absolute and relative risk

Absolute risk is the risk of developing a disease in a given population in a given time. For example, in the population of patients aged over 60 who have atrial fibrillation, their risk of suffering a stroke is 5% per year. Therefore, their absolute annual risk of stroke is 5%.

The absolute risk will be affected by treatment. In the population of atrial fibrillation patients aged over 60 years treated with warfarin, the risk of stroke is about 2% per annum. Therefore, treating the person with warfarin reduces their absolute risk to approximately 2%.

The absolute risk reduction is simply 5% minus 2%, making 3%. Therefore, warfarin reduces the absolute risk of stroke by 3% per annum. The patient on warfarin now has a 2% risk of stroke compared to the 5% they would have had untreated, i.e. 40% of the original risk. This is their relative risk. Their risk has gone down from 100% of the absolute risk to 40% of the absolute risk, i.e. a relative risk reduction of 60%.

Therefore, relative risk can be thought of as the ratio of the absolute risk in the population with the risk factor to the absolute risk in the control population without the risk factor.

Relative risk = absolute risk in risk population/absolute risk in control population

If the relative risk is greater than 1, then the risk factor increases stroke risk. If the relative risk is less than 1 then the 'risk factor' is actually protective.

Population-attributable risk

This describes the overall contribution a risk factor makes to stroke disease burden. The population-attributable or absolute risk is the proportion of disease for which the risk factor accounts.

This greatly depends on the prevalence of the risk factor in the population. This can be illustrated with hypertension. For example, elevation of systolic BP to greater than 180 mmHg confirms a greatly increased relative risk of stroke, which is much greater than the relative risk of stroke owing to a BP in the range 160–180 mmHg. However, such marked elevations of BP are rare, while more modest elevations are much more common.

Therefore, the population absolute risk associated with a BP elevation in the range 160–180 is greater than that due to BP elevation of greater than 180 mmHg.

Number needed to treat

The absolute risk allows a calculation for the number needed to treat. This is the number of patients needed to treat to prevent one additional bad outcome. It is calculated from the absolute risk reduction. It gives a good idea of the benefit of a treatment and is a simple and honest way to present the potential benefit of a treatment to a patient.

In the earlier example, treating patients aged over 60 years old who are in atrial fibrillation with warfarin reduces their risk of stroke by 3% per year:

- Therefore, treating 100 patients per year would save 3 from having a stroke
- Therefore, treating 33 patients per year would save 1 from having a stroke
- Therefore, the number needed to treat per year is 33 to prevent 1 stroke.

Alternatively:

- The absolute risk reduction is 3% per year
- Therefore, the absolute risk reduction would be 30% after 10 years
- Now, treating 100 people for 10 years would save 30 strokes
- Therefore, treating 3.3 people for 10 years would save 1 stroke
- Therefore, the number needed to save 1 stroke is 3.3 (for 10 years).

Odds ratio versus relative risk

Relative risk is used in prospective cohort studies, or prospective clinical trials to indicate the increased risk associated with a specific risk factor.

In cross-sectional (non-prospective) studies, the odds ratio (OR) is used instead to indicate the increased risk associated with a risk factor.

The difference is illustrated by the following example.

Consider the question: Does smoking cause stroke?

This can be answered in two ways:

1. It could be done by prospectively following up a whole population of people and identifying the smokers and non-smokers and see who develops stroke during follow-up. The absolute risk of having a stroke if you smoked and the absolute risk if you didn't could be calculated, and then the relative risk could be worked out. An easy concept but the downside of this is that it would take a long time (many years) to perform the study. This is because the population incidence of stroke is fairly low and a large number of patients and/or many years of follow-up are required to obtain sufficient endpoints (strokes)

2. Alternatively, a cohort of stroke patients could be collected who have been seen over a shorter period and how many of them smoked could be determined. This calculation would give the risk of being a smoker in an individual stroke population; it would not give the absolute risk of having a stroke from smoking. This sort of study is called a cross-sectional case-controlled study. It is relatively easy to do but does not allow relative risk calculation. Instead, it provides the OR.

Therefore, the OR is used because:
- it can be used in case-controlled studies
- it is relatively easy to manipulate mathematically
- it can be corrected for confounding variables in logistic regression models.

It may be possible to examine several other risk factors which produce different ORs. You could then look at the particular risk factor of interest and correct for all the others (logistic regression analysis) to see which risk factors are independent risk factors.

Let us use Table 1.3:
- The odds of having the risk factor if the patient suffered a stroke are 20:30, i.e. 2/3 (0.66)
- The odds of having the risk factor if the person didn't suffer a stroke are 10:40, i.e. 1/4 (0.25)
- The OR is 0.66/0.25, i.e. 2.64. An OR of greater than 1 suggests the risk factor plays a part in causing the stroke. Note this is *not* a relative risk of 2.64.

Table 1.3 Example of how to calculate an odds ratio (OR)

		The outcome (e.g. stroke event)	
		+	−
Risk factor exposure	+	a	B
	−	c	D
		a/c Odds of being exposed in cases	b/d Odds of being exposed in controls
		OR = a/c --- b/d	
		Stroke	
		Yes	No
	Risk factor	20	10
	No risk factor	30	40

Stroke risk factors

Risk factors for stroke: general considerations

Population-based prospective studies
- The most reliable identification of stroke risk factors comes from prospective cohort studies such as the Framingham Study.
- These give true population-based estimates and avoid referral bias.
- Stroke subtyping and characterization is often suboptimal because stroke cannot all be investigated in one hospital but may occur in the community or present to remote hospitals.
- Even in large prospective studies, the number of strokes during the follow-up period may be small.

Case–control studies
- Allow much more detailed evaluation of each individual stroke in a standardized fashion than population-based studies.
- Allow better differentiation between different stroke subtypes.
- However, they are subject to potential bias, both in patient and case-control selection.

In many studies, particularly population-based ones, there has been little or no division of stroke into cerebral haemorrhage and ischaemia, let alone any division of ischaemia into its different pathogenic subtypes. Because most strokes are due to infarction, most of these studies primarily tell us the risk factors for infarction rather than haemorrhage.

Because a large number of ischaemic strokes are related to the complications of atherosclerosis (e.g. carotid stenosis, embolism secondary to myocardial infarction, atrial fibrillation secondary to coronary heart disease), these studies have similar risk factor profiles to those of coronary heart disease. However, there do seem to be some differences, particularly in the importance of different risk factors for coronary heart disease and stroke.

More recent studies have included imaging, allowing differentiation of different stroke subtypes; this suggests that the risk factor profile of the different subtypes may vary.

A further problem with the population studies is that frequently the diagnosis of stroke is obtained from hospital records or death certification. Both may be unreliable.

Specific stroke risk factors

Many have been proposed and they are best thought of in terms of *modifiable* and *non-modifiable* risk factors for stroke. See Table 1.4.

Table 1.4 Risk factors for stroke

Non-modifiable	Modifiable
Older age	*Major—well described and/or most important:*
Male sex	Socioeconomic class
Ethnicity	Air pollution
Genetic predisposition	Obesity
	Physical inactivity
	Smoking
	Alcohol
	Hypertension
	Diabetes and metabolic syndrome
	Cholesterol
	Previous stroke or TIA
	Atherosclerosis
	Atrial fibrillation
	Structural cardiac abnormalities
	Minor—less well described and/or less important:
	Diet
	Homocysteine
	Recreational drug use
	Sleep-disordered breathing
	Thrombophilia
	Inflammation
	Infection
	Migraine
	Oral contraceptive pill use
	Hormone replacement therapy
	Other drugs

Non-modifiable stroke risk factors

Age

- Stroke incidence increases exponentially with age
- Each decade above 55 years leads to a doubling of stroke risk
- Under the age of 50, incidence of stroke is evenly represented between haemorrhagic and ischaemic subtypes, but the former declines with age, leaving an overall majority of 85% of all strokes being ischaemic in origin
- The lifetime risk of suffering stroke if a person lives to 85 years is approximately 1 in 4 for a man and 1 in 5 for a woman.

Gender

- Male sex confers an increased risk of ischaemic stroke (relative risk about 1.3 compared to female)
- Although stroke risk is higher in men than in women, more women die from stroke owing to their greater life expectancy
- Overall, women have more severe stroke, more significant stroke disability, and more post-stroke depression and dementia
- There is no clear genetic basis to explain the gender difference and the excess risk in men is less than that seen in ischaemic heart disease.

Ethnicity

There are ethnic differences in both stroke incidence and the relative frequency of stroke subtypes.

Black people

In the USA, relative risk of stroke is highest in Black Americans, who also have increased stroke mortality compared to Mexican Americans and white Americans. The CDC (℅ https://www.cdc.gov/mmwr/) estimated prevalence of stroke in the US in 2022 is:

- 5.3% American Indian or Alaska Native
- 4.3% Black Americans
- 2.8% Mexican Americans
- 2.7% white Americans

In the UK, data from the South London Stroke register have suggested the following:

- Incidence rates of first-ever stroke adjusted for age and sex are twice as high in Black people compared to white people
- This excess incidence cannot be accounted for by differences in social class in the age group 35–64 years
- Black people tend to have their first stroke at a younger age than white people
- Small-vessel cerebrovascular disease (lacunar stroke) and intracranial atherosclerosis are more common in Black than white patients
- In contrast, extracranial large-artery disease is less common in Black people
- Hypertension is common and often severe and this contributes to the small-vessel disease risk but does not explain it fully
- However, in general, Black patients in a south London population with first-ever stroke were more likely to survive than white patients (the

exceptions being in those aged <65 years and those with a prior Barthel score <15). This is likely to be related to their ischaemic stroke subtype which is mainly subcortical small volume stroke—as opposed to large-vessel atherosclerotic or cardioembolic stroke—associated with generally larger volume, cortical infarcts.

East Asian people
- Stroke is reportedly more common in East Asian countries, although with marked geographical variation within the region
- Northern China has an increased incidence of stroke of the order of 80% compared to white Americans, Japan (39%), and Taiwan (23%). Stroke is the second leading cause of death in China, Korea, and Taiwan, third in Japan and Singapore, sixth in the Philippines, and tenth in Thailand
- Stroke in patients of Chinese ethnic origin often has a greater incidence of intracranial atherosclerotic stenoses and primary haemorrhage (especially subarachnoid haemorrhage) compared to white European populations. A similar increase in these subtypes is found in Japan
- Multivariate analysis has suggested that hypertension is a more important risk factor in East Asian populations compared to white Americans but does not explain the variation in stroke incidence within the geographical region.

South Asian people
- South Asian people (from India, Pakistan, and Bangladesh) also have increased incidence of stroke
- In the UK, South Asian immigrants have particularly high levels of diabetes (sixfold greater than the rest of the population) and seem to have a predominantly small-vessel form of cerebrovascular disease
- Interestingly, South Asian people studied in Singapore have predominantly intracranial large-vessel stenoses as a cause of stroke.

Genetic predisposition
- Twin and family studies suggest that genetic factors contribute to the risk of stroke, although the degree of risk they contribute is uncertain.
- Having a first-degree family member with a history of stroke before the age of 65 is associated with a twofold increased risk of ischaemic stroke. Genetic predisposition to stroke may act either directly through vascular risk factors with their own genetic basis (e.g. hypertension and diabetes), independently of such factors or by modulating the effect of risk factors.
- Genetic factors are believed to be primarily polygenic (multiple genes having small effects) with interaction with environmental and other risk factors.
- In the past, many studies looked at genetic variants (polymorphisms) in candidate genes as risk factors. Results have been conflicting largely due to studies being underpowered. New chip technology allows screening of as many as 1 million or more single nucleotide polymorphisms (SNPs) spanning the whole chromosome in a genome-wide association scan (GWAS).

- Recent GWASs have identified a number of novel genetic associations with stroke. These are associated with odds ratios of 1.1–1.4. Most are associated with only one subtype of ischaemic stroke (large vessel, cardioembolic, or lacunar), emphasizing that different stroke subtypes have distinct pathophysiology.
- Methods can be applied to the GWAS chip data to derive heritability estimates for stroke and its subtypes, which provide further evidence that genetic predisposition is important in stroke.
- The differences in stroke mortality rates between, for example, eastern and western Europe, suggest that potentially modifiable factors may be more important than genetic differences for stroke susceptibility.
- The results of migrant studies also support this view. Japanese populations in the USA experience rates of stroke similar to the American white host population rather than to the indigenous Japanese population in Japan. However, it is likely that there are complex interactions between genetic and environmental influences, and environmental influences may only increase the risk of stroke in those with pre-existing genetic susceptibility.

Major modifiable stroke risk factors

Socioeconomic class

- Low socioeconomic class is associated with increased stroke risk
- Stroke mortality across Europe significantly correlates with GDP (a surrogate for the economic status of the country).

Air pollution

- Air pollutants include carbon monoxide, ozone, nitrous oxides, sulphur dioxides, and small particulate matter or PM (a mix of solid and liquid aerosol nanoparticles from fossil fuel combustion—measured as less than 10, 2.5, and 1 μm). Diesel exhaust fumes are rich in PM 2.5, for example.
- Both long (months to years) and short-term exposure to these pollutants increase ischaemic stroke risk and mortality (and other vascular and lung diseases). Possible mechanisms mediating this include the effects of exposure on vascular tone, endothelial function, inflammation, atherosclerosis, and thrombosis.
- Most studies have come from developed/high-income countries—with little evidence from Africa or the Middle East, where there are known high air pollution levels.
- Although the relative risk of air pollution and stroke is small at an individual level (but higher in those with otherwise increased stroke risk) due to the ubiquitous nature of air pollution the exposure is great and so the net effect at a population level is high. In the 2019 GBD Stroke Collaboration report it was estimated to be responsible for 16% of all stroke-related DALYs (see Fig. 1.4).

Obesity

- Obesity is associated with increased stroke risk, but much of this may be via other risk factors such as hypertension and diabetes
- There have been no trial data to demonstrate weight reduction reduces stroke risk, but weight reduction has been shown to reduce systolic BP by about 4 mmHg for every 5 kg reduction. Obesity also closely relates to type 2 diabetes

Evidence for obesity to be a risk factor is divided:

For:
- The Whitehall study showed that body mass index (BMI) was predictive of stroke in both smokers and non-smokers
- Increased weight seems to be associated with an increased stroke risk in a dose–response fashion. In the Korean Medical Insurance Corporation Study, adjusted relative risk for all stroke was approximately 1.04.

Against:
- Much of the association between BMI and stroke is reduced when confounding variables such as hypertension, diabetes, smoking, and exercise are taken into account. Therefore, obesity may not be an independent risk factor but be increasing via these risk factors
- In multivariate analysis that controls for other vascular risk factors, the relationship between obesity and stroke is attenuated but persists.

Physical inactivity

A sedentary or inactive lifestyle is an independent risk factor for stroke. At least 30 minutes of moderate exercise—such as continuous walking three times a week—has been shown to reduce the risk of recurrent stroke.

The mechanisms for this may include:

- improved risk factor (e.g. hypertension, diabetes) control
- an increase in plasma tissue plasminogen activator activity
- an increase in high-density lipoprotein (HDL) concentrations
- a decrease in fibrinogen levels and platelet activity.

Smoking

- The risk of ischaemic stroke in smokers is twice that of non-smokers
- The risk of haemorrhagic stroke in smokers is between two and four times higher than that of non-smokers
- Increased stroke risk is halved within 2 years of cessation and almost back to baseline within 5 years of smoking cessation.
- The INTERSTROKE Study estimated a global population-attributable risk of stroke of 12.4% associated with current smoking.

The mechanisms by which smoking increases stroke risk include:

- increased fibrinogen levels
- increased platelet aggregation
- increased haematocrit
- decreased HDL levels
- decreased blood vessel compliance
- increased inflammation, promoting atherosclerosis.

E-cigarettes and vaping have become common among young adults and as a tobacco-smoking substitute for those trying to give up. As well as nicotine, e-cigarettes and vapes cause propylene glycol and/or vegetable glycerine to be inhaled and enter the bloodstream, causing not only lung but also endothelial damage. The risk relationship with stroke remains uncertain, and epidemiological studies are in progress.

Alcohol

- Alcohol excess can increase stroke risk in a number of ways:
  - increasing hypertension
  - increasing large-vessel atherosclerotic cerebrovascular disease through dyslipidaemia
  - causing atrial fibrillation and cardiomyopathy, which may produce cardioembolic ischaemic stroke
  - causing a pro-atherogenic low-grade inflammatory response
- Earlier studies suggested a J-shaped curve, with a protective effect of small amounts of alcohol but it is now thought this was an artefact and there is a linear relationship between alcohol intake and stroke
- Binge drinking causes surges in BP and is particularly associated with increased haemorrhagic stroke risk

Hypertension

Hypertension is the strongest risk factor for all stroke. The relationship between risk of stroke and degree of hypertension is approximately linear

BP and risk of first stroke

7 prospective observational studies: 843 events, 405,500 individuals

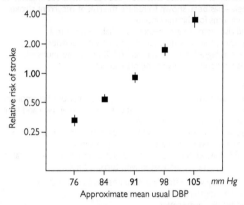

Fig. 1.2 Blood pressure and risk of first stroke.

Reproduced from *Lancet*, 335(8692), MacMahon S, Peto R, Cutler J, et al. Blood pressure, stroke, and coronary heart disease: Part 1, prolonged differences in blood pressure: prospective observational studies corrected for the regression dilution bias, pp. 765–774, Copyright (1990), with permission from Elsevier.

(Fig. 1.2). There is a similar association with high BP and premature death from stroke (Fig 1.3a).

- Increasing BP is strongly and independently associated with both ischaemic and haemorrhagic stroke.
- There appears to be no threshold BP below which the stroke risk plateaus, at least not over the normal range of BPs studied from 70 to 100 mmHg diastolic.
- The proportional increase in stroke risk associated with a given increase in BP is similar in both sexes and almost doubles with each 7.5 mmHg increase in diastolic BP.
- Although there are less data on the relationship between stroke and systolic BP, the association may be even stronger than for diastolic BP. Even 'isolated' systolic hypertension, with a normal diastolic BP, is associated with increased stroke risk.
- Approximately 40% of strokes can be attributed to a systolic BP of more than 140 mmHg.
- The causal nature of the relationship is strongly supported by the results of randomized controlled trials demonstrating that stroke can be prevented by treating BP this was seen most dramatically in the PROGRESS study where lowering BP in patients with conventionally 'normal' BP after stroke produced an almost 30% reduction in recurrent stroke incidence over 5 years.
- Optimal BP-lowering targets need to be individualized but the SPRINT study showed a reduction in cardiovascular disease (CVD) events in those

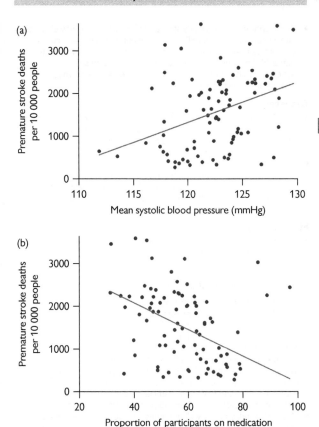

Fig. 1.3 a–b Graphs showing the linear relationship between blood pressure and premature stroke deaths.

Reproduced from *Lancet Global Health*, 10(8), Queran Lin *et al.*, Hypertension in stroke survivors and associations with national premature stroke mortality: data for 2.5 million participants from multinational screening campaigns, e1141–e1149. Available Open Access.

patients treated to a target of systolic BP below 120 mmHg compared to below 140 mmHg—but at a 'cost' of increased adverse events.
- Hypertension increases the risk of ischaemic stroke, both by promoting large-vessel atherosclerosis and intracranial small-vessel disease. It has been shown to be strongly associated with carotid stenosis, carotid plaque, and carotid intima–media thickness demonstrated using carotid ultrasound.

- Hypertension is a particularly strong risk factor for small-vessel disease with leukoaraiosis. About 80–90% of patients with lacunar stroke and leukoaraiosis have hypertension. It is also strongly related to white matter MRI hyperintensities in community populations.
- Hypertension is the major risk factor for cerebral haemorrhage and is most often associated with subcortical haemorrhage.

Diabetes

- Type 2 diabetes is associated with a relative risk of stroke in the order of 2–2.5 (and up to a six-times increase in some populations)
- Diabetes is a risk factor for carotid atherosclerosis and small-vessel cerebrovascular disease
- Aggressive BP control reduces stroke risk in diabetics
- The role of tight glycaemic control is still unproven in hyperacute stroke. In secondary prevention, glycosylated haemoglobin (HbA_{1c}) levels of 7% or lower are associated with reduced microvascular complications but no clear reduction in stroke.

Metabolic syndrome

- This is defined by the American Heart Association (AHA) as the presence of three or more of the following:
  - Elevated waist circumference:
    - Men ≥102 cm (40 inches)
    - Women ≥88 cm (35 inches)
  - Elevated triglycerides: ≥150 mg/dL (1.7 mmol/L)
  - Reduced HDL ('good') cholesterol:
    - Men <40 mg/dL (1.0 mmol/L)
    - Women <50 mg/dL (1.3 mmol/L)
  - Elevated BP: >130/85 mmHg
  - Elevated fasting glucose: ≥100 mg/dL (5.6 mmol/L).
- The WHO modified the definition to include hyperinsulinaemia
- Metabolic syndrome is highly prevalent in the USA: from the US National Health and Nutrition Examination survey (NHANES), it is estimated that over 37% (124 million) of Americans have it.
- Metabolic syndrome is a well-described risk factor for coronary and cardiovascular disease, but the relationship to stroke is as yet unclear.

Hypercholesterolaemia

- Increased total cholesterol and low-density lipoprotein (LDL) cholesterol are strong risk factors for ischaemic heart disease, while high levels of HDL cholesterol appear to be protective. The relationship to stroke appears to be weaker.
- This may be partly due to most studies including both haemorrhagic and ischaemic stroke. Those studies looking at ischaemic stroke separately have shown a similar relationship to that seen for ischaemic heart disease. In contrast, some studies have suggested low cholesterol levels increase cerebral haemorrhage risk.
- Reducing cholesterol with statin therapy reduces stroke in patients with established coronary disease (LIPID, WOSCOPS), patients at risk of

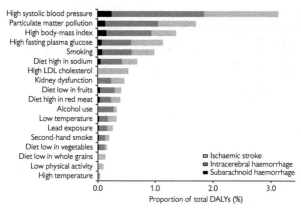

Fig. 1.4 Proportion of DALYs attributable to risk factors by pathological type of stroke for both sexes combined.

Reproduced with permission from 2019 GBD Stroke Collaborators Report on Stroke (2021) *Lancet Neurology*, 10: 785–820. Copyright © 2021 Elsevier.

stroke (ASCOT, HPS, HOPE-3), people with normal cholesterol but raised CRP (JUPITER), and those with symptomatic stroke disease (SPARCL).

- The HPS and JUPITER study showed a reduction in stroke even in those individuals with conventionally 'normal' cholesterol levels.
- SPARCL is the only randomized controlled trial to date which has taken a treatment group of stroke patients to assess the effect of statin treatment; it showed a 2.2% absolute risk reduction in all stroke with atorvastatin (see ➲ p. 274).
- Statin therapy has been shown to reduce carotid intima-media thickness and plaque in prospective studies and therefore, could be expected to be more effective in preventing stroke in large-artery stroke—a subgroup analysis from the SPARCL trial suggests this may be the case.
- No statin therapy trial has shown a definite increase in intracerebral bleeding as a side effect, but the benefit of statin therapy in reducing recurrent haemorrhagic stroke is uncertain.
- There is still doubt about the role of cholesterol reduction in the very elderly to reduce stroke risk alone. Some studies have suggested statins may increase ICH risk, but others have suggested a reduction in stroke risk.

Previous TIA/stroke

The recurrent stroke risk after TIA is highest in the first few days after TIA, making TIA a powerful predictor/risk factor for future stroke.

A risk stratification tool to identify individuals at high early risk of stroke after TIA has been developed between groups in California and Oxford. It is called the ABCD² score and is a derivation of the ABCD score (see Table 1.5).

- **A** (Age); 1 point for age ≥60 years
- **B** (Blood pressure ≥140/90 mmHg); 1 point for hypertension at the acute evaluation
- **C** (Clinical features); 2 points for unilateral weakness, 1 for speech disturbance without weakness
- **D** (Symptom duration); 1 point for 10–59 minutes, 2 points for ≥60 minutes
- **D** (Diabetes); 1 point.

Total scores range from 0 (lowest risk) to 7 (highest risk).
Stroke risk at 2 days, 7 days, and 90 days:
- Scores 0–3: low risk
- Scores 4–5: moderate risk
- Scores 6–7: high risk.

ABCD^2 is not a diagnostic score but a risk stratification score. To use it properly, first make a diagnosis then calculate the score. It is usefully predictive only for a few days.

Early (7-day) risk of stroke stratified according to ABCD^2 score at first assessment in the OXVASC TIA patient cohort

Atherosclerosis
- Atherosclerosis is associated with stroke because:
  - it may be the cause of the stroke itself, usually by artery-to-artery embolism
  - it is a marker of systemic atherosclerosis
- Therefore, risk factors for stroke are:
  - cardiac atherosclerosis (myocardial infarction, angina, or other ischaemic heart disease)
  - peripheral vascular atherosclerosis (e.g. intermittent claudication)
  - aortic atherosclerosis.

Table 1.5 Seven-day risk of stroke stratified according to ABCD^2 score at first assessment in the OXVASC validation cohort of patients with probable or definite TIA

	Patients (%)	Strokes (%)	% risk (95% CI)
ABCD2 score			
≤ 1	2 (1%)	0	0
2	28 (15%)	0	0
3	32 (17%)	0	0
4	46 (24%)	1 (5%)	2.2 (0–6.4)
5	49 (26%)	8 (40%)	16·3 (6.0–26.7)
6	31 (16%)	11 (55%)	35.5 (18.6–52.3)
Total	188 (100%)	20 (100%)	10.5 (6.2–14.9)

Reproduced from *Lancet*, 369(9558), Johnston SC, Rothwell PM, Nguyen-Huynh MN *et al.*, Validation and refinement of scores to predict very early stroke risk after transient ischaemic attack, pp. 283–292, Copyright (2007), with permission from Elsevier.

Results Published from the REACH registry (multicentre international database of 68 000 patients with either three or more risk factors for atherothrombosis or established coronary disease or stroke) suggest that stroke patients with concomitant peripheral vascular disease have twice the absolute risk of vascular death, myocardial infarction, or recurrent stroke at 1 year—emphasizing the need to consider global vascular risk in stroke patients.

Asymptomatic internal carotid artery stenosis
- The annual risk of stroke from an asymptomatic atherosclerotic internal carotid (ICA) stenosis of >50% is between 1% and 2.0% and the 5-year risk of ipsilateral stroke in 70-99% stenosis is in the order of 5–15% over 5 years.
- The risk of major complications (stroke/death) from carotid endarterectomy (CEA) in asymptomatic patients is about 3% in good units
- Two large prospective trials (ACAS and ACST) have shown a significant relative risk reduction in stroke (approximately 40%). However, due to the lower risk of stroke, the absolute risk reduction and overall population benefit is small (see ➲ Chapter 10)
- To make the benefit of operation easier to understand and more palatable, the statistics can be presented in a different way. Therefore:
  - 50 patients need to be treated to prevent one stroke over 2 years
  - 20 patients need to be treated to prevent one stroke over 5 years
  - 10 patients need to be treated to prevent one stroke over 10 years
  - 5 patients need to be treated to prevent one stroke over 20 years
  - The numbers needed to treat are approximately doubled when only disabling stroke is considered, which is probably most relevant for the patient
- The stroke risk in medically treated carotid stenosis appears to have fallen since the trials suggesting the benefit of operation may be even less (see ➲ Chapter 10, p. 297 for more on this topic).

Atrial fibrillation (AF)
- AF is the most common cause of cardioembolic stroke.
- Present in 5–6% of the population, it increases exponentially with age, with recent population studies suggesting a prevalence of over 20% in men over 80 years old (see Fig. 1.5).
- Paroxysmal or intermittent AF (PAF) has a similar associated stroke risk to persistent AF. Improved technology at detecting PAF has shown it to be very prevalent, particularly when sought post-stroke, where it may be identified in up to 23% of patients. As well as 24-hour Holter monitors and extended ambulatory Holter monitoring, implantable loop recorder (ILR) devices can be used to diagnose PAF. The question of how long a duration of AF is significant in the setting of PAF is also controversial but most authorities would accept an episode of 30 seconds or more to be relevant.
- The risk of first stroke in a patient aged >60 with AF is 5% per year.
- In a patient with stroke and AF the future stroke risk is 12% per year.

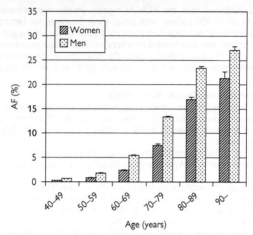

Fig. 1.5 Prevalence of atrial fibrillation (AF) in the general population in relation to age and sex.

Reproduced from *Stroke*, 44(11), Bjorck S *et al.*, Atrial fibrillation, stroke risk, and warfarin therapy revisited: a population-based study, pp. 3103–3108, Copyright (2013), with permission from Wolters Kluwer Health, Inc.

- AF causes over one-third of strokes in the over 80s—mainly large intracranial artery occlusions or striatocapsular infarcts.
- Consequently, patients with stroke due to AF tend to have severe neurological deficits and high associated mortality.
- Anticoagulation with warfarin to an international normalized ratio (INR) target 2.5 (range 2.0–3.0) has been shown to be superior in preventing stroke in comparison to aspirin, with a 60–70% relative risk reduction compared to 21% for aspirin alone. Direct-acting oral anticoagulants (DOACs) have shown similar benefits with improved safety compared to warfarin (see ➔ p. 289).
- In people aged under 60 years with non-valvular or 'lone' AF and no other vascular risk factors, the risk is lower, and aspirin alone is recommended as primary prevention.
- The risk of stroke in newly diagnosed AF can be estimated by using the CHA_2DS_2-VASc score (see Table 10.5, p. 290).

Structural cardiac abnormalities

Cardiomyopathy and ventricular thrombus

- Ischaemic or other forms of dilated cardiomyopathy can lead to mural thrombus within the left ventricle and cardioembolic stroke
- Following anterior myocardial infarction, mural thrombus may be managed by anticoagulation to prevent cardiac embolism. Where there is poor ventricular remodelling, a large akinetic segment or persistent reduced ejection fraction, long-term anticoagulation should be considered

- The incidence of stroke in heart failure patients seems to be inversely proportional to cardiac ejection fraction. There is, however, no randomized controlled trial evidence to date to support long-term anticoagulation over antiplatelet treatment in those patients in sinus rhythm with <30% ejection fraction.

Patent foramen ovale (PFO)

- PFO is caused by a failure of opposition of the two halves of the interatrial septum, resulting in more of a patent tract or tunnel than a 'hole in the heart' (see Fig. 1.6). This creates a potential communication between the left and right heart. Owing to high left-sided pressure, this usually has no physiological effect. However, if the defect is sizeable during a procedure such as 'Valsalva', where the right-sided atrial pressure increases above that of the left, venous blood from the right heart can mix with arterial blood on the left.
- PFO is a common normal variant, usually of no clinical significance. It is present *in utero*, allowing blood from the right side of the heart to cross to the left side. This allows oxygenated blood to pass from the mother's placenta to the arterial tree. In most cases, it closes at birth but fails to do so in between 17% and 35% of the general population.
- Evidence suggests it is a risk factor for stroke but only of minor significance on its own. PFO is present in about 22% of the population but in about 44% of an age-matched population with cryptogenic stroke. However, where the inferior interatrial septum is hypokinetic or floppy and tends to 'bow' or 'balloon' (so-called atrial septal aneurysm

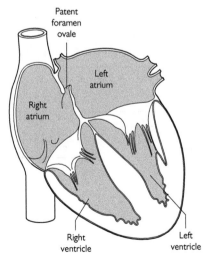

Fig. 1.6 Anatomy of a patent foramen ovale (PFO).

or ASA), a clot may form in the right atrium or in the ASA itself and the presence of PFO then leads to left-sided cardiac arterial embolism of the thrombus resulting in stroke.
- Although PFO and septal defects were originally only thought to be an issue in younger patients with apparent cryptogenic stroke, a recent study has identified that there is an increased prevalence in older (over 55 years) cryptogenic stroke patients, and cardiac embolism may in fact be the cause of stroke in this patient group too.
- Recent randomized controlled trials of transcatheter device closure against medical treatment have shown convincing benefit of intervention over medical treatment alone in stroke patients up to the age of 65 yrs, especially in 'high risk' PFOs where there is an associated aneurysmal interatrial septum and a large resting 'shunt'.
- High-risk PFO can best be assessed using such ECHO characteristics in combination with the Risk of Paradoxical Embolism (RoPE) score—which has been validated in the major RCTS of PFO closure— CLOSURE-I, RESPECT, and the PCT trial. High risk is associated with a RoPE score of 7 or more (low is less than 7); see Table 1.6.

Table 1.6 Risk of paradoxical embolism (RoPE) score calculator

Patient characteristic	Points
NO history of hypertension	+1
NO history of diabetes	
NO history of TIA stroke	+1
Non-smoker	+1
Cortical infarct on imaging	+1
Age (years)	
18–29	+5
30–39	+4
40–49	+3
50–59	+2
60–69	+1
~0 or older	+0
Total RoPE score	0–10

Minor modifiable stroke risk factors

Diet

- Numerous cohort studies have confirmed an inverse association between fruit/vegetable intake and stroke incidence and mortality
- Other studies have found that low potassium intake and low serum potassium are associated with increased stroke mortality. Potassium and magnesium supplementation and diets high in fibre may reduce stroke risk. In an 8-year study of 44 000 men, these factors were found to reduce risk of stroke by 38%
- Cross-sectional and case–control studies have generally shown an inverse association between consumption of fish and fish oils and stroke risk. In the Nurses Health Study, a significant decrease in the risk of thrombotic stroke (relative risk, 0.49; 95% confidence interval, 0.26–0.93) was observed among women who ate fish at least twice a week compared to women who ate fish less than once per month, after adjustment for age, smoking, and other cardiovascular risk factors. No association was observed between consumption of fish or fish oil and haemorrhagic stroke
- Salt ingestion is related to high BP and restriction of dietary salt intake can produce falls in BP in the region of 10 mmHg or more.
- The role of the gut microbiome is of current interest in prevention of cardiovascular health and reduced gut microbiome diversity is seen more prominently in stroke patients than healthy controls, and is associated with worse outcome. Studies are ongoing both in primary prevention of stroke and heart disease and in early stroke care.

Current 'healthy eating recommendations' for stroke risk prevention include the following:
- At least five portions of fruit and vegetables daily
- Six servings of grains daily
- 30 g fibre daily
- Limited salt (<3 g daily)
- Limited saturated fats and cholesterol
- Twice-weekly servings of oily fish, such as tuna or salmon.

Hyperhomocysteinaemia

- Very high levels of serum homocysteine occur in the autosomal recessive condition homocystinuria, and are associated with an increased risk of stroke and other arterial thrombosis at an early age
- Considerable evidence suggests more modestly elevated homocysteine is associated with an increased stroke risk in the general population
- This association could act via multiple mechanisms, including impaired endothelial function, promoting atherogenesis and increasing thrombosis
- Meta-analysis of genetic association studies of genes increasing homocysteine supports a causal relation between homocysteine and stroke
- Homocysteine levels are under both genetic and dietary control

- A number of enzymes control its synthesis, including methylene tetrahydrofolate reductase (MTHFR) (see Fig. 1.7)
- Low vitamin B_{12} and, to a greater extent, low folate levels are associated with high homocysteine levels
- Folate supplementation reduces homocysteine levels
- Raised homocysteine can be treated. Once vitamin B_{12} deficiency has been excluded, oral vitamin B compound (incorporating vitamins B_6 and B_{12}) and folic acid 5 mg are given
- Although there is evidence that high homocysteine contributes to stroke risk, two trials (VISP and VITATOPS) looking at vitamins to reduce homocysteine levels showed no significant benefit, although there was a possible benefit in the lacunar stroke subgroup in VITATOPS.
- A primary prevention trial in China found vitamin therapy to reduce homocysteine reduced stroke risk in previously stroke-free hypertensive individuals
- Elevated homocysteine appears to be a particularly strong risk factor for small-vessel disease stroke.

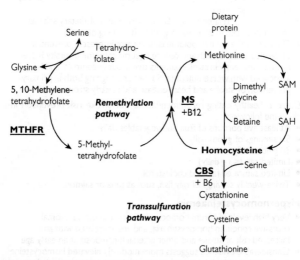

Fig. 1.7 Schematic diagram of homocysteine synthesis.

Sleep-disordered breathing/obstructive sleep apnoea (OSA)

- OSA is very common among stroke patients (estimated at 50–75%)
- OSA probably has a small effect in increasing the risk of stroke
- Stroke often occurs during sleep (up to one in three strokes) and there is controversy over whether snoring and OSA have a causative association with stroke

- OSA has been associated with hypertension and increased cardiovascular events
- OSA can also cause reduced cerebral autoregulation, blood hypercoagulability, and also arrhythmias can occur during periods of oxygen desaturation
- A recent observational study suggested that independent of age, sex, and established stroke risk factors, patients with established OSA have an increased relative risk of stroke of 2 compared to controls
- Successful treatment of OSA can reduce BP and there is emerging evidence to suggest that stroke risk may also be reduced
- Treating OSA with continuous positive airway pressure (CPAP) has shown some functional benefits in previously untreated stroke patients with OSA.

Inflammation and C-reactive protein

- Highly sensitive C-reactive protein (hs-CRP) is an assay of one of the acute phase proteins released by the liver that increase during systemic inflammation.
- Raised CRP has been associated with atherosclerosis in both coronary and carotid arteries, although much of this association disappears after conventional risk factors are accounted for.
- A level of hs-CRP of 3 mg/L or above is thought to be high risk for atherosclerotic disease. Levels of greater than 10 mg/L usually have non-cardiovascular causes excluded (autoimmune, cancer, infection, and other causes of inflammation).
- It has been suggested that testing CRP levels in the blood may be an additional way to assess cardiovascular and stroke risk, although there is currently no evidence to support this as a screening test.
- CRP may be predictive of recurrent stroke and survival after stroke.
- However, the prognostic significance of a CRP rise after stroke is not clear.
- Atherosclerosis can be thought of as a chronic inflammatory process, which may be accelerated by systemic inflammation of which hs-CRP is a marker. Increasing evidence suggests that some conventional risk factors may increase atherosclerosis via inducing a chronic pro-inflammatory state. These include smoking, alcohol excess, and obesity (adipose tissue secretes cytokines).
- Recent trials have shown drugs that reduce inflammation (such as colchicine and canakinumab, a therapeutic monoclonal antibody targeting interleukin-1β), reduce recurrent events in coronary artery disease, where the major pathology is atherosclerosis. Whether such anti-inflammatory approaches have a similar therapeutic effect in secondary prevention of ischaemic stroke is being investigated.

Infections

(HIV infection is covered on ➔ p. 350. and COVID-19 on p. 348)
  Infections may cause stroke in two possible ways:

1. Acute infection precipitating acute stroke
Case–control studies have found that recent infections (within 7 days) are more common in stroke patients. They may induce a hypercoagulable state and/or endothelial dysfunction.

2. Chronic infection and inflammation and atherosclerosis

Cytomegalovirus (CMV), *Chlamydia pneumoniae*, *Helicobacter pylori*, and Gram-negative bacteria associated with periodontal infection have all been isolated in atherosclerotic plaque. It may well be that chronic inflammation associated with such low-grade infection—rather than the bacteria itself—is responsible for inducing atherosclerotic disease.

Migraine

- Migraine can be associated with stroke in two ways:
  1. Stroke occurs during a migraine attack
  2. As a risk factor for stroke
- Stroke during a migraine attack (migrainous stroke) is very rare and more common in migraine with aura
- Epidemiological studies have shown migraine is a risk factor for stroke
- The stroke risk is highest for migraine with aura. The relative risk of migraine causing stroke is 1.5–2.0 while migraine with aura is up to 6
- There is an interaction between smoking, migraine (particularly with aura), and the combined oral contraceptive (COC) pill. Women who smoke, take the COC pill, and suffer migraine with aura have an increased stroke risk of up to tenfold
- Recent-onset migraine with aura is thought to be associated with the greatest stroke risk
- In terms of primary prevention, there is no evidence to suggest that migraine prophylaxis reduces stroke risk.

Contraceptive use/pregnancy

- The relative risk of stroke is approximately doubled in users of the COC pill
- However, the absolute risk remains very low. This is because the incidence of ischaemic stroke in women aged under 35 is very low: three in 100 000
- More recent studies with low-dose oestrogen (<50 μg) suggest the risk is even less with modern COC
- There is no increased risk of haemorrhagic stroke and no increase in stroke mortality in COC users. COCs should not generally be prescribed to young women with established vascular risk and a family history of venous thromboembolism (VTE)
- There is no, or a much smaller increased risk in women who take the progestogen-only contraceptive pill.

Hormone replacement therapy (HRT)

- HRT also increases the relative risk of stroke by about 2. However, it is taken by older women and their absolute risk of stroke is higher. Therefore, the potential population-attributable risk is higher.
- Therefore, current advice is to use HRT for 5 years only and to continue only in older women where the unpleasant menopausal symptoms outweigh their risk of stroke.
- Prior to recent trial data, it was thought that HRT may protect against cardiovascular risk and stroke, and this led to trials assessing this hypothesis which, to many people's surprise, demonstrated that they

actually increased risk. The Heart & Estrogen-progestin Replacement Study (HERS) showed no effect of HRT on stroke primary prevention. HRT in the secondary prevention Women's Estrogen for Stroke Trial (WEST), however, increased the risk of recurrent fatal stroke and worsened the neurological and functional deficit of recurrent stroke in a stroke population.

- Data from 257 194 women in the UK Biobank have suggested that the risk of stroke is highest in the first year of use of both HRT and the COC pill.
- HRT should not be used in primary stroke prevention for women with other vascular risk factors.

Recreational drug use

A number of commonly used recreational drugs increase the risk of stroke; these include amphetamines and cocaine. They are covered in detail on ➔ p. 347.

Other drugs

There has been concern over other drugs increasing stroke risk. These include the following.

Cyclooxygenase (COX)-2 inhibitors and NSAIDs

- Nonsteroidal anti-inflammatory drugs (NSAIDs) are one of the most commonly used medications worldwide. Their main mechanism of action is via inhibition of the cyclooxygenase (COX) enzyme, which has into 2 isoforms (COX-1 and COX-2).
- COX-1 is a housekeeping enzyme that is expressed under normal physiological condition, while COX-2 expression is inducible under an inflammatory state.
- Traditional NSAIDs such as ibuprofen have been used as analgesics. However, these nonselective NSAIDs have adverse effects associated with inhibition of the COX-1 enzyme, particularly gastrointestinal irritation and ulceration.
- Specific COX-2 inhibitors have higher specificity and were marketed as a safer alternative to conventional NSAIDs. Clinical trials showed they had a better gastrointestinal safety profile compared with traditional NSAIDs.
- However, post-licensing studies found selective COX-2 inhibitors were associated with an increased stroke and myocardial infarction risk.
- Traditional NSAIDs such as ibuprofen and naproxen have also been associated with a smaller, but significantly increased risk of stroke and myocardial infarction, even with short-term use as recognized by FDA warnings in 2005, and a strengthened warning in 2015. They should be used with caution in patients with stroke.

Atypical antipsychotic medication

- Evidence from randomized trials shows a small increased risk of stroke in patients with dementia and agitation treated with the atypical antipsychotics risperidone and olanzapine. However, this is based on a small number of events and a small increase in relative risk with wide confidence intervals. A large observational study failed to find any increased risk and probably limits the size of the effect to no more than two extra strokes per 1000 person-years of treatment. The mechanism for this small increase in stroke risk is unclear

- Nevertheless, atypical neuroleptic drugs are not recommended for the treatment of behavioural problems in dementia, although they may be used under supervision for short periods of time. The licence has not been affected outside their use in dementia patients
- A recent case-controlled study argued in fact that the risk is similar in all antipsychotic medications and highest in patients on treatment with dementia.

Relative contribution of different stroke risk factors

The relative risks associated with different risk factors for stroke are shown in Table 1.7. These are representative figures derived from different studies of each risk factor.

It is important to remember that risk factors frequently coexist and often have more than summative effects on stroke risk, e.g. diabetes, hypertension, and the presence of peripheral vascular disease is associated with a more than 12-fold increase in stroke risk.

The Framingham stroke risk profile (➜ see Table 1.8, p. 39) estimates 10-year predicted stroke risk according to common risk factors.

Table 1.7 Relative contribution of different stroke risk factors

Risk factor	Relative risk for stroke
Age (55–64 years versus >75 years)	5
Male sex	1.3
Afro-Caribbean	2
Social class (I versus V)	1.6
Air pollution 1.2	
Physical activity (little or none versus some)	2.5
Smoking (current status)	2
Alcohol (>60 g per day)	1.6
Blood pressure 160/95 vs. 120/80 mmHg	7
Diabetes mellitus	2
Previous TIA (symptomatic ICA stenosis >70%)	5(10)
Ischaemic heart disease	3
Heart failure	5
Atrial fibrillation	5
Oral contraceptives	2

Framingham stroke risk

The Framingham stroke risk tables can be used to calculate stroke risk in an individual person. The tables shown apply to individuals not in AF.

The risk score is calculated from the first table; there are separate tables for men (Table 1.8) and women (Table 1.9). This risk score is than converted into a stroke risk over the next 10 years using the conversion table (Table 1.10).

Table 1.8 Table for calculating Framingham risk score in men, not in atrial fibrillation

Risk score	Points 0	+1	+2	+3	+4	+5	+6	+7	+8	+9	+10
Risk score for men aged 55–85 years											
Age (years)	54–56	57–59	60–62	63–65	66–68	69–72	73–75	76–78	79–81	82–84	85
Untreated SBP	97–105	106–115	116–125	126–135	136–145	146–155	156–165	166–175	176–185	186–195	196–205
Treated SBP	97–105	106–112	113–117	118–123	124–129	130–135	136–142	143–150	151–161	162–176	177–205
Diabetes	No		Yes								
Current smoker	No			Yes							
CVD	No				Yes						
ECG LVH	No					Yes					

Reproduced from Stroke, 25(1), D'Agostino RB, Wolf PA, Belanger AJ, Kannel WB, Stroke risk profile: adjustment for antihypertensive medication. The Framingham Study, pp. 40–43; Copyright (1994), with permission from Wolters Kluwer Health, Inc.

CVD, history of myocardial infarction, angina, intermittent claudication or heart failure; ECG, electrocardiogram; LVH, left ventricular hypertrophy; SBP, systolic blood pressure (mmHg).

Table 1.9 Table for calculating Framingham risk score in women, not in atrial fibrillation

Risk score	Points 0	+1	+2	+3	+4	+5	+6	+7	+8	+9	+10
Risk score for women aged 55–85 years											
Age (years)	54–56	57–59	60–62	63–64	65–67	68–70	71–73	74–76	77–78	79–81	82–84
Untreated SBP	95–106	107–118	119–130	131–143	144–155	156–167	168–180	181–192	193–204	205–216	
Treated SBP	95–106	107–113	114–119	120–125	136–131	132–139	140–148	149–160	161–204	205–216	
Diabetes	No			Yes							
Cigarettes	No			Yes							
CVD	No		Yes								
ECG LVH	No				Yes						

Reproduced from *Stroke*, 25(1), D'Agostino RB, Wolf PA, Belanger AJ, Kannel WB, Stroke risk profile: The Framingham Study, pp. 40–43, Copyright (1994), with permission from Wolters Kluwer Health, Inc.

SBP = systolic blood pressure (mmHg); CVD = history of MI, angina, intermittent claudication, or heart failure; LVH = left ventricular hypertrophy

Table 1.10 Table for converting Framingham risk scores to 10-year probability of stroke: conversion of points from risk factor profiles to probability of stroke over 10 years

Points	10-year probability (%), men	10-year probability (%), women	Points	10-year probability (%), men	10-year probability (%), women	Points	10-year probability (%), men	10-year probability (%), women
1	3	1	11	11	8	21	47	43
2	3	1	12	13	9	22	52	50
3	4	2	13	15	11	23	57	57
4	4	2	14	17	13	24	63	64
5	5	2	15	20	16	25	68	71
6	5	3	16	23	19	26	74	78
7	6	4	17	27	23	27	79	84
8	7	4	18	32	27	28	84	
9	8	5	19	37	32	29	88	
10	10	6	20	42	37	30		

Further reading

Global burden of stroke

Feigin VL, Brainin M, Norrving B, et al. (2025). World Stroke Organization: Global Stroke Fact Sheet 2025. *International J of Stroke* **20**(2), 132–144.

Martin SS, Aday AW, Almarzooq ZI, et al. (2024). Heart disease and stroke statistics: a report of US and global data from the American Heart Association. *Circulation* **149**, e347–e913.

Stroke subtyping

Adams HP, Bendixen BH, Kappelle LJ (1993). Classification of subtype of acute ischemic stroke. Definitions for use in a multicenter clinical trial. TOAST. Trial of Org 10172 in Acute Stroke Treatment. *Stroke* **24**, 35–41.

Goldstein LB, Jones MR, Matchar DB, et al. (2001). Improving the reliability of stroke subgroup classification using the Trial of ORG 10172 in Acute Stroke Treatment (TOAST) criteria. *Stroke* **32**, 1091–1098.

Incidence and prevalence

GBD 2019 Stroke Collaborators (2021). Global, regional, and national burden of stroke and its risk factors, 1990–2019: a systematic analysis for the Global Burden of Disease Study 2019. *Lancet Neurol* **20**, 795–820.

Li L, Scott CA, Rothwell PM (2022). Association of younger vs older ages with changes in incidence of stroke and other vascular events, 2002–2018. *JAMA* **328**, 563–574.

Economic cost of stroke care

Lorio A, Garcia-Rodriguez C, Seifi A (2024). Two decades of stroke in the United States: a healthcare economic perspective. *Neuroepidemiology* **58**, 143–150.

Patel A, Berdunov V, Quayyum Z, King D, Knapp M, Wittenberg R (2020) Estimated societal costs of stroke in the UK based on a discrete event simulation. *Age Ageing* **49**, 270–276.

Non-modifiable stroke risk factors

Ethnicity

De Silva DA, Woon FP, Lee MP, et al. (2007). South Asian patients with ischemic stroke: intracranial large arteries are the predominant site of disease. *Stroke* **38**, 2592–2594.

Howard VJ. (2013). Reasons underlying racial differences in stroke incidence and mortality. *Stroke* **44**(6 Suppl 1), S126–S128.

Markus HS, Khan U, Birns B, et al. (2007). Differences in stroke subtypes between Black and white patients with stroke—The South London Ethnicity and Stroke Study. *Circulation* **116**, 2157–2164.

Genetic predisposition

Debette S, Markus HS (2022). Stroke genetics: discovery, insight into mechanisms, and clinical perspectives. *Circ Res* **130**, 1095–1111.

Mishra A, Malik R, Hachiya T, et al. (2022). Stroke genetics informs drug discovery and risk prediction across ancestries. *Nature* **611**, 115–123.

Major modifiable stroke risk factors

Physical inactivity

Ghozy S, Zayan AH, El-Qushayri AE, et al. (2022). Physical activity level and stroke risk in US population: a matched case-control study of 102,578 individuals. *Ann Clin Transl Neurol* **9**, 264–275.

Li J, Siegrist J (2012). Physical activity and risk of cardiovascular disease—a meta-analysis of prospective cohort studies. *Int J Environ Res Public Health* **9**, 391–407.

Air pollution

Kulick ER, Kaufman JD, Sack C (2023). Ambient air pollution and stroke: an updated review. *Stroke* 54, 882–893.

Alcohol

Smyth A, O'Donnell M, Rangarajan S, et al. (2023). Alcohol intake as a risk factor for acute stroke. The INTERSTROKE Study. *Neurology* **100**, e142–e153.

Smoking

Klein AP, Yarbrough K, Cole JW (2021). Stroke, smoking and vaping: the no-good, the bad and the ugly. *Ann Public Health Res* **8**, 1104.

Wang X, et al. (2024) Tobacco use and risk of acute stroke in 32 countries in the INTERSTROKE Study: a case–control study. *eClinicalMedicine* **70**, 102515.

Hypertension

Lewington S, Clarke R, Qizilbash N, *et al.* (2002). Age-specific relevance of usual blood pressure to vascular mortality: a meta-analysis of individual data for one million adults in 61 prospective studies. [Published correction appears in] *Lancet* **360**, 1903–1913.

PROGRESS Collaborative Group (2001). Randomised trial of a perindopril-based blood-pressure-lowering regimen among 6,105 individuals with previous stroke or transient ischaemic attack. *Lancet* **358**, 1033–1041.

Metabolic syndrome

Hirode G, Wong RJ (2020). Trends in the prevalence of metabolic syndrome in the United States, 2011–2016. *JAMA* **323**(24), 2526–2528.

Kernan WN, Inzucchi SE, Viscoli CM, *et al.* (2002). Insulin resistance and risk for stroke. *Neurology* **59**, 809–815.

Lakka HM, Laaksonen DE, Lakka TA, *et al.* (2002). The metabolic syndrome and total and cardiovascular disease mortality in middle-aged men. *JAMA* **288**, 2709–2716.

Hypercholesterolaemia

Prospective Studies Collaboration (2007). Blood cholesterol and vascular mortality by age, sex and blood pressure: a meta-analysis of individual data from 61 prospective studies with 55 000 vascular deaths. *Lancet* **370**, 1829–39.

The Stroke Prevention by Aggressive Reduction in Cholesterol Levels (SPARCL) Investigators (2006). High-dose atorvastatin after stroke or transient ischemic attack. *N Engl J Med* **355**, 459–559.

Atherosclerosis

MRC Asymptomatic Carotid Surgery Trial (ACST) Collaborative Group (2004). Prevention of disabling and fatal strokes by successful carotid endarterectomy in patients without recent neurological symptoms: randomised controlled trial. *Lancet* **363**, 1491–1502.

Atrial fibrillation

Björck S, Palaszewski B, Friberg L, Bergfeldt L (2013). Atrial fibrillation, stroke risk, and warfarin therapy revisited: a population-based study. *Stroke* **44**, 3103–3108.

Sposato LA, Cipriano LE, Saposnik G, *et al.* (2015). Diagnosis of atrial fibrillation after stroke and transient ischaemic attack: a systematic review and meta-analysis. *Lancet Neurol* **14**, 377–387.

Structural cardiac abnormalities

Turc G, Calvet D, Guérin P, Sroussi M, Chatellier G, Mas JL; CLOSE Investigators (2018). Closure, anticoagulation, or antiplatelet therapy for cryptogenic stroke with patent foramen ovale: systematic review of randomized trials, sequential meta-analysis, and new insights from the CLOSE study. *J Am Heart Assoc* **17**(7), e008356.

Minor modifiable stroke risk factors

Diet

Guo N, Zhu Y, Tian D, Zhao Y, Zhang C, Mu C, Han C, Zhu R, Liu X (2022). Role of diet in stroke incidence: an umbrella review of meta-analyses of prospective observational studies. *BMC Med* **24**(20), 194.

Lakkur S, Judd SE (2015). Diet and stroke: recent evidence supporting a mediterranean-style diet and food in the primary prevention of stroke. *Stroke* **46**, 2007–2011.

Peh A, O'Donnell JA, Broughton BR, Marques FZ (2022). Gut microbiota and their metabolites in stroke: a double-edged sword. *Stroke* **53**(5), 1788–1805.

Hyperhomocysteinaemia

Hankey GJ, Eikelboom JW, Yi Q, et al. (2012). VITATOPS trial study group. Antiplatelet therapy and the effects of B vitamins in patients with previous stroke or transient ischaemic attack: a post-hoc subanalysis of VITATOPS, a randomised, placebo controlled trial. *Lancet Neurol* **11**, 512–520.

Huo Y, Li J, Qin X, et al.; CSPPT Investigators (2015). Efficacy of folic acid therapy in primary prevention of stroke among adults with hypertension in China: the CSPPT randomized clinical trial. *JAMA* **313**, 1325–1335.

Wang X, Qin X, Demirtas H, et al. (2007). Efficacy of folic acid supplementation in stroke prevention: a meta-analysis. *Lancet* **369**, 1876–1882.

Obstructive sleep apnoea

Koo DL, Nam H, Thomas RJ, Yun CH (2018). Sleep disturbances as a risk factor for stroke. *J Stroke* **20**, 12–32.

Yaggi HK, Concato J, Kernan WN, et al. (2005). Obstructive sleep apnea as a risk factor for stroke and death. *N Engl J Med* **353**, 2034–2041.

Inflammation and CRP

Parikh NS, Merkler AE, Iadecola C (2020). Inflammation, autoimmunity, infection, and stroke: epidemiology and lessons from therapeutic intervention. *Stroke* **51**, 711–718.

Infections

Elkind MSV, Boehme AK, Smith CJ, Meisel A, Buckwalter MS (2020). Infection as a stroke risk factor and determinant of outcome after stroke. *Stroke* **51**, 3156–3168.

Hormone replacement therapy

Chang CL, Donaghy M, Poulter N (1999). Migraine and stroke in young women: case-control study: the World Health Organization collaborative study of cardiovascular disease and steroid hormone contraception. *BMJ* **318**, 13–18.

Johansson T, Fowler P, Ek WE, Skalkidou A, Karlsson T, Johansson Å (2022). Oral contraceptives, hormone replacement therapy, and stroke risk. *Stroke* **53**(10), 3107–3115.

Viscoli CM, Brass LM, Kernan WN, et al. (2001). A clinical trial of estrogen-replacement therapy after ischemic stroke. *N Engl J Med* **345**, 1243–1249.

Other drugs

Kearney PM, Baigent C, Godwin J, et al. (2006). Do selective cyclo-oxygenase-2 inhibitors and traditional non-steroidal anti-inflammatory drugs increase the risk of atherothrombosis? Meta-analysis of randomised trials. *BMJ* **332**, 1302–1308.

Zivkovic S, Koh CH, Kaza N, Jackson CA (2019). Antipsychotic drug use and risk of stroke and myocardial infarction: a systematic review and meta-analysis. *BMC Psychiatry* **19**, 189.

Neuroanatomy

Introduction

Stroke is a disease affecting the brain. Therefore, there is no escaping having to understand some neuroanatomy. However, stroke is a very practical subject and with a relatively simple understanding of the neuroanatomy and vascular anatomy, it is not difficult to localize the lesion and the arterial territory involved in many cases of stroke.

The most important aspects of neuroanatomy to understand are:

- the motor system
- the sensory system
- the visual system
- the brainstem
- cortical function
- neuroanatomy of stroke subtypes
- neuroanatomy of vascular territories.

Basic neuroanatomy principles

Some simple principles:

First, decide the side affected:

- The right side of the brain normally controls the left side of the body (and vice versa)
- The exception is the cerebellum, which controls the same side of the body.

Second, decide the level of the lesion:

- The nervous system is arranged in a series of ascending levels
- You should learn enough neuroanatomy to be able to work out the level of the lesion.

These two principles allow you to think of the body as a grid and to pinpoint the lesion. After that, using a knowledge of the cerebral arterial territories, one can work out which vascular territory is involved.

Motor system

The motor system is an efferent system. It runs from the brain down and is organized as follows (see Fig. 2.1).

Motor cortex

- Located in the precentral gyrus in the frontal lobe
- Different parts of the body are laid out in a homunculus (see Fig. 2.8)
- As this is a relatively large area, small infarcts here may cause paralysis of an isolated region such as the hand or arm
- Complete paralysis of one side occurs if the infarct involves the whole motor cortex (or corticospinal tract—see next). This is the case for many middle cerebral artery infarcts.

Corticospinal tract

- The motor fibres from the cortex descend in this tract, which passes through the centrum semiovale and the 'fan-shaped' corona radiata, on down through the internal capsule into the brainstem, and on to the spinal cord. Disruption at any of these sites may cause motor deficit (hemiparesis).

Centrum semiovale

- Here the corticospinal track fibres are gathered together from the cortex into smaller bundles Therefore, infarcts here cause more extensive symptoms than similar-sized infarcts in the motor cortex
- Infarcts in the corticospinal tracts usually cause hemiparesis, which involves at least two areas of the body (e.g. face and arm or arm and leg)
- Lacunar infarcts are common at this site.

Internal capsule

- This is rather small and runs through the basal ganglia
- It is boomerang-shaped with an anterior and a posterior limb
- Motor fibres run in the posterior limb
- The fibres are tightly packed which means lacunar infarcts here cause paralysis of a whole side (complete hemiparesis) or at least two areas of the body (e.g. arm and leg, or face and arm)
- Lacunar infarcts are common at this site.

Brainstem

- The motor fibres run through the brainstem
- The cranial nerve nuclei are in close proximity to the motor pathways
- Therefore, infarcts here may cause quadriparesis as well as affect several cranial nerves.

Pyramids

- Here the fibres cross over to the other side.

Spinal cord

- The motor fibres run down in the cord until they reach their exit level
- They terminate at the anterior horn cell (the junction of the upper motor neuron and the lower motor neuron).

Peripheral nerve

- Here the motor fibres run out to the muscle.

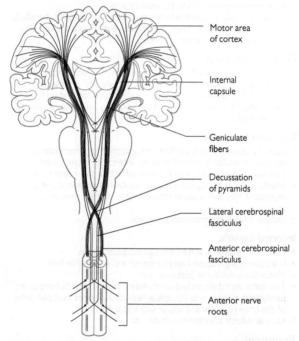

Fig. 2.1 Diagram of the motor system. The corticospinal fibre tracts start from the cortex, run through the internal capsule, and cross over in the pyramids (the pyramidal tracts). They then descend towards the anterior horn cells in the spinal cord. The nerve down to the ending on the anterior horn cell is the 'upper motor neuron'. From the anterior horn cell to the end muscle is the 'lower motor neuron'.

Sensory system

The sensory system is an afferent system. It runs from the periphery up to the brain and is organized as follows (see Fig. 2.2).

Peripheral nerves

- These arise from sensory receptors in the skin or end-organs
- Some fibres are myelinated and fast conducting (e.g. joint position sense)
- Some fibres are unmyelinated and slow conducting (e.g. some pain fibres)
- The main peripheral sensory nerves enter the dorsal spinal cord.

Spinal cord

- Most fibres run up the same side of the spinal cord in the dorsal columns. These carry sensation for light touch, vibration, and joint position sense
- Some fibres cross over straight away. These are spinothalamic fibres and run in the spinothalamic tract. They carry the sensations of pain and temperature.

Brainstem

- Here, the fibres from the dorsal columns (light touch, vibration, and joint position sense) cross over to the other side and run up in a tract called the medial lemniscus.

Thalamus

- This is the big group of nuclei where the sensory fibres end
- The fibres and nuclei in the thalamus are very tightly packed
- The thalamus relays the sensory information to the sensory cortex
- Because fibres are closely packed, a small infarct here usually results in complete hemisensory loss (i.e. affecting the face, arm, and leg).

Primary sensory cortex

- This lies in the postcentral gyrus of the frontal lobe on either side
- Like the motor cortex, it is very extensive
- Therefore, infarcts may involve only part of the sensory cortex and result in sensory loss in only one limb or part of limb (e.g. arm or leg or face alone).

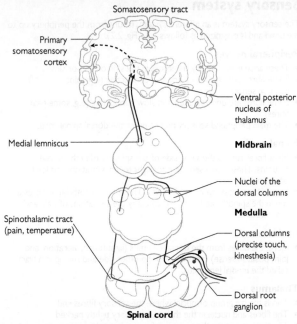

Fig. 2.2 Schematic diagram of the sensory pathway.

Somatosensory tract

Primary
somatosensory
cortex

Ventral posterior
nucleus of thalamus

Medial lemniscus

Midbrain

Nuclei of the
dorsal columns

Medulla

Spinothalamic tract
(pain, temperature)

Dorsal columns
(precise touch,
kinesthesia)

Dorsal root
ganglion

Spinal cord

Visual system

The visual system is organized as follows.

The retina

- Detects light and converts this into transmissible electrical impulses
- The visual world is split into left and right. Half of each retina detects the left field, and the other half of each retina detects the right visual field
- Retinal ischaemia may cause temporary monocular visual loss (amaurosis fugax) or permanent blindness (e.g. central retinal artery occlusion).

Optic nerve

- This runs from each eye to the optic chiasm
- A lesion here will cause blindness of one eye. The other eye will be unaffected.

Optic chiasm

- Here fibres from each optic nerve partially cross over (see Fig. 2.3)
- The important point is that the visual world is split into left and right
- A lesion affecting the whole chiasm will cause complete blindness
- A lesion pushing on the centre of the chiasm and affecting the central crossing fibres (e.g. a pituitary tumour) will cause a bitemporal hemianopia.

Optic tract

- Each optic tract carries information from one visual field
- Lesions here will cause visual disturbance, affecting the same field in *both* eyes
- If the whole optic tract on one side is damaged, the entire hemifield may become blind; a homonymous hemianopia.

Optic radiation

- Each optic radiation stretches back from the lateral geniculate nucleus to the visual cortex
- The radiation is actually quite wide. Therefore, small infarcts may affect only a small part of one radiation. This may damage the bottom (or top) half of the left or right visual field. This causes a quadrantanopia.

Visual cortex

- This occupies the occipital cortex
- Complete infarction of one side will produce a homonymous hemianopia.

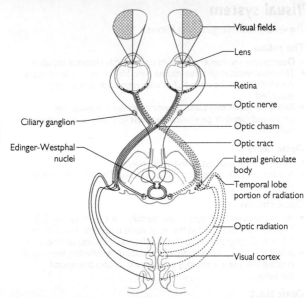

Fig. 2.3 The optic pathways. For visual field defects arising from lesions at different locations, see Fig. 5.2.

Labels on figure:
- Visual fields
- Lens
- Retina
- Optic nerve
- Ciliary ganglion
- Optic chasm
- Edinger-Westphal nuclei
- Optic tract
- Lateral geniculate body
- Temporal lobe portion of radiation
- Optic radiation
- Visual cortex

Brainstem

The brainstem contains:
- a large number of cranial nerve nuclei and their interconnections
- the descending motor and ascending sensory pathways
- cerebellar connections.

It can appear confusing. However, if one localizes the site and side of the lesion by knowing which cranial nerves it is affecting, and which ascending and descending pathways are involved, it becomes easier.

Think of the brainstem as a grid. If you know what each cranial nerve does, it is quite easy to localize lesions to the brainstem (Table 2.1).

Table 2.1 Cranial nerves and their functions

Nerve	Function
Olfactory (I)	Olfaction (smell)
Optic (II)	Vision
Occulomotor (III)	Eye movements and pupillary responses
Trochlear (IV)	Eye movements: superior oblique. "Look at your nose"
Trigeminal (V)	Facial sensation and muscles of mastication
Abducens (VI)	Eye movements: lateral rectus. "Look to the side"
Facial (VII)	Facial movement
Auditory (VIII)	Hearing and balance
Glossopharyngeal (IX)	Pharyngeal sensation
Vagus (X)	Muscles of larynx and pharynx
Accessory (XI)	Trapezius and sternocleidomastoid
Hypoglossal (XII)	Tongue movement

The site of origin of the cranial nerves in the brainstem is shown in Fig. 2.4. On subsequent pages, cross-sectional views of the brainstem at the different levels are shown.

When localizing a lesion, first work out which of the following are affected:
- Cranial nerves
- Motor pathway
- Sensory pathway
- Cerebellar function.

Then refer to these diagrams and it is usually possible to localize the lesions.

Examination of the individual cranial nerves is covered in Chapter 5, p. 116.

Figs 2.4 and 2.5 show the positions of the cranial nerve nuclei in the brainstem.

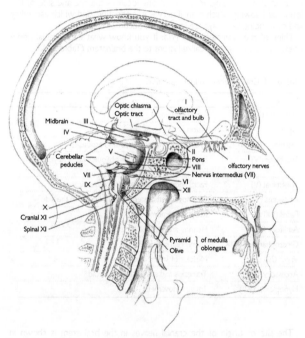

Fig. 2.4 Origin of the cranial nerves from the brainstem.

Reproduced from MacKinnon P, Morris J, *Oxford Textbook of Functional Anatomy*, Vol. 3, Copyright (2005), with permission from Oxford University Press.

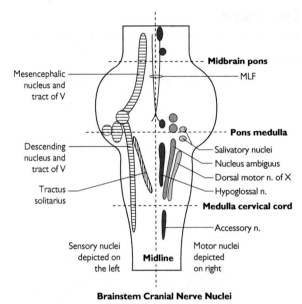

Mesencephalic nucleus and tract of V

MLF

Midbrain pons

Descending nucleus and tract of V

Tractus solitarius

Pons medulla

Salivatory nuclei

Nucleus ambiguus

Dorsal motor n. of X

Hypoglossal n.

Medulla cervical cord

Accessory n.

Sensory nuclei depicted on the left

Midline

Motor nuclei depicted on right

Brainstem Cranial Nerve Nuclei

Fig. 2.5 Longitudinal diagram of the brainstem showing the cranial nerve nuclei and the position of the major tracts.

Cerebellum

- The cerebellum is located inferior to the tentorium cerebelli. The anatomy and blood supply are shown in Figs 2.6 and 2.7
- It coordinates muscle activity and balance
- It is split into three lobes:
  - flocculonodular lobe (archicerebellum) supports equilibrium
  - anterior lobe (paleocerebellum) supports muscle tone
  - posterior lateral lobes (neocerebellum) support coordination.

The motor tracts are doubly crossed so affect the ipsilateral side. Major cerebellar tracts are:
- spinocerebellar, connecting the spinal cord
- vestibulospinal, connecting the vestibular system
- corticopontocerebellar, connecting the cortex and pons
- dentatorubrothalamic connecting to the red nucleus and thalamus.

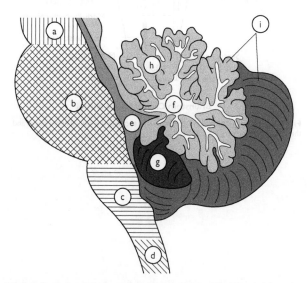

Fig. 2.6 Cerebellum and surrounding regions; sagittal view of one hemisphere. a, midbrain; b, pons; c, medulla; d, spinal cord; e, fourth ventricle; f, arbor vitae; g, tonsil; h, anterior lobe; i, posterior lobe.

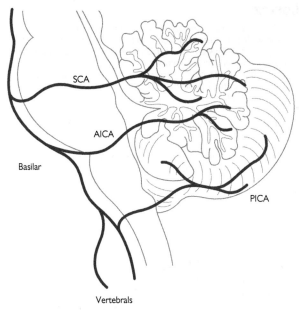

Fig. 2.7 Blood supply to the cerebellar regions. AICA, anterior inferior cerebellar artery arises from the basilar artery; PICA, posterior inferior cerebellar artery arises from intracranial vertebral artery; SCA, superior cerebellar artery.

Cortex

- Different functions are localized in specific cortical regions
- A knowledge of where in the cortex different functions are localized is important to allow one to localize a brain infarct and subsequently determine which arterial territory is involved
- Fig. 2.9 shows how different areas of the cortex control different functions,illustrating how infarcts in different regions may produce particular symptoms
- Large infarcts will affect multiple regions.

Fig. 2.8 shows the motor homunculus; how the motor function are spread out over the cortex. Because the function are so spread out, a small infarct in the motor cortex may cause hand weakness alone. To paralyse the whole side would require a large infarct. From Fig. 2.9, you can see it is impossible to paralyse the whole motor cortex alone; other areas such as the sensory cortex must also be involved. In contrast, where the motor fibres are closely packed in the internal capsule, a small lesion can damage them all and cause an isolated complete hemiplegia (pure motor stroke lacunar infarct).

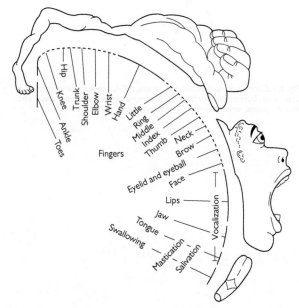

Fig. 2.8 The motor homunculus.

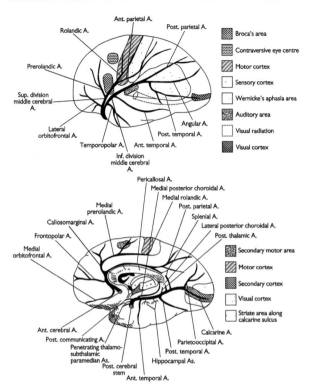

Fig. 2.9 Images showing lateral (upper figure) and medial (lower figure) views of the cerebral cortex. The different cortical regions are shown although it is not necessary to learn all their names. However, it is important to remember the location of the areas controlling the major functions which are shown in different shadings. The major arteries supplying the cortex are also shown. © Hugh Markus.

Vascular anatomy and stroke syndromes

Introduction

Stroke is a disease of blood flow. Therefore, it is important to understand the blood supply of the brain (see Figs 3.1 and 3.2). Most ischaemic stroke is embolic. Emboli may arise anywhere from the heart and the arterial tree connecting the heart to the brain.

The circulation is conventionally split into:
- anterior circulation: carotid artery distribution
- posterior circulation: vertebral and basilar artery distribution.

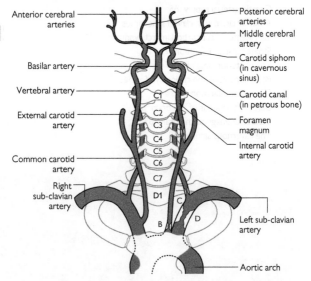

Fig. 3.1 The arterial supply of the brain with common sites of atheroma shown.

The anterior circulation

This comprises the territory supplied by the carotid arteries.
- The left carotid arises from the aorta
- The right carotid arises from the brachiocephalic artery.

The internal carotid artery is divided into four portions (Fig. 3.2):
- Cervical
- Petrous
- Cavernous
- Cerebral.

Cervical carotid artery

- This runs from the bifurcation of the common carotid to the carotid canal within the petrous portion of the temporal bone
- Behind it is the superior cervical ganglion of the sympathetic trunk and the superior laryngeal nerve. The close proximity to the sympathetic fibres means a carotid dissection with an expanding artery often causes unilateral Horner's syndrome
- The glossopharyngeal, vagus, accessory, and hypoglossal nerves lie between the artery and the internal jugular vein. The hypoglossal artery is particularly vulnerable during carotid endarterectomy
- There are no branches.

Petrous carotid artery

- The carotid curves upward through the petrous bone to enter the skull cavity
- The artery is surrounded by the carotid plexus, which contains sympathetic fibres from the superior cervical ganglion.

Cavernous carotid artery

- The artery runs through the cavernous sinus
- The artery is surrounded by the sympathetic fibres
- It lies close to cranial nerves III, IV, Va and Vb, and VI
- An important branch is the ophthalmic artery. Emboli passing into this artery are common in carotid stenosis and cause amaurosis fugax (transient monocular blindness) or occasionally permanent blindness.

Cerebral carotid artery

- The artery penetrates the dura mater and passes between the second and sixth cranial nerves
- Terminal branches include the:
  - anterior cerebral artery
  - middle cerebral artery—this supplies a very large part of the cerebral cortex
  - posterior communicating artery
  - anterior choroidal artery.

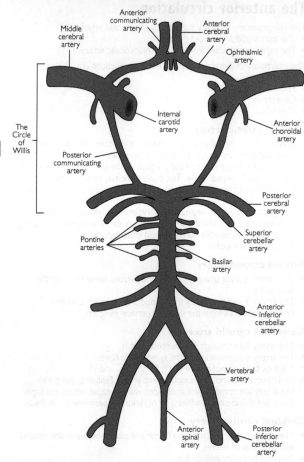

Fig. 3.2 The circle of Willis and the major intracranial arteries.

Carotid arterial supply

The anterior cerebral artery (ACA)

The ACA is a major termination of the carotid artery (Fig. 3.3). It has several branches.

- Anteromedial ganglionic branches are small arteries arising at the start of the ACA which supply part of the corpus callosum and head of caudate
- Inferior branches supply the orbital surface of the frontal lobe and the olfactory lobe
- Anterior branches supply a part of the superior frontal gyrus and send twigs over the edge of the hemisphere to the superior and middle frontal gyri and upper part of the anterior central gyrus
- Middle branches supply the corpus callosum, the cingulate gyrus, and the medial surface of the superior frontal and upper part of the anterior central gyrus
- Posterior branches.

The ACA lies close to the opposite ACA and is linked by the anterior communicating artery.

The anterior communicating artery (Acom)

The Acom connects the two ACAs. Its length averages about 4 mm. It is very variable and sometimes both ACAs arise from the same side.

The middle cerebral artery (MCA)

The MCA is the largest branch of the internal carotid. It runs laterally in the Sylvian fissure to the insula where it divides into several branches over the lateral surface of the hemisphere.

The branches include the:

- lenticulostriate branches from the MCA itself, which supply the basal ganglia, internal capsule, and thalamus
- inferior lateral frontal which supplies the inferior frontal gyrus (Broca's area)
- ascending frontal which supplies the anterior central gyrus
- ascending parietal which supplies posterior frontal and superior parietal lobule
- parietotemporal which supplies the supramarginal and angular gyri, and the posterior parts of the superior and middle temporal gyri
- temporal branches, two or three in number, which supply the temporal lobe.

The posterior communicating artery (Pcom)

The Pcom connects the internal carotid to the posterior cerebral artery. It is frequently larger on one side. It may be so large that the posterior cerebral artery appears to arise from the internal carotid rather than from the basilar. It gives off a few small branches.

The anterior choroidal artery

The anterior choroidal artery is a small branch which arises from the internal carotid near the Pcom. It supplies the choroid plexus and hippocampus.

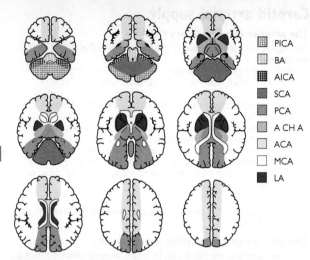

Fig. 3.3 Territories of the main cerebral arteries supplying the supratentorial structures. © Hugh Markus. PICA, posterior inferior cerebellar artery; BA, basilar artery; AICA, anterior inferior cerebellar artery; SCA, superior cerebellar artery; PCA, posterior cerebral artery; AChA, anterior choroidal artery; ACA, anterior cerebral artery; MCA middle cerebral artery; LA, lenticulostriate artery.

Anterior circulation clinical syndromes

By combining a knowledge of arterial anatomy, which brain regions are supplied by the different arteries (see Fig. 3.3), and which functions are located in which brain region (see Fig. 3.4), one can work out the consequences of occlusion of a particular artery.

Remember, deficits can arise from:
- involvement of cortical regions controlling specific functions (see Fig. 3.5a)
- involvement of ascending or descending connections (Fig. 3.5b)
- involvement of subcortical and brainstem nuclei (Fig. 3.5b).

Ophthalmic artery
- Emboli from an internal carotid stenosis often pass down this artery
- Occlusion causes uniocular loss of vision
- Often transient when it is called amaurosis fugax
- Can result in permanent loss of vision
- Tight carotid stenosis can occasionally be associated with 'positive' retinal symptoms with glaring or flashing white lights owing to haemodynamic compromise.

Anterior cerebral artery
- Leg and trunk weakness
- Leg more affected than arm and sparing of the face
- Bilateral ACA infarction may cause weakness of both legs and gait apraxia (both ACAs can arise from a single ICA as a normal variant).

Middle cerebral artery
- Contralateral hemiplegia
- Eye deviation towards the side of the infarct (owing to disruption of frontal eye fields)
- Contralateral hemianopia
- Contralateral sensory loss
- Aphasia (dominant hemisphere)
- Neglect
- Anosagnosia (non-dominant hemisphere)
- Apraxia
- Movement disorders such as chorea and dystonia.

Anterior choroidal artery
- Contralateral hemiparesis,
- Contralateral sensory loss
- Homonymous hemianopia

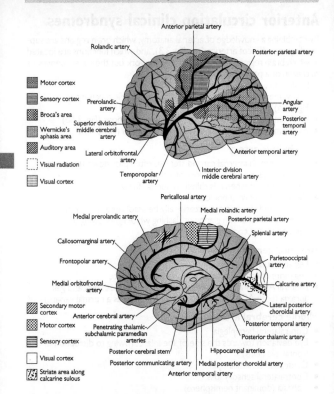

Fig. 3.4 Cortical brain regions supplied by the middle cerebral artery (upper figure) and anterior and posterior cerebral arteries (lower figure). © Hugh Markus.

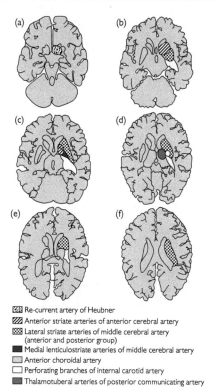

Re-current artery of Heubner
Anterior striate arteries of anterior cerebral artery
Lateral striate arteries of middle cerebral artery
(anterior and posterior group)
Medial lenticulostriate arteries of middle cerebral artery
Anterior choroidal artery
Perforating branches of internal carotid artery
Thalamotuberal arteries of posterior communicating artery

Fig. 3.5a Vascular supply of supratentorial subcortical regions. © Hugh Markus.

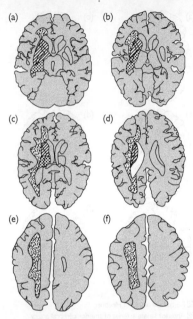

(a)   (b)

(c)   (d)

(e)   (f)

White matter medullary branches territory
Lenticulostriate territory
Anterior choroidal artery territory

Fig. 3.5b Vascular supply of supratentorial subcortical regions. © Hugh Markus.

Supratentorial subcortical infarct syndromes

Specific types of subcortical infarcts include:
- lacunar infarcts
- striatocapsular infarcts.

Lacunar infarcts

- These are the most common type of subcortical infarcts occurring because of the occlusion of perforating end-arteries supplying the white matter, deep grey matter nuclei, and brainstem
- Named after the small lakes or 'lacunae' of infarction, they cause
- Conventionally defined as being <1.5 cm in maximum diameter
- Symptoms occur due to disruption of white matter tracts
- Because the fibres are packed together closely in the descending and ascending tracts, if they affect the motor pathways and cause weakness usually the face, arm, and leg are affected together. Sometimes only two body parts are affected. However, it is unusual for a single body part (e.g. arm or hand alone) to be affected. MRI studies have shown that these syndromes are more commonly caused by small cortical infarcts (see Fig. 3.6).

Common 'classical' lacunar syndromes

- Pure motor stroke—hemiparesis (most common)
- Pure sensory stroke—hemisensory loss
- Sensorimotor stroke—hemiparesis and hemisensory loss
- Ataxic hemiparesis—ataxia and hemiparesis on the same side
- Clumsy hand and dysarthria syndrome.

A large number of atypical syndromes may also occur.

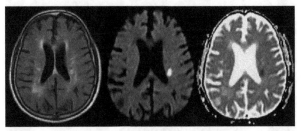

Fig. 3.6 MRI of an acute lacunar infarct. From left to right the scans show FLAIR and diffusion-weighted (DWI) images and an apparent diffusion coefficient (ADC) map. An acute lacunar infarct in the left corona radiata can be seen as high signal on DWI and corresponding low signal on the ADC map. It is in the corona radiata and resulted in right hemiparesis owing to disruption of the corticospinal tract. © Hugh Markus.

Striatocapsular infarction

These are infarcts in the striatocapsular region which includes the corpus striatum and internal capsule. They are typically comma-shaped (see Fig. 3.7) and are larger than the upper limit for lacunar infarcts (>1.5 cm).

They arise from transient occlusion of the MCA, usually due to an embolus. This results in ischaemia in both:
- the territory of the perforating arteries coming off the MCA
- the regions of the cortex supplied by the MCA.

The perforating arteries arising from the trunk of the MCA (lentostriatal branches) are end-arteries with no collateral supply. Therefore, the area supplied by them (the striatocapsular region) rapidly dies if the MCA is occluded by thrombus preventing flow into these perforating arteries. In contrast, the cortical regions receive some collateral supply and can survive for longer. If recanalization and reperfusion occurs before cortical infarction occurs, then the only region infarcted is the striatocapsular region.

Clinical features

Clinical features are caused by:
- infarction in the striatocapsular region, causing hemiparesis and hemisensory loss; as these areas are infarcted, these deficits are usually permanent
- ischaemia in cortical regions, e.g. dysphasia, neglect, hemianopia; as these areas are reperfused, the deficit is usually transient although it may take a few days to recover.

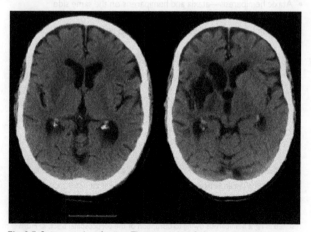

Fig. 3.7 Striatocapsular infarction. The scan on the left shows an early striatocapsular infarction with low density in the striatocapsular region. On the late scan on the right a much more well-developed area of infarction can be seen. © Anthony Pereira.

Causes

Striatocapsular infarction is usually due to either embolism from the heart or carotid artery or sometimes associated with MCA stenosis.

It often occurs in patients who are thrombolysed, when the treatment results in reperfusion and sparing of the cortex while infarction has already occurred in the region supplied by the perforating vessels.

This is an important diagnosis to be aware of because:

- cardiac embolic sources with echocardiogram and ECG monitoring, and carotid stenosis should always be carefully sought
- it is not caused by small-vessel disease
- the symptoms and signs owing to transient cortical ischaemia usually improve rapidly.

The posterior circulation

This comprises the vertebrobasilar circulation.
- The two vertebral arteries combine to form the basilar artery
- The basilar artery terminates in the two posterior cerebral arteries
- The anterior and posterior circulations are joined by the circle of Willis (see ➲ Fig. 3.2, p. 64).

The vertebral artery

- First branch of the subclavian artery
- It ascends through the foramina in the transverse processes of the upper six cervical vertebrae
- It then winds behind the atlas
- It enters the skull through the foramen magnum
- At the lower border of the pons it meets the vessel of the opposite side to form the basilar artery.

The vertebral artery may be divided into four parts (see Fig. 3.8):
- **V1**—the first part runs upward and backward behind the internal jugular and in front of the transverse process of the seventh cervical vertebra
- **V2**—the second part runs upward through the foramina in the transverse processes of the upper six cervical vertebrae, and pursues an almost vertical course as far as the transverse process of the atlas
- **V3**—the third part exits the foramen of the transverse process of the atlas and curves backwards behind the atlas and enters the vertebral canal by passing beneath the posterior atlanto-occipital membrane
- **V4**—the fourth part pierces the dura mater and inclines to the front of the medulla oblongata. At the lower border of the pons it unites with the vessel of the opposite side to form the basilar artery.

V1–3 are extracranial. V4 is intracranial.

The most common site of atheromatous stenosis is at the origin, i.e. in the V1 section. Sometimes the origin itself is referred to separately as the V0 section.

Asymmetry is common between the vertebral arteries—unlike the carotids. Around 15% of the population have a hypoplastic or atretic single vertebral artery (<2 mm in diameter). This may be clinically significant if the dominant vessel becomes diseased.

The branches of the vertebral artery

(See Fig. 3.9.)

Posterior spinal artery

This arises at the side of the medulla oblongata. Passing backward, it descends and is reinforced by a succession of small branches which enter the vertebral canal, and it continues to the cauda equina.

Anterior spinal artery

This arises near the termination of the vertebral and, descending in front of the medulla oblongata, unites with its fellow of the opposite side at the foramen magnum to form a single descending trunk which stretches down to the cauda equina.

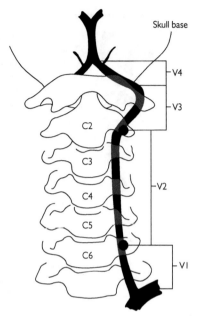

Fig. 3.8 The four segments of the vertebral artery.

Posterior inferior cerebellar artery (PICA)
The PICA is the largest branch of the vertebral arising from the intracranial portion and winds back around the upper part of the medulla oblongata. It supplies part of the brainstem and cerebellum.

Basilar artery
This is a single trunk formed by the junction of the two vertebral arteries: it extends from the lower to the upper border of the pons, lying in its median groove under cover of the arachnoid. It ends by dividing into the two posterior cerebral arteries. Its branches include:
- pontine vessels which come off at right angles from either side of the basilar artery and supply the pons
- the anterior inferior cerebellar artery
- the internal auditory artery
- the superior cerebellar artery.

Perforating arteries
End-arteries come off the intracranial vertebral and basilar arteries and supply the brainstem—occlusion of these results in brainstem lacunar infarcts.

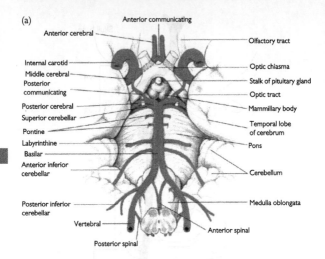

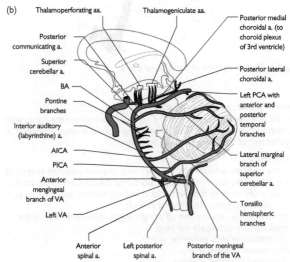

Fig. 3.9 The blood supply of the brainstem. (a) Anterior posterior view and (b) lateral view.

Reproduced from MacKinnon P, Morris J, *Oxford Textbook of Functional Anatomy*, Vol. 3, Copyright (2005), with permission from Oxford University Press.

Posterior cerebral arteries

These are the large terminal branches of the basilar artery. They are linked to the anterior circulation through the Pcom arteries. Their branches supply:

- posterior choroidal branches to the choroid plexus
- a considerable portion of the thalamus
- the temporal lobe cortex
- the occipital lobe.

An embryonic/normal variant seen in approximately 5% of the population is that the PCA arises directly from the ICA. This is clinically relevant as, in such circumstances, carotid stenosis can cause posterior circulation stroke symptoms.

Posterior circulation clinical syndromes

Ischaemia in the posterior circulation can present with symptoms caused by damage to functions controlled by the:
- the occipital cortex
- thalamus
- brainstem nuclei
- descending motor and ascending sensory pathways
- cerebellum
- the MRI in Fig. 3.10 shows multiple infarcts.

Posterior cerebral artery infarction

The following areas may be involved:

Parieto-occipital involvement
- Unilateral occipital infarction produces homonymous hemianopia
- Sparing of the macula may occur because of collateral vascular supply to the occipital pole
- Bilateral infarctions of the occipital lobes produce cortical blindness:
  - Anton syndrome, patients have realistic visual hallucinations
- Balint syndrome:
  - Bilateral parieto-occipital infarction
  - Simultanagnosia (patient identifies specific parts of a scene but cannot describe the entire picture), optic ataxia (a loss of hand–eye coordination) and apraxia of gaze.
- Pure alexia may result from infarction of the dominant occipital cortex.

Thalamus
- Thalamic infarction may present with confusion or memory disturbance and, if isolated, the diagnosis of stroke is sometimes missed. It often improves, particularly if the infarction is unilateral
- Pure hemisensory loss (infarction of the ventral posterolateral nucleus of the thalamus)
- Bilateral thalamic ('butterfly') infarction may cause an obtunded or comatose patient and/or severe memory dysfunction
- The artery of Percheron is a rare variant where a single thalamo-perforating artery arises from one P1 segment and bifurcates to supply both paramedian thalami. Occlusion results in bilateral paramedian thalamic infarcts with or without mesencephalic infarctions
- Thalamic infarction can be associated with post-stroke pain affecting one side of the body.

Other features
- Occlusion of the posterior choroidal artery may produce hemianopia, hemidysaesthesia, and memory disturbance
- In some cases, the posterior limb of the internal capsule is supplied from the PCA and infarction then results in hemiparesis
- Infarction of the medial temporal lobe or medial thalamic nuclei may result in permanent anterograde amnesia (normally bilateral infarction needed).

(a)   (b)

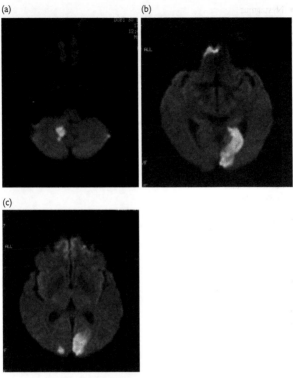

(c)

Fig. 3.10 Diffusion-weighted MRI showing multiple infarcts in the posterior circulation territory involving the (a) right cerebellum, (b) left cortical PCA territory, and (c) both occipital poles. © Hugh Markus.

Brainstem infarcts

From Fig. 3.11, it can be seen that there are many nuclei and tracts densely packed in the brainstem. Therefore, infarction here tends to be accompanied by other features and damage to the cranial nerves:
- Vertigo
- Diplopia
- Sensorineural hearing loss
- Facial numbness or paraesthesias
- Dysphagia
- Dysarthria
- Syncope (loss of consciousness)

- Nystagmus
- Limb and trunk ataxia
- Contralateral pain and temperature loss
- Ipsilateral limb and trunk numbness.

Two important brainstem syndromes are:

Lateral medullary infarct (Wallenberg syndrome)
- Ipsilateral facial pain and numbness
- Ipsilateral ataxia (falling to side of lesion)
- Vertigo, nausea, and vomiting
- Contralateral pain and temperature loss
- Nystagmus
- Ipsilateral Horner's syndrome.

Basilar artery occlusion
- Decreased level of consciousness
- Locked-in state
- Tetraplegia
- Horizontal gaze palsy
- Bifacial and oropharyngeal palsy.

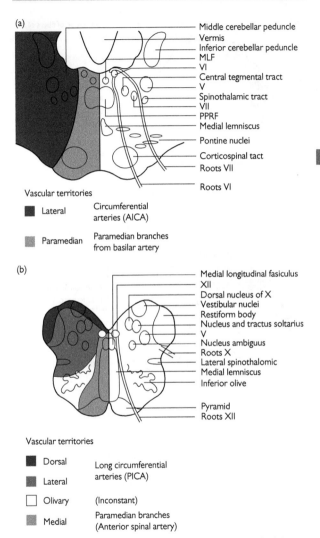

Fig. 3.11 Arterial supply of the pons (a) and medulla (b). Arterial supply of the lower (c) and upper (d) midbrain.

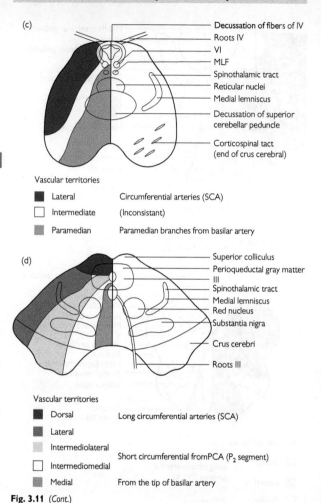

(c)

Decussation of fibers of IV
Roots IV
VI
MLF
Spinothalamic tract
Reticular nuclei
Medial lemniscus
Decussation of superior cerebellar peduncle
Corticospinal tact (end of crus cerebral)

Vascular territories

■ Lateral   Circumferential arteries (SCA)

□ Intermediate   (Inconsistant)

▨ Paramedian   Paramedian branches from basilar artery

(d)

Superior colliculus
Perioqueductal gray matter
III
Spinothalamic tract
Medial lemniscus
Red nucleus
Substantia nigra
Crus cerebri
Roots III

Vascular territories

■ Dorsal   Long circumferential arteries (SCA)

▨ Lateral

▤ Intermediolateral

□ Intermediomedial   Short circumferential fromPCA (P₂ segment)

▨ Medial   From the tip of basilar artery

Fig. 3.11 (Cont.)

Cerebellar infarction

This presents with ataxia. In addition, brainstem nuclei and their connections are also frequently infarcted, resulting in cranial nerve deficits, and involvement of ascending sensory and descending motor pathways in the brainstem is common; this results in hemiparesis and/or hemisensory loss.

Syndromes associated with infarction in specific cerebellar artery territories (Fig. 3.12) include the following.

Superior cerebellar artery infarct

- Ipsilateral ataxia
- If upper brainstem/cortex is involved:
  - hemianopia (or cortical blindness)
  - memory loss
  - confusion
  - contralateral hemiparesis.
- If brainstem is involved
  - ipsilateral Horner's syndrome
  - contralateral loss of pain sensation
  - contralateral sixth palsy
  - tremor.

Anterior inferior cerebellar artery

- Vertigo
- Dysarthria
- Ipsilateral facial palsy
- Ipsilateral Horner's syndrome
- Ipsilateral ataxia
- Ipsilateral hearing loss
- Contralateral pain loss
- Gaze palsy.

Posterior inferior cerebellar artery

- Wallenberg syndrome (see ➲ Brainstem infarcts, p. 123).

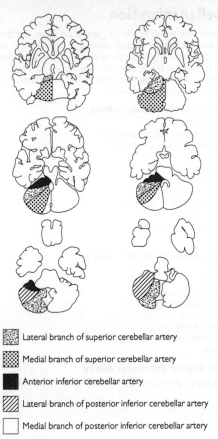

Lateral branch of superior cerebellar artery

Medial branch of superior cerebellar artery

Anterior inferior cerebellar artery

Lateral branch of posterior inferior cerebellar artery

Medial branch of posterior inferior cerebellar artery

Fig. 3.12 Arterial supply of the cerebellum.

Border zone areas of the brain

These regions of the brain are at the extremities of the vascular supply i.e. the regions which receive the lowest perfusion. Reduction in perfusion pressure either caused by systemic hypotension, and/or by tight stenoses, particularly if the collateral supply is poor, may result in border zone (or watershed) infarction.

The classical border zone areas are:
- cortical (dark grey in Fig. 3.13 and 3.14):
  - anterior border zone where the ACA supply meets the MCA
  - posterior border zone where the MCA supply meets the PCA.
- subcortical (light grey in Fig. 3.13 and 3.14):
  - internal border zone which is found at the extremity of the arterial arcades supplying the white matter of the centrum semiovale (see Fig. 3.15).

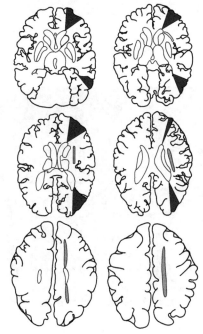

Fig. 3.13 The cerebral arterial border zone regions.

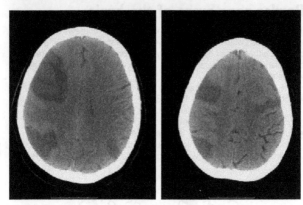

Fig. 3.14 Two slices of a CT brain scan in a patient who suffered cardiac arrest. The hypodense areas are regions of infarction. They are visible in the anterior and posterior border zones. © Hugh Markus.

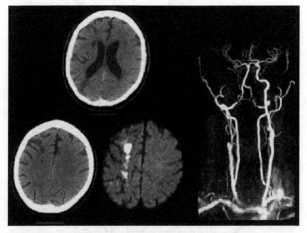

Fig. 3.15 The figure shows imaging from a patient who has suffered an acute right hemisphere infarct. The MRI (diffusion) image clearly shows the new infarcts, which appear bright on the DWI image, in the right internal border zone region. The CT scans show low density in the anterior and posterior cortical watershed areas and low density in the corona radiata comparable to the MRI. The MRA show an occluded right internal carotid artery. © Hugh Markus.

Venous drainage of the brain

The venous drainage of the brain is through the cerebral venous sinuses (see Fig. 3.16). They are:

- Situated between the two layers of the dura mater and are lined by endothelium continuous with that which lines the veins
- Devoid of valves
- Occlusion of the cerebral sinuses occurs in cerebral venous thrombosis (see Chapter 12).

The superior sagittal sinus

- This occupies the convex margin of the falx and runs from anterior to posterior
- There are usually three lacunae on either side of the sinus: a small frontal, a large parietal, and an occipital
- Most of the cerebral veins from the outer surface of the hemisphere open into these lacunae, and numerous arachnoid granulations (Pacchionian bodies) project into them from below
- It receives many dural draining veins and the superior cerebral veins.

The inferior sagittal sinus

- This runs in the posterior part of the free margin of the falx cerebri
- It ends in the straight sinus
- It receives several veins from the falx cerebri.

The straight sinus

- This is situated at the junction of the falx cerebri with the tentorium cerebelli
- It runs downward and backward from the end of the inferior sagittal sinus
- Its terminal part communicates with the confluence of the sinuses (sometimes called the Torcula)
- Besides the inferior sagittal sinus, it receives the great cerebral vein (great vein of Galen) and the superior cerebellar veins.

The transverse sinuses

- One, often the right, is the direct continuation of the superior sagittal sinus, while the other is a continuation of the straight sinus
- Each passes lateral and forward in the attached margin of the tentorium cerebelli
- It then leaves the tentorium and curves downward to reach the jugular foramen, where it ends in the internal jugular vein
- The portion which occupies the groove on the mastoid part of the temporal bone is sometimes termed the *sigmoid sinus*
- They receive the blood from the superior petrosal sinus
- They receive some of the inferior cerebral and inferior cerebellar veins.

The occipital sinus

- This is the smallest of the cranial sinuses
- It is situated in the attached margin of the falx cerebelli.

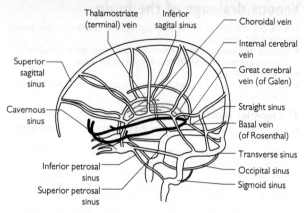

Fig. 3.16 The major cerebral venous sinuses.

The confluence of the sinuses

- This is the dilated extremity of the superior sagittal sinus
- It receives blood from the occipital sinus
- It connects across the midline to the opposite transverse sinus.

The cavernous sinuses

These structures (see Fig. 3.17) are anatomically important because thrombosis here results in a specific syndrome (see Chapter 12).

- They are so named because they present a reticulated structure
- They are traversed by numerous interlacing filaments
- They extend from the superior orbital fissure to the apex of the petrous portion of the temporal bone
- Each opens behind into the petrosal sinus
- On the medial wall of each sinus is the internal carotid artery
- Near the artery is the abducens nerve
- On the lateral wall are the oculomotor and trochlear nerves, and the ophthalmic and maxillary divisions of the trigeminal nerve are separated from the blood by the lining membrane of the sinus
- The cavernous sinus receives the superior ophthalmic vein through the superior orbital fissure
- It communicates with the transverse sinus by means of the superior petrosal sinus with the internal jugular vein through the inferior petrosal sinus
- The two sinuses also communicate with each other by means of the anterior and posterior intercavernous sinuses.

The superior petrosal sinus

- Small
- Connects the cavernous with the transverse sinus
- It joins the transverse sinus where the latter curves downward on the inner surface of the mastoid part of the temporal bone.

The inferior petrosal sinus

- It joins the cavernous sinus to the superior bulb of the internal jugular vein
- The inferior petrosal sinus receives the internal auditory veins and also veins from the medulla oblongata, pons, and undersurface of the cerebellum.

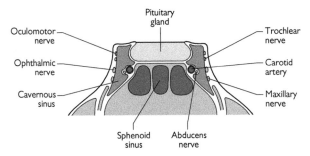

Fig. 3.17 Cross-sectional view through the cavernous sinus.

History-taking in the stroke patient

General principles of history-taking in the stroke patient

Stroke is defined as a sudden-onset focal neurological deficit lasting for 24 hours or more, or leading to earlier death attributed to a vascular cause.

Some newer definitions would classify symptoms lasting less than 24 hours as a stroke if there was an accompanying new brain infarct.

General points about history-taking

Make the patient central

Stroke affects people of all ages but is more common in older people. It can be very challenging to get a coherent history. By definition, stroke is sudden onset: one moment a person is well, and the next they are not. Acute stroke patients are often frightened, drowsy, disorientated, dysphasic, or confused as a result of the stroke or other comorbidity. Therefore, the history, the most vital part of clinical evaluation, may be very difficult.

Always start by allowing the patient to give their version of events. If allowed to speak, most patients will not talk for more than a couple of minutes and often that amount of time will provide all the information you need to make a diagnosis.

It cannot be overstated how important it is to get even a small amount of history from a patient. For example, it may provide a clue to the initial chest pain from the heart attack that led to the stroke—the heart attack that you are just about to miss because the stroke seems so obvious!

Always take a collateral history

This is particularly important in stroke patients, many of whom have communication or cognitive problems that limit their ability to give a complete history.

Therefore, consider talking to:
• witnesses who saw the event
• ambulance personnel who brought the patient to the emergency department
• family members who may provide important information on the patient's premorbid state and whether there were pre-existing cognitive problems
• the family doctor, who may provide important information on past medical history, particularly if an informant is unavailable.

Scheme of history-taking in stroke

Skilful history-taking should not take more than a few minutes, but it is important to have in mind a scheme of what you are looking for to help you find it.
• First, make the diagnosis
• Second, look for a cause
• Third, look for the risk factors.

Making the diagnosis

Key points to determine are:
- Is it a stroke?
- Could it be a mimic?
- What vascular territory is affected?

Some useful principles in stroke diagnosis

- The attack on the brain happens suddenly
- The brain stops working. A loss of function (e.g. weakness or visual field defect) rather than a gain of function (e.g. involuntary movement or positive visual phenomena) usually occurs
- The symptoms the patient experiences will parallel the underlying pathological process: the symptoms are 'telling' you the pathology
- An important feature of the history is the time course of symptoms, which indicates the time course of the pathological process.

Transient ischaemic attack (TIA)

TIA is defined as a sudden-onset focal neurological deficit which is fully recovered within 24 hours, i.e. it has a similar presentation to stroke and a similar pathophysiology

- TIA is defined as a sudden-onset focal neurological deficit which is fully recovered within 24 hours, i.e. it has a similar presentation to stroke and a similar pathophysiology
- Although patients with TIA recover within 24 hours, the average length of TIA is about 15 minutes and most last less than 1 hour
- With MRI it has been shown that many TIAs which last longer than an hour are associated with new infarction on DWI MRI and according to some newer definitions, would now be considered a stroke
- During the acute phase, particularly within the first 4½ hours when decisions on thrombolysis are being made, TIA and stroke cannot be differentiated
- Patients with TIA may not present for several days or weeks after the event, as transient symptoms are often ignored by patients. Then, obtaining a history of only 15 minutes of illness can be difficult.

Time of onset

- Re-perfusion therapies of thrombolysis and thrombectomy are time-dependent with regards to outcome and it is important to establish a time of onset of stroke.

Consider the time courses of disease

There are several time courses seen in neurology and keeping them in the back of your mind when tackling the history will help distinguish stroke from its mimics.

Sudden onset

Few pathological processes are sudden in onset, the main ones being:
- stroke
- epilepsy
- trauma.

Subacute

Here symptoms build up either over hours or days or perhaps weeks. The underlying pathology here may be:
• infectious
• inflammatory
• metabolic
• malignant.

Chronic and progressive

Symptoms which progress relentlessly over months or years are usually due to:
• malignancy
• degenerative disease, e.g. Alzheimer's disease or motor neuron disease.

Relapsing and remitting

A good example of this is multiple sclerosis.

The 'normal' stroke history

Stroke is almost always sudden in onset. If the symptoms are not sudden onset, then you should be very wary of diagnosing stroke.

The normal history for stroke is a sudden-onset loss of function of something. Most commonly, this will be loss of power down one side.

In a minority of cases stroke can progress after onset with new or worsening symptoms and signs; this is called early neurological deterioration (END). However, even in such cases the first symptoms are usually sudden onset.

Sometimes there are a multiplicity of symptoms which appear confusing. The way to tackle this is to deal with each symptom individually and try to work out the time course of the start of each symptom.

Differentiating stroke/TIA from mimic conditions

The main differential diagnoses of TIA in the emergency department are:
• blackouts/syncope
• epilepsy
• migraine with aura
• metabolic, particularly hypoglycaemia.

Isolated loss of consciousness

This is seldom due to stroke or TIA. Loss of consciousness in stroke occurs with:
• massive supratentorial stroke
• brainstem stroke—other posterior circulation neurological signs are almost always present (e.g. eye signs, ataxia, vertigo, vomiting)
• seizures (complicating the stroke).

Epileptic seizures

These may occur secondary to the acute stroke, but seizures in the absence of stroke can also present as a stroke mimic.
• Seizures are usually sudden onset
• There may be an aura that patients may recognize from previous attacks
• The aura is normally quite short

- The patient will lose consciousness
- The most common seizure type is the generalized tonic/clonic fit. This is aptly named as the patient will exhibit a tonic stage where the body goes stiff, usually in extension, followed by a clonic phase when all four limbs shake rhythmically
- Most seizures last only a couple of minutes
- The patient may bite their tongue or be incontinent during the seizure
- They will usually be confused and disorientated afterwards
- Post-ictal neurological symptoms and signs may occur—most commonly Todd's paresis, a hemiparesis which can last hours to days. This is more common in patients with previous stroke
- A careful eyewitness history is very helpful for diagnosis.

Migraine with aura

A typical migraine attack with aura accompanied by severe unilateral headache, nausea, and vomiting is easy to differentiate from stroke. However, migraine can present with aura alone and this can present diagnostic difficulty.

- The time course for migraine aura is that it usually develops over 5–20 minutes and lasts less than 60 minutes
- Migraine aura may precede or accompany the headache or occur in isolation
- The most common aura is visual; typically the patient may notice flashing lights, zigzag lines, or castellations moving across the visual field. Other aura symptoms include sensory (e.g. tingling in the arm) and dysphasic (difficulty finding words)
- There is what is termed a characteristic 'march' of symptoms: the visual phenomenon occurs first followed by the other phenomena, one subsiding while the next one starts. Similarly, sensory symptoms may march along the limb.

What vascular territory is affected?

Occlusion of a cerebral artery will result in ischaemia in the territory of that artery. Therefore, all symptoms and signs will be caused by malfunction of brain regions supplied by the affected artery. The pattern of symptoms (and signs) will help identify which arterial territory is affected. This may be of clinical importance, e.g. identifying a symptomatic carotid stenosis requiring urgent endarterectomy.

Initially try to determine whether the stroke has affected the anterior or posterior circulation. More details on vascular anatomy and associated stroke syndromes are given in ➔ Chapter 3. Some symptoms and signs (e.g. hemiparesis) may be caused by both anterior and posterior circulation ischaemia, while others are specific to one arterial circulation. This is detailed as follows and illustrated in Table 4.1.

Anterior circulation stroke

- Eighty per cent of cerebral blood flow and therefore 80% of ischaemic stroke
- Anterior cerebral artery:
  - may be asymptomatic
  - if hemiparesis, the leg is affected more
  - aphasia may occur with expressive difficulties or mutism

- Middle cerebral artery:
  - hemiparesis: face and arm are often more affected
  - hemianopia: optic radiation passes through MCA territory
  - aphasia: expressive and/or receptive (dominant hemisphere)
  - apraxia: present with infarction in either hemisphere
- Do check handedness of patients. Most patients are right-hand dominant and left hemisphere language dominant. In those who are left-hand dominant, 50% will still be left hemisphere language dominant.

Posterior circulation stroke
- Sometimes termed vertebrobasilar territory infarction or vertebrobasilar insufficiency; the latter term is better not used
- Most ischaemic stroke is embolic or due to small-vessel disease
- Haemodynamic insufficiency is a much rarer cause
- The vertebral arteries unite to form the basilar artery, which terminates in the posterior cerebral arteries. These vessels supply the brainstem, pons, cerebellum, occipital lobes, and, to a varying degree, the posterior thalamus
- Common clinical features of posterior circulation ischaemia include

Brainstem and cerebellar involvement:
- Vertigo
- Vertigo
- diplopia
- nausea and vomiting
- unsteadiness and ataxia
- deafness
- dysarthria
- hemiparesis—but will spare face if below pons
- hemisensory loss
- loss of consciousness
- bilateral or crossed weakness/sensory disturbance

Posterior cerebral artery involvement:
- hemianopia
- cortical blindness (owing to basilar occlusion and disruption of both posterior cerebral arteries)
- confusion/amnesia (branches supplying posterior thalamus).

A good rule of thumb is that at least *two* symptoms and signs should be present to make one suspect posterior circulation infarction.

A crucial point is that hemiparesis may be caused by a lesion anywhere along the motor pathway from the motor cortex to the cervical cord. However, only if it is in the brainstem would it become accompanied by vertigo, diplopia, nausea, and vomiting.

Isolated vertigo is rarely due to stroke or TIA and is far more commonly caused by peripheral labyrinthine disturbance. However, it is important to determine whether the onset was truly sudden and probe for other brainstem symptoms in these cases.

Table 4.1 Symptoms and signs associated with anterior and posterior circulation stroke

Symptom/sign	Anterior circulation	Posterior circulation
Hemiparesis	Yes	Yes
Hemisensory loss	Yes	Yes
Hemianopia	Yes	Yes
Slurred speech	Yes	Yes
Neglect	Yes	No
Aphasia	Yes	No
Apraxia	Yes	No
Drowsy	Yes	Yes
Loss of consciousness	No	Sometimes
Diplopia	No	Yes
Nystagmus	No	Yes
Ataxia	No	Yes
Nausea/vomiting	No	Yes
Vertigo	No	Yes
Crossed signs	No	Yes
Quadriparesis	No	Yes

What caused the stroke: clues from the history

Stroke describes a syndrome which can be caused by many different pathologies. A key question, which is of major importance later when planning management, is 'What has caused this stroke in this person?'; i.e. is it embolism from a carotid artery, cardioembolism, small-vessel disease, dissection, etc.

This is *not* the same as asking for risk factors, although the two do overlap. Go through the normal history.

Past medical history

- Previous stroke or TIA
- Heart disease:
  - past myocardial infarct (MI)
  - recent chest pain suggesting recent MI (or thoracic root aortic dissection)
  - atrial fibrillation
  - rheumatic fever as a child
  - valvular heart disease or valve replacement
  - symptoms of heart failure
  - palpitations
  - pacemaker
- Peripheral vascular disease
- Diabetes
- Recent injury (e.g. to the neck). Ask if the patient has had any trauma of the head or neck in the last few weeks and investigate whether they have noticed any neck pain or pain behind the eye that may identify dissection
- Evidence of thrombophilia (e.g. DVT, PE, recurrent miscarriages).

Drug history

- Triangulate the drug history with the past history. For example, patients may have forgotten past seizures but they may still be on an antiepileptic
- Oral contraceptive pill
- Hormone replacement therapy
- Illicit drug use, e.g. cocaine.

Family history

This must be taken in full. A full family history is important for two reasons.
- It may detect rare monogenic causes of stroke (➔ p. 326)
- Family history is a risk factor for 'sporadic' stroke.

This should be taken in a systematic fashion.
- For first-degree relatives (parent and siblings) ask:
  - are they are alive—if so, what age?
  - if dead—age and cause of death
  - have they had stroke—if so, at what age?
  - have they had MI—if so, at what age?

- have they had other neurological disease (e.g. stroke in the young can be misdiagnosed as multiple sclerosis; vascular dementia is often misdiagnosed as Alzheimer's disease).
- For more distant relatives, ask if any had stroke, MI, dementia, or other neurological diseases and if so, record age of onset and death
- It helps to record family history on a family tree visually using standard symbols (Fig. 4.1).

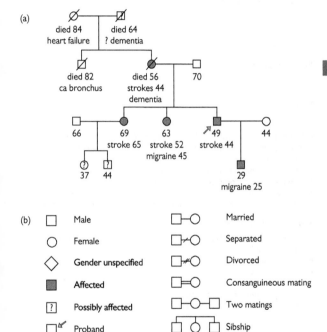

Fig. 4.1 (a) An example of a family tree from a family with CADASIL, an autosomal dominant form of stroke (➔ p. 328). (b) Standard symbols illustrated are used to indicate the status of individuals.

Reproduced from Markus H, *Stroke Genetics*, Copyright (2003), with permission from Oxford University Press.

Risk factors

History of risk factors

Next, move on to the risk factors. This will be identified by both history and examination and investigation. Ask about:
- hypertension
- diabetes
- angina
- peripheral vascular disease
- high cholesterol
- smoking
- alcohol
- family history of stroke.

Social history

It is very important to have some idea of the person who now has the disease.
- Do they work; if so, what is their job?
- Do they drive?
- Do they have a partner?
- Who do they live with—what is their social support network?
- Are they in receipt of social services or reliant on others for domestic or personal care?
- What are their hobbies or pastimes?
- What sort of accommodation do they live in?
- Also, you must not be shy about asking if they take recreational drugs or are at risk of HIV or sexually transmitted diseases such as syphilis.

Functional enquiry

Lastly, go through the functional enquiry. This is a good chance to catch anything missed.
- Cardiovascular system
- Respiratory system
- Abdominal system
- Urinary system and continence
- Problems with skin or joints. Previous level of mobility/falls.

Summary

- Stroke is almost always sudden in onset
- Determine the time of onset
- The time course of symptoms is essential.

First, make the diagnosis:
- Is it a stroke?
- Could it be a mimic?
- What vascular territory is affected?

Second, look for a cause, e.g.:
- Heart disease
- Drug use.

Third, look for the risk factors:
- Hypertension
- Diabetes
- Smoking
- Heart disease
- Cholesterol
- Age
- Family history.

Make sure you take as much history from the patient as possible.

Find out about the patient's premorbid state and home situation, and determine what the immediate problems are for the patient.

Take an eyewitness report if available.

Always take a collateral history.

It may be helpful to talk to the family doctor.

Examination of the stroke patient

Introduction

The examination must seek specific information to:
- understand the anatomy of the disease
- form a diagnosis
- plan management
- anticipate possible complications.

The neurological examination provides information to aid diagnosis:
- Where is the lesion and does it fit into an arterial territory?
- Is there evidence of single or multiple lesions?
- Is the stroke in an arterial territory supplied by the carotid or vertebral artery?
- Has the stroke damaged or spared the cerebral cortex?
- Is this a lacunar syndrome?

The systemic examination is an equally important part of the evaluation of the stroke patient. Like the neurological examination, it must be directed to look for signs that may identify the cause of the stroke and it may identify aetiological factors such as:
- atrial fibrillation
- hypertension and hypertensive end-organ damage
- complications of diabetes mellitus
- carotid bruits
- cardiac murmurs
- absent peripheral pulses
- cigarette tar-stained fingers.

The examination will also assess the degree of neurological impairment and disability. In the acute setting, the NIH Stroke Scale (NIHSS) is most frequently used (see ➲ p. 546) as a standardized examination to assess stroke severity and has become an integral part in the assessment of a suspected stroke.

In the non-acute setting, other scales to describe the degree of disability, such as the Modified Rankin (mRS) (see ➲ p. 560) and the Barthel scales are more often used.

The examination is important in planning individualized management and rehabilitation. How has a stroke affected the person in front of you and what issues will they immediately be confronted with on the stroke unit?
- Is swallowing impaired?
- To what extent is communication affected?
- Is there neglect?
- Is the patient continent?
- Is there function left in the hands/arms?
- Can the patient sit/stand/walk?

Neurological examination

Follow a conventional neurological examination. Start at the top and work down.

Components of the neurological examination
- Inspection
- Conscious level
- Speech and language
- Higher mental function
- Cranial nerves
- Peripheral nervous system
- General examination.

Inspection

This is an important part of any examination. Stand back and look at the patient for a few moments. It can pay dividends. For example, you may see focal twitching of a limb and make a diagnosis of seizure.

It is best to have a system for inspection. We do the following:
- Is the patient alert or drowsy?
- Is the patient having absences?
- Is the speech abnormal?
- Is the head normal size and shape? Is there evidence of head injury?
- Is there pallor or cyanosis?
- Is there abnormal facial asymmetry?
- Is there eye deviation to one side or a squint?
- Are the limbs normal length? A fractured limb may be apparent from observation
- Are all limbs moving spontaneously or is there a particular pattern of lack of movement (e.g. hemiplegia/paraplegia/tetraplegia)?
- Is there resting tremor or jerking of any limbs?

Higher mental function and conscious level

Higher mental function

Many trainees find this difficult to assess. It is best to examine using a systematic approach, as described next. If some parts cannot be examined due to aphasia, other cognitive deficits, or reduced conscious level, record this and move on.

Examination of higher mental function should be considered as examination of different parts of the brain itself. For example, Broca's aphasia would indicate damage to the dominant frontal lobe.

Domains which should be assessed include:
- conscious level
- speech: dysarthria or dysphonia or aphasia
- orientation (time, place, and person)
- memory
- neglect
- ability to think and calculate
- ability to mime simple tasks
- ability to read, write, and copy drawn shapes.

Conscious level

This should be assessed using the Glasgow Coma Score (GCS). This gives some indication of the size of stroke and has some predictive value regarding the long-term outcome. Unconscious patients have a much worse prognosis.

Glasgow Coma Score
- This scale is widely used to assess, and monitor, conscious level
- It is scored between 3 and 15, 3 being the worst, and 15 being the best (see Table 5.1)
- It contains three domains: best eye response, best verbal response, and best motor response
- It is better to think about the composition of the GCS rather than just a number
- Remember, all dysphasic patients will have a reduced GCS but may not be drowsy.

Orientation

Test this by asking the current time, current place, and if the patient can identify an appropriate person (e.g. doctor or nurse). Identify if they are aphasic or confused (see ➲ Speech and language, p. 108). The two are frequently confused.

Table 5.1 Glasgow Coma Score

Best eye response (maximum 4 points)	
No eye opening	1
Eye opening to pain	2
Eye opening to verbal command	3
Eyes open spontaneously	4
Best verbal response (maximum 5 points)	
No verbal response	1
Incomprehensible sounds	2
Inappropriate words	3
Confused	4
Orientated	5
Best motor response (maximum 6 points)	
No motor response	1
Extension to pain	2
Flexion to pain	3
Withdrawal from pain	4
Localizing pain	5
Obeys commands	6

Speech and language

Listening carefully to spontaneous speech during history-taking may already have identified a speech problem. Specific questions during the examination will then allow the nature of the speech problem to be fully determined (see Fig. 5.1 for the anatomy).

Speech problems can be divided into:
- dysarthria
- dysphonia
- aphasia.

Dysarthria

- This describes slurred speech
- The commonest cause of this is weakness of the face, and a facial palsy may be apparent
- Patients can be very difficult to understand but usually one can discern that their words are appropriate but slurred
- They will be able to use 'yes' and 'no' correctly and consistently—either verbally or by head nods/shakes or gesture
- With experience, one can distinguish:
  - lower motor neuron (bulbar) dysarthria with air escape through the nose
  - upper motor neuron, pseudobulbar, spastic dysarthria; the patient sounds as though they are speaking with a boiled sweet in their mouth
  - cerebellar dysarthria has a characteristic 'mon-o-syl-lab-ic' quality
  - Parkinsonian, extrapyramidal dysarthria: quiet, monotonous, and slow
  - Remember mild dysarthria may pre-exist or be due to ill-fitting dentures or the effects of drugs and alcohol.

Dysphonia

- A problem with sound production
- Speech articulation is normal, as is the content but the sound is abnormal (e.g. bovine cough) or hypophonic
- May be caused by vocal cord paralysis.

Aphasia

- This is a problem with language
- The terms aphasia and dysphasia are both used but aphasia is increasingly seen as the preferred terminology
- Examination for aphasia includes testing spontaneous speech, fluency, naming, and repetition. Also remember to test comprehension, reading, and writing
- Aphasia is normally split into expressive or receptive problems
- Usually in stroke, both coexist. Where there is no verbal output and no understanding of language, the condition is termed global aphasia.

Receptive aphasia

- Caused by a lesion in the dominant temporal lobe affecting Wernicke's area, superior temporal gyrus posterior to the Sylvian fissure
- To test a receptive aphasia, start by testing comprehension

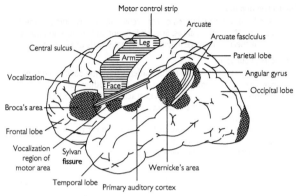

Fig. 5.1 Diagram of the speech areas.

- Ask the patient to perform a single-stage command such as to touch their nose or put a hand on their head. Then move on to a more complex command; e.g. give them a two-stage command ('touch your nose and then your ear'), asking them not to start acting the command until you have finished the full command or use a complex task such as ordering objects on the bedside table
- Patients with a severe receptive aphasia tend to be fluent in their speech but use the wrong words. Sometimes this can manifest as real words used in the wrong context or made-up words (neologisms) or just plain gibberish
- If the patient is truly receptively aphasic, they will be distant and unable to communicate either verbally or by writing or by using behavioural cues (e.g. pointing to the mouth to indicate hunger).

Expressive aphasia

- Caused by a lesion in the dominant dorsal frontal lobe affecting Broca's area
- An impairment of speech production or the ability to 'think of words'
- Comprehension is better. In pure forms or as patients understand that what they are saying is wrong, they frequently become frustrated
- Communication with these patients can be improved by tailoring the consultation to simple 'yes' and 'no' closed questions and by using cues and gestures
- If receptive abilities are preserved, there is a greater capacity for recovery
- Nominal aphasia is a subtype of expressive aphasia. It is the inability to identify names of objects. This is most easily tested by asking the subject to name different parts of a watch or pen or object by the bedside.

Conduction aphasia

- Caused by subcortical lesions of the arcuate fasciculus which connect Broca's and Wernicke's areas. Speech is fluent and comprehension is intact but there is a severe inability to repeat words or phrases.

Transcortical aphasias

- The important feature here is that patients have the ability to *repeat* words although they may not be able to speak otherwise
- The transcortical motor aphasia is characterized by reasonable understanding of speech but difficulty in producing words. Speech is effortful and halting
- The transcortical sensory aphasia looks very similar to a receptive aphasia but with intact repetition.
- Transcortical aphasia indicates a subcortical lesion.

Apraxia of Speech (Verbal apraxia)

- This is when there is difficulty in producing the movements required to phonate and articulate speech in the absence of any weakness or paralysis
- Apraxic speech causes issues with generating the sound of speech as well as rate and rhythm of speaking
- It is often caused by damage to the inferior frontal and pre-central dominant cortex (MCA territory) and so often coexists with a degree of aphasia as well as contralateral upper limb weakness.

Apraxia and agnosia

Apraxia

Here there is loss of ability to perform a previously learned or well-practised motor task. For example, the loss of the ability to walk in spite of normal power, sensation, and coordination may be described as gait apraxia.

Types of apraxia to consider:

- Gait apraxia, where walking is very abnormal although the legs may move well enough in the bed
- Dressing apraxia, where the patient's dressing routine becomes disordered
- Ideomotor apraxia, where a patient cannot mime a response to your command but may do the movement spontaneously (e.g. 'scratch your nose')
- Ideational apraxia, where the patient cannot plan a series of movements and cannot perform a three-part command
- Constructional apraxia, where the patient cannot copy.

Apraxia normally indicates a dominant hemisphere parietal lesion. However, the inability to copy interlocking shapes indicates a deficit in the right parietal lobe.

In stroke it is unusual to have a pure apraxia. More commonly in a MCA infarct, apraxia coexists with aphasia and hemiparesis.

It is helpful to have a list of examination routines to use if you think the patient is apraxic. We ask the patient to:

- make a fist
- scratch their nose
- imitate combing their hair
- imitate using scissors to cut something
- imitate how they would pay for their shopping
- mimic the examiner interlocking the fingers of both hands
- copy two interlocking shapes drawn by the examiner.

Agnosia

This is the failure to recognize objects in spite of normal working afferent input (e.g. normal sensation or vision).

Forms of agnosia to consider:

- Visual agnosia—here patients can see an object and describe it but may not be able to say what it is
- Prosopagnosia—here one cannot recognize a famous face
- Anosagnosia—here a stroke patient may not realize they have had a stroke or that the affected limbs are weak (this usually indicates a right parietal lesion causing left-sided anosognosia)
- Astereognosis—here a patient will not be able to distinguish coins of differing value placed in their hand. Sensation in the hand must be preserved and the hand must retain some dexterity.

Location of lesion in agnosias

- Usually indicates a parietal lesion
- Visual agnosia may be attributed to a parieto-occipital lesion

- Anosagnosia is caused by a frontoparietal lesion. The patient may deny they have any (obvious) weakness
- A form of visual anosagnosia (Anton syndrome) is seen in patients with bilateral occipital infarction; these patients have bilateral cortical blindness but may deny that they are blind.

Neglect and inattention

Here patients fail to recognize or attend to stimuli on one side of the body.

- A patient may completely ignore (neglect) one side of their body and things/people on this side
- Neglect may indicate a lesion of either parietal lobe but is classically described with right-sided lesions
- It is important to detect as it has implications for rehabilitation, e.g. the patient may only attend to people and stimuli on one side. It is associated with worse outcomes from rehabilitation.

Inattention should be tested for as part of the neurological examination. It may be:

- sensory
- visual
- auditory.

Neglect and inattention may be assessed by the following:

- Careful observation during history-taking and examination
  - You may notice the patient is not attending to one side
- Systematic examination:
  - To test for inattention, stimuli are presented to both sides simultaneously and the patient fails to identify the stimulus on the affected side
  - First, it is essential to determine that the patient can detect the stimulus when presented to the affected side alone, i.e. if they have a hemianopia, it is not possible to test for visual inattention
  - Therefore, to detect visual inattention, move a finger in one hemifield, then the other. If they can detect both, then move fingers in both simultaneously. If they have visual inattention, they will not notice it in the neglecting field on bilateral simultaneous presentation
  - For sensory inattention, touch both hands in turn and then both simultaneously
  - Similarly, for auditory inattention, snap one's fingers simultaneously by each ear having first ensured adequate hearing on each side.

Memory and frontal tests

Memory

During normal examination, a screen, including memory tests, is performed, such as the abbreviated mental test score (aMTS), the MiniMental Test Examination (MMSE), or the Montreal Cognitive Assessment (MoCA, which can be downloaded from ℛ http://www.mocatest.org/). This is useful for identifying gross deficits and dementia. If deficits are uncovered, more detailed testing is required, and this is often performed with the assistance of a neuropsychologist.

The simple schema suggested here for bedside testing relies on memory being subdivided into the following subtypes.

Episodic memory

This is the ability to recall 'episodes in one's life'. For our purposes, we can think of it as the ability to learn new memories and recall them after minutes or days. It is split into the following:
- Anterograde memory, the ability to remember new things. Ask the patient to repeat the names of three objects (e.g. apple, pen, tie) and then recall them after 5 minutes
- Retrograde memory, the recall of past events

It usually indicates damage to the prefrontal cortex and hippocampus, and may be profound if bilateral.

Working memory

Working memory is the temporary storage of information while manipulations are performed on the memorized information.
- This can be assessed by determining digit span backwards
- It is often caused by disruption of cortical–subcortical circuits due to subcortical stroke or leukoaraiosis.

Semantic memory

This is the recall of meanings and general knowledge. Test historical data (e.g. the years of World War II, the name of the last prime minister).

Implicit memory

This is the recall of learned patterns (e.g. riding a bicycle depends on procedural memory, a form of implicit memory).

Calculation

Ask the patient to subtract 7 serially from 100 (or 3 from 20 for an easier task). This tests concentration and memory as well as calculation.

Frontal and executive tests

The frontal lobes are involved in planning and execution of tasks. Lesions of the frontal lobes may, therefore, produce problems with executive tasks (i.e. the ability to carry out a task). Cortical lesions often only result in these deficits if they are bilateral. Executive deficits are common in subcortical vascular disease, particularly bilateral lacunar stroke and/or leukoaraiosis caused by small-vessel disease. This is due to the disruption of white matter pathways and the disruption of frontocortical projections. These are not well detected by screening tests such as the MMSE and aMTS designed for memory impairment, and require tests focusing on executive function such as the Brief Memory and Executive Test (BMET; freely downloadable from ℘ www.bmet.info).

Frontal lobe lesions may be identified by the following features.

As well as using cognitive batteries such as the BMET there are simple bedside tests for executive function such as Trails B—the patient is asked to connect numbers and letters alternately in ascending order (e.g. 1, A, 2, B,3, C) and the accuracy and speed with which they do it is recorded.

Perseveration

Patients may continue to repeat a past movement when asked to do something else. They have difficulty changing sequence. This can be demonstrated using Luria's hand sequence task. The patient is asked to tap with their fist, palm, and the side of their hand in sequence. Patients with frontal dysfunction have difficulty with this or when asked to change the sequence.

Utilization behaviour

Here, handing the patient an object may stimulate them to use it no matter how inappropriate. For example, patients may put on a second or even third (!) pair of spectacles.

Emotional lability

Inappropriate laughing and crying often in response to the most minor stimuli or even no stimulus at all.

Inaccurate cognitive estimates

The patient loses the ability to reason and may guess wildly inaccurately. For example, one can ask:
• How high is Nelson's column (185 feet, 56 metres)?
• How fast does a race horse run (not 100 mph)?
• How many elephants are there in England?

Clues from the history of executive dysfunction

• Loss of motivation: 'sits in front of the TV all day'
• Loss of ability to multi-task
• Loss of planning ability.

In addition to these tests, there are frontal release signs indicating bilateral frontal damage or disconnection:
• Grasp reflex—stroke the patient's palm with the handle of the tendon hammer. The patient may grasp it and not be able to let go
• Rooting reflex—here, stroking the side of the mouth will make the subject turn their head towards the stimulus. The subject may also start sucking
• Palmar mental reflex—here, a contraction of the mentalis muscle of the chin is elicited following a brief scratch of the thenar side of the palm.

Examination of the cranial nerves

There are 12 cranial nerves (see Table 5.2).

Table 5.2 Cranial nerves

	Name	Function	Clinical
I	Olfactory	Sense of smell	Anosmia
II	Optic	Vision and direct pupillary light reflex	Blindness, loss of direct pupillary light reflex
III	Oculomotor	Medial rectus, superior rectus, inferior rectus, inferior oblique levator palpebrae	Dilated, fixed pupil, ptosis, ipsilateral gaze fixed 'down and out'
IV	Trochlear	Superior oblique intorts eye and rotates down and out	Weakness of down gaze. Can't look at your nose
V	Trigeminal	Ophthalmic, maxillary, mandibular branches	Loss of sensation in the face, eyes, nose, and mouth. Loss of corneal reflex. Deviation of the jaw to the ipsilateral side
VI	Abducens	Lateral rectus muscle	Esotropia
VII	Facial	Facial movement, taste, salivation, and lacrimation	Facial palsy, loss of blink, loss of taste from the anterior two-thirds of the tongue
VIII	Acoustic (vestibulocochlear)	Balance and hearing	Vertigo, tinnitus, and deafness
IX	Glossopharyngeal	Taste, salivation, and swallowing	Loss of pharyngeal and gag reflex, loss of taste from posterior third of tongue
X	Vagus	Larynx and swallowing	Dysarthria
XI	Spinal accessory	Larynx and muscles in the neck	Difficulty in turning the neck; drooping shoulder
XII	Hypoglossal	Tongue movement	Ipsilateral tongue paralysis

Examination of the cranial nerves should encompass:

- Visual acuity and visual fields
- Eye movements
- Pupillary responses, corneal reflex, and fundoscopy
- Facial movement (expression and biting)
- Facial sensation
- Hearing
- Palatal and tongue movement and gag reflex

Shoulder shrug, head turning, and neck flexion.

Cranial nerve I (olfactory)

- Unmyelinated fibres going from the olfactory epithelium in the nose, through the cribriform plate of the ethmoid bone to the olfactory bulb
- Seldom affected in stroke
- Damage causes loss of smell (sometimes manifesting in the patient's perception as loss of taste)
- Test by getting the patient to identify the smell of fruit.

Cranial nerve II (optic)

- Connects the retina to the superior colliculi and lateral geniculate nuclei (see Fig. 5.2)
- There is a decussation at the optic chiasm
- The lateral fibres continue on the ipsilateral side
- The nasal fibres decussate to the opposite side
- Proximal to the decussation, damage results in blindness in one eye
- Distal to the decussation and in the ensuing optic radiation which terminates in the occipital cortex, damage results in loss of information for the right or left visual field and hence hemianopia
- The pupillary light reflex fibres bypass the geniculate body and go to the pretectal area, then to the Edinger Westphal nucleus and the parasympathetic fibres run with the third nerve: the arc for the consensual pupillary reflex.

The examination of the optic nerve includes:

- Acuity, using the Snellen chart
- Visual fields to confrontation (do each eye separately)
- Colour, with an Ishihara chart (sensitive to optic neuropathy or demyelination)
- Fundoscopy—ideally with a pan ophthalmoscope (papilloedema, vessel changes, e.g. hypertension, retinopathy, emboli)
- Pupil examination—shine a bright torchlight into each eye separately. Look for the response to direct light and then the consensual response to light directed into the contralateral eye. Next, ask the patient to follow your finger as it is moved back and forth. Observe the pupil constrict as the finger nears the patient's nose and the pupil dilate as it is moved away again
- Sympathetic dysfunction produces Horner's syndrome where the pupil is small but reacts to light. This is accompanied by partial ptosis and is common in carotid dissection

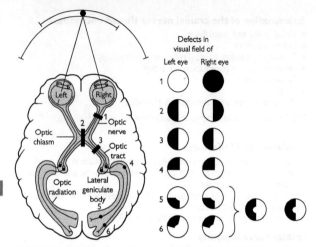

Fig. 5.2 The anatomy of the visual pathway showing the visual field defects which result from lesions at different sites. 1, Unilateral blindness; 2, bitemporal hemianopia; 3, homonymous hemianopia; 4, superior quadrantanopia; 5, 6, inferior and superior quadrantanopias with macular sparing. Reproduced from Manji H, *Oxford Handbook of Neurology*, Copyright (2006), with permission from Oxford University Press.

Reproduced from *Lancet*, 304(7872), Teasdale G, Jennett B, Assessment of coma and impaired consciousness: A practical scale, pp. 81–83, Copyright (1974), with permission from Elsevier.

- Parasympathetic dysfunction produces a large and poorly reacting pupil
- Damage to the ciliary ganglion or short ciliary nerves produces a tonic pupil where the pupil reacts very slowly to light and then may remain contracted. The response to accommodation is rapid
- Marcus–Gunn pupil: this is demonstrated by the swinging flashlight test. The abnormal pupil appears to dilate (paradoxically) when the light is switched back to the abnormal eye. It is seen in a relative afferent pupillary defect.

Cranial nerve III (oculomotor)

This comes from its nucleus in the midbrain. It supplies:
- the pupil constrictors (damage causes a dilated pupil)
- levator palpebrae superioris (damage causes ptosis)
- superior, inferior, and medial rectus and inferior oblique (damage causes ophthalmoplegia).

In a complete palsy, the eye will often be in a down and out position. Damage to the nerve or its nucleus causes diplopia in more than one direction of gaze. Also, as the medial rectus is involved, adduction of the eye is difficult.

Cranial nerve IV (trochlear)

This comes from the midbrain and runs over the trochlea pulley. It controls the superior oblique and tips the eye down and in. It enables you to look at the end of your nose.

- Lesions result in the eye drifting out
- If the right superior oblique is affected, the diplopia is worse when the eye tries to look to the left or the head is tilted to the right
- Often, if asked to look down, the patient notes diplopia with two images, one above the other. If the two images are horizontal, they appear angulated, like an arrowhead, and it points towards the bad side
- If the patient's head is tilted towards the shoulder on the side of a superior oblique palsy, the separation of the images increases (Bielschowsky sign).

Cranial nerve V (trigeminal)

This nerve has a long nucleus. The nucleus lies in the midbrain and pons with part of it reaching down to the cervical region (the spinal tract of the trigeminal nerve). It provides sensation from the face and innervates the muscles of mastication. There are three divisions of the trigeminal nerve:

- Ophthalmic (V_1)—damage results in sensory loss over the forehead
- Maxillary (V_2)—damage results in loss of sensation over the cheek
- Mandibular (V_3)—damage results in loss of sensation in the jaw back towards the ear.

In stroke, if complete paralysis of the trigeminal nerve occurs, this results in sensory loss over the ipsilateral face and weakness of the muscles of mastication. Attempted opening of the mouth results in deviation of the jaw to the paralysed side.

Cranial nerve VI (abducens)

The nucleus of the nerve is located in the paramedian pontine region in the floor of the fourth ventricle. It innervates the lateral rectus which abducts the eye.

- Damage results in failure of abduction of the eye and diplopia on lateral gaze
- Abducens nerve palsy may result from raised intracranial pressure and pressure on the nerve as well as pontine stroke.

Cranial nerve VII (facial)

The nucleus of the nerve lies in the floor of the fourth ventricle (facial colliculus).

- The fibres wind around the nucleus of the sixth nerve
- The facial nerve exits the cranial cavity through the stylomastoid foramen
- It sends branches to the muscles that control facial expression
- It also innervates a small strip of skin at the back of the pinna and around the external auditory canal
- The nervus intermedius conducts taste sensation from the anterior two-thirds of the tongue
- It also supplies autonomic innervation to the salivary and lacrimal glands

- Lower motor neuron lesions occur in Bell's palsy
- Upper motor neuron lesions occur in stroke.

These are sometimes confused, resulting in Bell's palsy being diagnosed as stroke. They can usually easily be differentiated:
- A lower motor neuron facial palsy paralyses the whole side of the face.
- In an upper motor neuron lesion, the forehead is spared.

Isolated facial palsies are not uncommon in stroke. Exceptionally, a brain-stem stroke affecting the facial nerve can cause a lower motor neuron facial palsy but this is very rare.
Other tricks to help the differentiation:
- If the lesion is proximal to the nerve to the stapedius, hyperacusis, loss of taste in the anterior two-thirds of the tongue, loss of lacrimation, and facial weakness occur
- If the lesion is distal to the nerve to the stapedius but before the chorda tympani, loss of taste in the anterior two-thirds of the tongue and facial weakness occur
- If the lesion is distal to the nerve to the chorda tympani, facial weakness occurs.

Cranial nerve VIII (vestibulocochlear)

This arrives in the brainstem at the pontomedullary junction. It serves hearing and vestibular function.

Hearing

- Tested by whispering numbers into one of the patient's ears while covering the other ear and asking the patient to repeat the numbers heard
- Alternatively, hold a tuning fork close to each ear and ask the patient to say when they cannot hear it any longer. If you can still hear it but they cannot, then there is a problem
- If hearing loss is identified, then one has to distinguish conductive loss from sensorineural loss. There are two common tests used:
  - *Rinne's test*—a vibrating tuning fork is placed at the opening of the ear canal (air conduction) and then on the mastoid bone (bone conduction). It is normally louder when heard at the mouth of the ear canal. If there is a conductive problem (such as damage to the ossicles), sound is better heard when the tuning fork is placed on the mastoid bone
  - *Weber's test*—the tuning fork is placed on the forehead in the midline. Normally sound is heard equally in the centre. In conductive hearing loss, sound is better heard in the 'bad' ear. If the patient is deaf in one ear, it will be heard in the good ear.

Therefore, to test hearing quickly:
1. Can you hear this tuning fork?
2. Which side is louder? (Weber's test)
3. Is it louder in front or behind the ear? (Rinne's test).

Vestibular function

The vestibular nerve links the utricle and saccule (linear acceleration) and the cristae in the ampullae of the semicircular canals (angular acceleration) with the vestibular nucleus. This is a complex nucleus. The superior, lateral, medial, and inferior nuclei project to the:

- Pontine gaze centre through the medial longitudinal fasciculus
- Cervical and upper thoracic levels of the spinal cord through the medial vestibulospinal tract
- Lumbosacral regions of the ipsilateral spinal cord through the lateral vestibulospinal tract
- Ipsilateral flocculonodular lobe, uvula, and fastigial nucleus of the cerebellum through the vestibulocerebellar tract.

Hallpike (Bárány) test

Here, the patient reclines from the sitting position with the head turned to one side and hanging over the end of the bed. If positive, the patient experiences nystagmus after a latent period. The nystagmus increases to a crescendo and then dissipates. The test is repeated on the other side. A positive test shows an abnormality in the peripheral vestibular function. It is particularly useful in detecting benign positional vertigo, which is commonly mistaken for TIA.

Head Impulse–Nystagmus–Test of Skew (HINTS) test

A set of bedside tests that can help differentiate whether acute vertigo and dizziness are central or peripheral in origin.

Head Impulse Test

- Sit facing the patient and gently hold their head, moving it from side to side while they look at you.
- Their eyes should be still. The vestibulo-ocular reflex (VOR) is intact.
- Then rapidly turn their head about 20 degrees to the right.
- If the VOR has been disrupted, the eyes will turn with the head and then there will be a corrective saccade back to the centre.
- Repeat turning the head to the other side.
- If either are abnormal, it suggests a peripheral problem. If the head impulse test is normal, it suggests a central cause.
- In the typical stroke population, this test can be uncomfortable so ensure that the patient can move their neck smoothly and does not complain of significant cervical arthritis. Only small movements are usually needed to demonstrate a corrective saccade.

Nystagmus

- Watch the patient's eyes while they look straight ahead. Try to avoid their fixating on any particular object. Then ask them to turn their eyes left or right.
- Unidirectional, horizontal nystagmus is likely to be peripheral.
- Bidirectional, vertical, or rotatory nystagmus is more likely to be central.

Skew

- Ask the patient to look at you.
- Then cover each of their eyes alternating using your hand.
- If there is a skew defect, their uncovered eye will make a vertical corrective saccade.
- If this is the case, the problem is likely to be central.

The three tests together comprise HINTS and can be used to deduce the likelihood that a patient has a posterior circulation stroke or peripheral vestibular disturbance.

Sometimes a fourth item, unilateral hearing loss, is added to make HINTS+. Hearing loss may indicate cochlear infarction usually from an AICA stroke.

Remember: Always look in the ears of a dizzy patient

This is an excellent 📹 video demonstrating The HINTS 'plus' exam in Vertigo,

https://www.youtube.com/watch?v=84waYROlI4U

(SOURCE: Peter Johns, Assistant Professor, Department of Emergency Medicine, University of Ottawa)

Cranial nerve IX (glossopharyngeal)

The nucleus lies in the medulla closely apposed to the nuclei of cranial nerves X and XI (nucleus ambiguous).

- It provides sensory innervation of the posterior third of the tongue and the pharynx
- The motor side supplies the pharyngeal muscles
- Glossopharyngeal nerve lesions cause loss of taste and sensation in the posterior third of the tongue.

Cranial nerve X (vagus)

This nerve has a long course.

- It supplies the pharyngeal muscles and the larynx
- It innervates smooth muscle in the trachea, bronchi, oesophagus, and gastrointestinal tract
- Stretch afferents from the aortic arch and carotid sinus travel in the nerve of Herring to join the glossopharyngeal nerve, terminating in the nucleus ambiguous, and thence the dorsal nucleus of the vagus, resulting in parasympathetic control of blood pressure.

It is examined by testing pharyngeal and palatal sensation with an orange stick:

- The gag reflex occurs when the posterior wall of the pharynx is touched. The response of retraction of the tongue and elevation of the palate is lost if cranial nerves IX and X are damaged
- You should touch either the right or left side of the palate. If only one side is affected, the good side contracts and pulls the uvula over
- In the palatal reflex, touching the soft palate will result in elevation of the soft palate on that side.

Cranial nerve XI (spinal accessory)

- The cranial part of the nerve stems from the nucleus ambiguous and joins the vagus nerve to form the recurrent laryngeal nerve which innervates the larynx
- The spinal portion of the nerve arises from motor nuclei in the upper five cervical segments, enters the skull through the foramen magnum, and exits through the jugular foramen:

- It supplies sternocleidomastoid and trapezius. Remember, the
  sternocleidomastoid pushes the face towards the other side
- Therefore, weakness of head turning to the left is due to paralysis of
  the right sternocleidomastoid.

Cranial nerve XII (hypoglossal)

- This nucleus lies in the lower medulla
- The nerve exits the skull through the hypoglossal canal
- It supplies the muscles of the tongue
- Ask the patient to protrude their tongue. Deviation to one side
  indicates paralysis on the same side. The good side pushes the tongue
  across.

Eponymous cranial nerve syndrome details

The important thing is to localize the lesion and determine the arterial territory affected rather than to identify rare eponymous syndromes. A number
of syndromes were described before the advent of the ability to localize
brainstem infarcts accurately with MRI. We list them in Table 5.3 for those
interested.

Table 5.3 Eponymous cranial nerve syndromes

Weber	Oculomotor palsy and contralateral hemiplegia from corticospinal tract damage
Claude	Oculomotor palsy with contralateral cerebellar ataxia and tremor
Benedikt	Oculomotor palsy with contralateral cerebellar ataxia, tremor, and hemiplegia from corticospinal tract damage
Nothnagel	Ocular palsies, paralysis of gaze, and cerebellar ataxia. This is at the level of the superior cerebellar peduncles
Parinaud	Supranuclear paralysis of upward gaze and accommodation with fixed pupils
Millard–Gubler and Raymond–Foville	This is at the level of the facial nerve (and abducens). There is a facial palsy and contralateral hemiplegia with a gaze palsy to the side of the lesion sometimes
Avellis	Paralysis of soft palate and vocal cord and contralateral hemianaesthesia with a Horner's syndrome. It is at the level of the spinothalamic tracts
Jackson	Tongue paralysis with contralateral hemiplegia
Wallenberg	This affects the lateral medulla at the level of nerves IX, X, and XI, and spinal V. Ipsilateral V, IX, X, and XI palsies, Horner's syndrome, cerebellar ataxia. Contralateral loss of pain and temperature

Peripheral nervous system examination

The scheme for testing the peripheral nerves is as follows:
- Inspection
- Tone
- Power
- Sensation
- Reflexes and plantar responses.
- Coordination
- Gait.

Think as you go along how the signs will help localize the lesion.

Peripheral nervous system examination—inspection

Involuntary movements

These include the following:
- Seizures—always stop and look for evidence of seizures. They may manifest as subtle chewing movements or blinking or jerking of the arms
- Fasciculations are random muscle twitches seen under the skin. They may indicate serious neuromuscular disease such as motor neuron disease
- Myoclonus is a very brief muscle jerk. It may be focal or generalized
- Dystonia is abnormal, prolonged muscle contraction where part of the body adopts an abnormal posture
- Hemiballismus is a violent flinging movement of one side of the body. It is associated with lesions of the subthalamic nucleus
- Chorea comprises short movements that flit from different parts of the body. Often the patient looks fidgety
- Asterixis is where there are brief, jerky downward movements of the outstretched, pronated, dorsiflexed hands when the eyes are closed. It usually signifies a metabolic encephalopathy.

Muscle bulk

In a stroke patient, muscle bulk will usually be normal. Wasting suggests a lower motor neuron problem or a chronic upper motor neuron problem with disuse atrophy. There should be a system of inspection, e.g. start at the top and work down. Look at the temples; look at the tongue; look for the pattern of wasting. Wasting can be:
- unilateral
- symmetrical
- proximal
- distal wasting affecting the small muscles of the hands.

Pronator drift

Pronator drift is a very good way of bringing out subtle pyramidal abnormalities. Ask the patient to hold their arms outstretched in front of them with the palms facing upwards. Look for any dysmetria on one side that may indicate a cerebellar lesion. The patient should hold the position for at least 30 seconds and a drift of one side down and into pronation may be observed. If present, follow up with examination of the limb for evidence of weakness which may be slight and otherwise overlooked; look for slowing of fine finger movements (e.g. ask them to move their fingers as though playing a scale on the piano).

Peripheral nervous system examination—tone

Muscle tone is the steady state of partial muscle contraction. It is assessed by passive movement.

- Hypotonia is defined as decreased tone (lower motor neuron lesions, early acute stroke, and spinal shock)
- Hypertonia may manifest as spasticity or rigidity:
  - Spasticity with the clasp-knife phenomenon
  - Rigidity with increased tone associated with extrapyramidal lesions; it may result in a cogwheel (stepwise) or lead-pipe (uniform) resistance to passive movement
  - Clonus is seen in upper motor neuron lesions. It can be elicited by recreating a muscle stretch reflex manually. For example, with the knee relaxed and bent and the ankle in the neutral position, the examiner briskly dorsiflexes the foot. If clonus is present, this will generate a rhythmic, oscillation of the foot. We think of clonus as 'sustained' (abnormal and seemingly never-ending) or unsustained (probably normal)
  - Gegenhalten, where resistance increases in flexion and extension (commonly seen in advanced dementia).

Peripheral nervous system examination—power

The MRC grading scale is simple and useful to describe weakness severity. Category 4 is a large category, from mild weakness to disabling weakness. It is sometimes subdivided into 4− and 4+.

0. No movement
1. Flickers of movement
2. Weak but can move with gravity eliminated
3. Weak but can move against gravity
4. Weak but can move against resistance
5. Full strength.

The pattern of weakness following stroke is often in a pyramidal distribution: power in the arm muscle flexors is greater than in the extensors; the reverse is true in the legs. In mild stroke, weakness may only be manifest in finger abduction and hip flexion.

Peripheral nervous system examination—sensation

This comprises light touch, pin-prick, joint position sense, vibration, and astereognosis.

- Look for hemisensory loss. This is the commonest and normally caused by a hemispheric lesion
- Look for crossed signs. This is seen in a brainstem stroke
- If the patient is diabetic, there will usually be a stocking neuropathy
- Always think about cord compression.

If the signs seem to stop at the neck you *must* look for a sensory level and you *must* go all the way up to the head. The common mistake is only to look for a sensory level on the chest and abdomen and forget to go up the neck.

Peripheral nervous system examination—reflexes
(See Table 5.4.)

Primitive reflexes
These include the glabellar tap, rooting, snout, sucking, and palmomental reflexes. They are termed frontal release signs and are seen in cases of dementia.

Jaw jerk
This is elicited by placing the examiner's index finger on the patient's lower jaw and then striking it with the reflex hammer. An exaggerated reflex indicates the presence of a suprapontine lesion. When the rest of the examination findings are normal, it may indicate physiological hyperreflexia.

Table 5.4 Anatomical basis of the different reflexes

Reflex	Afferent	Centre	Efferent
Corneal	Trigeminal (C5)	Pons	Facial (C7)
Pharyngeal	Glossopharyngeal (C9)	Medulla	Vagus
Abdominal (upper)	T7, T8, T9, T10	T7, T8, T9, T10	T7, T8, T9, T10
Abdominal (lower)	T10, T11, T12	T10, T11, T12	T10, T11, T12
Cremasteric	Femoral	L1	Genitofemoral
Plantar	Tibial	S1, S2	Tibial
Anal	Pudendal	S4, S5	Pudendal
Deep reflexes			
Jaw	Trigeminal	Pons	Trigeminal
Biceps	Musculocutaneous	C5, C6	Musculocutaneous
Triceps	Radial	C6, C7	Radial
Supinator	Radial	C6, C7, C8	Median
Patellar	Femoral	L2, L3, L4	Femoral
Achilles	Tibial	S1, S2	Tibial
Visceral			
Light	Optic	Midbrain	Oculomotor
Carotid sinus	Glossopharyngeal	Medulla	Vagus

Superficial reflexes

The most important superficial reflex is the plantar reflex. This may be elicited by stroking the lateral aspect of the sole with a sharp(ish) object such as a key or end of the tendon hammer. The normal response is plantar flexion of the big toe. Dorsiflexion of the big toe and fanning of the other toes suggests an upper motor neuron lesion.

Deep tendon reflexes

These are monosynaptic spinal segmental reflexes. When present, the cutaneous input, motor output, and descending cortical control must be intact. You are looking for asymmetry of the sides.

- Biceps—musculocutaneous nerve C5, C6
- Brachioradialis—radial nerve C6
- Triceps—radial nerve C7
- Knee jerk—femoral nerve L2–4
- Ankle jerk—tibial nerve S1, S2.

Important points to remember

- After stroke (resulting in an upper motor neuron lesion), reflexes are increased. However, in the acute phase they may not be increased
- Determining physiologically increased reflexes from pathologically increased reflexes can be difficult. They are pathological if:
  - there is asymmetry
  - there is spreading of the reflex to other muscles not being directly stimulated
  - there is also sustained clonus
- plantar responses are extensor.

Coordination and gait

Coordination

Look for both lateralizing cerebellar signs (indicating damage to one side of the cerebellum or its brainstem connections) and truncal ataxia.

Lateralizing cerebellar signs:

- Tapping the outstretched arms while the eyes are closed may lead to rebound of the affected arm
- Patients may not be able to match the position of one arm in space using the other, a sign termed dysmetria
- Finger–nose test—ask the patient to point to their nose and then to your finger. Make sure they stretch out their arm to full extension to reach your finger. Intention tremor and past pointing indicate a cerebellar lesion
- Heel–shin test—ask the patient to place their heel on their knee and slide it down the shin
- Remember if a limb is weak that it is very difficult to test coordination
- Ataxia and mild hemiparesis on the same side suggest the ataxic hemiparesis lacunar syndrome. This is caused by a small infarct in the internal capsule, the pons, or in between.

Truncal ataxia

- This may be evident on walking but more subtle deficits can be detected by testing heel-to-toe tandem gait. Ask the patient to walk with one foot directly in front of the other.
- If the patient cannot walk, sit them up in bed and see if they can maintain balance when pushed gently to one side.

Gait

It is important to look at gait if at all possible. There are several gaits to identify.

Hemiparetic gait

The shoulder is adducted, the elbow flexed, and the forearm pronated with the wrist and fingers flexed. In the leg, the knee is extended and then plantar-flexed. To walk, the patient circumducts the affected leg.

Ataxic gait

The patient spreads their legs to widen the base of support and compensate for the lack of balance. This is a wide-based gait. If you are not sure, ask the patient to walk heel-to-toe (tandem gait) and this should magnify the ataxia. Subtle ataxia may be missed unless the patient is assessed (if possible) while seated, standing, and walking.

Shuffling gait

The patient shuffles, taking small steps. This is seen in Parkinson's disease where the patient's steps may become faster and faster (festinant) and in subcortical cerebrovascular small-vessel disease where it is thought to be a type of gait apraxia ('marche a petit pas'). It is commonly associated with other aspects of dysexecutive function such as poor sequencing and planning and is a cause of falls. To test if it is apraxia, ask the patient to mime walking or cycling while lying on the bed. They should be able to do this without a problem.

High stepping
This is caused by bilateral foot drop usually owing to severe peripheral neuropathy. This sort of gait can normally be heard.

Spastic gait
Here the legs are very stiff and there is little bending of the knees when walking. If very bad, there is adductor spasm and the legs are pulled together as the patient walks. The knees may knock together or even cross (a scissoring gait).

Antalgic gait
This is basically a limp caused by a unilateral painful leg. The patient puts most weight on the good leg.

Examination of the unconscious patient

Trainees often find this difficult but if a systematic approach is taken, a useful assessment can be made.

- Remember to look for neck stiffness, which is essential in the unconscious patient
- Observe the patient's response to pain by squeezing the trapezius muscle. The responses may be:
  - decorticate posturing—adduction of the arms, flexion of the forearms, wrists, and fingers
  - decerebrate posturing—adduction of the arms, extension and pronation of the forearms, and extension of the legs.
- Pupil responses are tested as usual
- Visual fields may be tested by moving your fingers into the visual field suddenly. There may be a sudden closure of the eyelid to threat
- Look at the resting position of the eyes:
  - This is particularly important in the drowsy or comatose patient
  - Deviation to one side often indicates a frontal lesion, ipsilateral to the side of eye deviation (the eyes 'look towards' the sound limb)
  - A skew deviation indicates a pontine lesion
  - Absence of the 'doll's eye reflex' is an ominous sign of severe brainstem damage but Guillain–Barré syndrome or myasthenia gravis may mimic it
  - If a patient cannot follow the examiner's hand or other target, ask them to follow their own hand as you guide it back and forth to assess eye movement
  - Failure of gaze to one side indicates a lesion of the pontine gaze centre.
- Extraocular muscles may be evaluated by inducing eye movements via reflexes:
  - The doll's eye reflex, or oculocephalic reflex, is produced by moving the patient's head side to side or up and down
  - The eyes will normally remain stationary in spite of the head moving
  - The afferent arc consists of the vestibular apparatus and neck proprioception
  - The efferent part consists of cranial nerves III, IV and VI, and eye muscles
  - The two parts join in the pons and medulla
  - If this reflex is damaged, turning the head from side to side moves the eyes in the same manner
  - In caloric testing, cold water is infused into the patient's ear: The patient's eyes turn towards the ear of injection (the same effect as turning the patient's head away from the injection) with nystagmus towards the contralateral ear. An absent reflex indicates severe damage in the medulla or pons or nerves that control eye movements.
- The corneal reflex tests the afferent trigeminal nerve pathway and the efferent facial nerve pathway
- The gag reflex tests nerves IX and X.

The motor system is assessed by testing for:
- Spasticity—it takes some practice to be able to elicit spasticity:
  - The speed of the movement is important. For example, examine the forearm and arm around the elbow joint. Extending the flexed forearm at moderate speed will normally result in a 'catch' as the tone suddenly seems to increase
  - Continued traction on the forearm will result in an equally sudden 'give' in the resistance: the 'clasp knife' phenomenon
  - If the manoeuvre is too slow, the 'catch' will be missed. Too fast and the limb will appear rigid. This clasp-knife phenomenon is best seen in arm flexors and leg extensors
  - Withdrawal responses to pain may be asymmetric, indicating a hemiparesis.
- Reflexes may be increased (but early on may be reduced)
- Plantar responses may be extensor.

Criteria for 'brainstem death' are discussed in ➲ Chapter 17.

Examination of swallowing

This must be performed in all patients. It is best to test the overall action of swallowing. Relying on the presence or absence of the gag reflex is very misleading. Many units have local swallowing screening protocols which should be applied. However, a simple test is to observe whether aspiration occurs when a patient sips water from a cup. The patient must be alert and able to sit up or be so positioned.

Swallowing is divided into four stages:
1. Oral preparatory stage—here food and liquid entering the mouth are retained in the mouth while moving from side to side and being chewed
2. Oral stage—here food and liquid move from the front to the back of the mouth
3. Pharyngeal stage—here food and liquid move through the throat into the oesophagus. This is the stage where the airway has to be protected from aspiration
4. Oesophageal stage—here food and liquid move through the oesophagus to the stomach.

To assess swallowing, the patient must be conscious and alert long enough to swallow. Then perform the following:
• Sit the patient upright in a comfortable position
• Give them 5 mL of water
• Ask them to hold the water in their mouth momentarily (observe for dribbling)
• Then allow to swallow
• After each swallow, ask the patient to talk and cough
• Look out for signs of poor or unsafe swallowing:
  • coughing or choking on swallowing
  • 'wet' voice or cough after swallowing
  • water pooling in mouth
  • absent swallow
  • reduced laryngeal elevation
  • evidence of respiratory distress.

If the swallow looks unsafe, then ensure the patient is kept 'nil by mouth' until further assessed by a speech therapist

An algorithm for ongoing management of an unsafe swallow is given on ➔ p. 445.

A poorly coordinated swallow is often due to swallowing apraxia—where the automatic components of swallowing are largely intact but those under voluntary control are unable to integrate. In this diagnosis, as with other forms of apraxia, there should be no examinable motor or sensory deficit to explain this.

General examination

A thorough general examination is essential and may identify possible aetiological factors for stroke as well as possible complications. Relevant abnormalities include the following.

Cardiovascular

- Blood pressure
- Arrhythmias, particularly atrial fibrillation
- Evidence of cardiac failure
- Valvular heart disease
- Peripheral sign of endocarditis
- Peripheral pulses/evidence of peripheral vascular disease
- Complications of diabetes in the feet.

Respiratory

- Pneumonia, especially following aspiration
- Pleural effusion or pleural rub.

Abdominal

- Signs of chronic liver disease
- Organomegaly, especially liver (metastases)
- Enlarged bladder (urinary retention).

Skin

- Rashes, e.g. facial photosensitive rash of SLE
- Livedo reticularis
- Evidence of pressure sores over bony prominences.

Musculoskeletal

- Hypermobility or other evidence of collagen vascular disease, e.g. Ehlers–Danlos type IV associated with cervical dissection
- Inflammatory arthritis associated with a vasculitis
- Arthritis that may have functional consequences and hamper rehabilitation.

Chapter 6

Investigation of the stroke patient

Investigation of the stroke patient

Investigation of acute stroke patients can be categorized into five sections:
1. Emergency investigation of the patient
2. Investigation to confirm or refute the diagnosis of stroke
3. Investigation of the aetiology of stroke
4. Investigation of risk factors (see E Chapters 1 and 10)
5. Anticipation of complications of stroke.

This chapter provides an overview of stroke investigation. ➲ Chapter 7 provides details on imaging in stroke.

Emergency investigation of the patient

It is *impossible* to distinguish between infarction and haemorrhage on clinical grounds alone. Therefore, urgent brain imaging is essential.

Imaging
- A brain scan should be performed as soon as possible after admission
- Aspirin or other specific treatment is not normally given until the result of the admission scan is known.

Blood tests
- Full blood count
- Electrolytes (renal disease)
- Blood glucose
- Clotting screen (if haemorrhage is suspected).

Cardiac test
- ECG (myocardial infarction or atrial fibrillation).

Radiology tests
- Chest X-ray (heart failure or suspected pneumonia).

Other tests
- Sometimes a blood gas analysis is necessary.

Investigation to confirm or refute the diagnosis of stroke

Brain imaging with either CT or MRI is the key investigation here.

Computed tomography

CT scanning is usually the most easily available:

- It is cheap
- Widely accessible
- Non-invasive
- It can reliably identify intracerebral haemorrhage early
- However, it may be difficult to identify early cerebral infarction
- Posterior fossa and brainstem lesions may not be visible
- It may not detect small infarcts, particularly lacunar infarcts
- It cannot differentiate between old infarcts and old intracerebral haemorrhage (once blood has been resolved and an area of infarction remains)
- CT can incorporate other techniques to provide vital information beyond the plain scan (see ➲ Chapter 7)
- CT angiography (CTA) has become an essential additional investigation to identify arterial occlusion for mechanical thrombectomy
- CT perfusion (CTP) can identify salvageable penumbral tissue and provide clues that a medium or distal intracranial vessel occlusion is present.

For most ischaemic stroke patients, we do CT and CTA. In cases where we are assessing whether there is still salvageable tissue (i.e. an ischaemic penumbra), for reperfusion therapy we also do CTP.

- CT Venography (CTV) is used to investigate the cerebral vein and venous sinuses and can demonstrate a Cerebral Venous Sinus Thrombosis.

Magnetic resonance imaging

MRI offers better resolution as well as a number of other advantages. A typical examination uses several sequences, each of which contributes different information.

- It is much better at visualizing the posterior fossa
- It is more sensitive to small infarcts, particularly lacunar infarcts
- The most useful sequence in acute stroke is diffusion-weighted imaging (DWI). This becomes positive within minutes or a couple of hours of stroke onset, and the new stroke appears bright ('light bulb' sign on the DWI image). It therefore allows:
  - Early detection of ischaemia
  - Differentiation of old infarction from recent infarction; the latter appears as a bright region on DWI imaging for 2–3 weeks after stroke onset. This is particularly useful in a patient with an old stroke in whom you want to know if they have had a new stroke or merely an exacerbation of existing deficit, as, for example, can happen following a seizure.

- Sometimes very small lesions in the brainstem may be missed (especially if MRI performed in the first 24 hours after stroke), but over 95% of acute ischaemic infarcts can be competently and quickly diagnosed with this modality
- MRI with gradient echo (GE) or susceptibility-weighted imaging (SWI) is exquisitely sensitive to paramagnetic compounds such as hemosiderin and is therefore very sensitive to both new and old haemorrhage; an old bleed results in deposition in the brain of hemosiderin from in the red blood cells. Blood appears as signal loss—a 'black hole'
- GE or SWI allows one to determine whether an old lesion was initially caused by infarction or haemorrhage. This can be impossible to differentiate using CT
- GE and SWI can also detect cerebral microbleeds.

Similar to CT, MRI can also be used to study vessels (MR angiography (MRA)) and assess cerebral and perfusion (MR perfusion).

MRI can also suppress the signal from blood—so-called 'black blood' sequences. This allows study of the vessel wall, helping to differentiate between inflammatory causes (such as vasculitis) form atheroma as an underlying cause of intracranial vessel stenosis.

In many ways, it makes more sense to use MRI first rather than CT as diffusion-weighted changes are so apparent that they make diagnosis relatively easy for the non-specialist. However, availability often means CT is the first-line approach, and some acute stroke patients find MRI difficult to tolerate.

Brain imaging is covered in more detail in ➲ Chapter 7.

Investigation into the aetiology of stroke

The aetiology of stroke is:
- ischaemic (80%), of which 60–80% is embolic
- haemorrhagic (up to 20%).

In ischaemic stroke, it is important to look for a source of embolism or site of thrombosis. Emboli can arise anywhere in the arterial tree from the heart to the brain. Common sites are the:
- carotid artery at the bifurcation of internal and external carotid
- vertebral artery, particularly at its origin
- intracranial vessels, particularly in certain ethnic groups (e.g. Chinese, African American)
- heart
- aortic arch.

Potential embolic sources can be detected by:
- imaging of the extracerebral vessels with duplex ultrasound, computed tomography angiography (CTA), or magnetic resonance angiography (MRA)
- imaging of the intracerebral vessels with CTA or MRA
- cardiac investigation:
  - ECG and prolonged cardiac rhythm monitoring
  - echocardiography (transoesophageal echocardiography (TOE) also allows detection of aortic atheroma)
  - cardiac MRI is now becoming a more important investigation into structural heart disease.

Imaging of the extracerebral and intracerebral arteries is covered in Chapter 7. The aortic arch outside of cases of suspected aortic root dissection (see Chapter 11) is not normally routinely imaged, although there is research currently looking specifically at management of aortic arch atherosclerotic embolism.

A variety of blood tests and other tests may be required in stroke patients—these are listed in Table 6.1.

Table 6.1 A list of investigations in the stroke patient

	In all patients	Selected patients
All strokes	*Blood tests:*	
	Full blood count (esp. platelet) ESR hsCRP Urea and electrolytes Glucose, HbA$_{1c}$ Liver function tests Thyroid function	
	Other tests:	
	ECG Brain CT or MRI Chest X-ray Urinalysis	
Cerebral infarction	*Blood tests:*	*Blood tests:*
	Lipids	Sickle cell screen
		Thrombophilia, including anticardiolipin antibody and lupus anticoagulant
		Homocysteine and vitamin B$_{12}$ Drug screen (urine + blood) Syphilis serology HIV Autoantibody screen Blood cultures Genetic tests (e.g. CADASIL, Fabry) Clopidogrel resistance testing
	Other tests:	*Other tests:*
	Imaging of extracranial arteries	Echocardiography
		24-hour ECG or more prolonged monitoring Imaging of intracerebral arteries MRA/CTA Cerebral angiography Temporal artery biopsy CSF examination

Table 6.1 (Contd.)

	In all patients	Selected patients
Cerebral haemorrhage	*Blood tests:*	*Blood tests:*
	Clotting screen	Sickle cell screen
		Drug screen
		Other tests:
		Imaging of intracerebral arteries MRA/CTA
	Anti-factor Xa level for apixaban, rivaroxaban, and edoxaban if necessaryDilute thrombin time assay (dTT) for dabigatran	Cerebral angiography

Cardiac investigation

ECG

- 12-lead ECG should always be performed
- Left ventricular hypertrophy measured by voltage criteria can be a marker of hypertensive end-organ damage or a racial variant. An abnormal ECG may also indicate a source of cardiac embolism, e.g. evidence of an old myocardial infraction
- A 'baseline' ECG is helpful should complications arise after stroke; these include myocardial infarction or pulmonary embolus
- Occasionally, subarachnoid bleeding can induce ECG changes which mimic acute myocardial ischaemia
- It is helpful to be able to monitor the cardiac rhythm continuously for a few days after stroke, seeking atrial fibrillation or paroxysmal tachycardia or bradycardia
- Ward cardiac telemetry, 24-hour ECG, or longer-term cardiac monitoring devices such as an implantable loop recorder (ILR) may identify paroxysmal atrial fibrillation. ILR are small subcutaneously implanted devices (typically the size of a matchstick) that can monitor and record heart rhythm continuously. Modern battery life enables monitoring for up to 4 years with either patient prompted or routine downloading of recordings using Bluetooth
- An abnormal 12-lead ECG should generally be further investigated with echocardiography.

Echocardiography

This may identify a potential embolic source. Some units perform it in most patients while others argue that, while it may detect abnormalities relatively frequently, it does not often alter management. Therefore, they do not perform it routinely. If access is limited, we would recommend performing transthoracic echocardiography (TTE) in cases with:

- cardiac abnormality on examination or ECG
- ischaemic stroke aged under 65 years
- strokes or cerebral infarcts on imaging in multiple territories. This suggests a cardiac or aortic arch embolic source
- a cerebral infarct that looks as if it may be embolic (e.g. a wedge-shaped cortical infarct or subcortical striatocapsular infarct) and no other obvious embolic source.

Transoesophageal echocardiography

- This has a greater sensitivity than TTE. In particular, it is better at looking for left atrial abnormalities, a PFO, vegetations in infective endocarditis, and aortic arch atheroma
- A specialized probe containing an ultrasound transducer at its tip is passed into the patient's oesophagus
- It does have disadvantages:
  - The patient must fast
  - The technique requires a team of medical personnel and takes longer to perform

- It is uncomfortable for the patient and usually requires sedation
- There are some risks associated with the procedure: oesophageal perforation occurs in 1 in 10 000.

Cardiac MRI

- This can provide detailed information about the anatomical structure and blood flow within the cardiac chambers
- Left atrial and ventricular thrombus may be visible
- Valve vegetations may be detected in endocarditis
- It can show a PFO but is not as good as TOE.

Investigations to anticipate complications

Complications after stroke include:
- infections (pneumonia, urinary tract infection, cellulitis)
- myocardial infarction or arrhythmia
- electrolyte imbalance
- re-feeding syndrome
- deep vein thrombosis and pulmonary embolus
- aspiration due to impaired swallowing.

Patients should be monitored with regular:
- temperature
- blood pressure
- continuous cardiac monitoring looking for arrhythmias
- O_2 saturation and respiratory rate
- full blood count
- urea and electrolytes
- CRP
- liver function tests (always check before starting statin therapy and remember to check again 6–12 weeks after to exclude significant transaminitis).

It may be helpful to perform a:
- chest X-ray as a baseline investigation in a stroke patient who is likely to be hospitalized for a long time
- videofluoroscopy or fibreoptic endoscopic examination of swallowing in anticipation of the patient needing a percutaneous endoscopic gastrostomy (PEG).

Clopidogrel resistance

- About 20–30% of patients have some degree of clopidogrel resistance
- This means that clopidogrel may not provide effective stroke prevention for them
- Clopidogrel is a prodrug activated by Cytochrome P450 and irreversibly binds to P2Y12 ADP receptors on platelets. Normally, ADP binds the activating glycoprotein GPIIb/IIIa complex and causes platelet aggregation. Clopidogrel, once activated, stops this
- CYP2C19 is the gene that codes for the Cytochrome P450 enzymes that activate clopidogrel
- Some people have loss of function variant of this gene and are rendered clopidogrel resistant
- It is possible to identify these people either through gene testing or bedside testing for clopidogrel resistance
- It can be considered particularly in patients presenting with ischaemic stroke while on clopidogrel and is important to know in advance of elective procedures such as carotid or vertebral artery stenting. If found—an alternative drug such a ticagrelor or prasugrel can be considered in combination with aspirin.

Further reading

Imaging

Radiopaedia is an excellent resource for learning about imaging in stroke. Available online at: https://radiopaedia.org/articles/ischaemic-stroke

Cardiological Investigation

Doehner W, Scheitz JF (2020). Stroke as interdisciplinary disease: what the practising cardiologist can do. *e-Journal of Cardiology Practice*, 18. Available online at: https://doi.org/10.37461/escejcp.18.8

Chapter 7

Imaging in stroke

Introduction

Imaging plays a central role in diagnosis of stroke, planning treatment, and identification of the underlying pathophysiology.

Functions of imaging

Imaging in stroke has a number of major functions:

Diagnosis
- Identification of infarction
- Identification of haemorrhage
- Identification of structural stroke mimics.

Examination of the vasculature and vascular lesion leading to the stroke syndrome
- Detection of stenosis or occlusion
- Identification of collateral supply
- Detection of aneurysms and other vascular malformations.

Planning treatment
- Selecting patients for thrombolysis.

Imaging can also provide information on:
- brain perfusion and haemodynamics
- plaque and arterial wall morphology
- circulating cerebral embolism.

Methods

Methods of imaging the brain include:
- computed tomography (CT) techniques
- magnetic resonance (MR) techniques
- single-photon emission computed tomography (SPECT)
- positron emission tomography (PET).

The former two are the most widely used, the latter two have little applicability in normal stroke clinical practice.
Methods of imaging the cerebral vessels include:
- ultrasound
- CT angiography
- MR angiography
- intra-arterial angiography.

Computed tomography (CT)

Brain CT scanning was first introduced in 1971 (first scan) at Atkinson Morley Hospital in Wimbledon, UK by the radiologist Jamie Ambrose and the scientist Godfrey Hounsfield who later went on to win the Nobel Prize for the development.

- It is the most widely available method of brain imaging
- The patient lies on a table
- A beam of X-rays revolves around the patient delimiting a slice through the subject (usually axial)
- The X-ray beam is attenuated by passing through the patient's tissues
- The exit beam is detected
- Computerized algorithms then reconstruct the image of the slice
- The slice thickness can be varied
- Changing the window level changes the contrast appearance, making structural identification easier (e.g. differentiating grey and white matter or bone) (see Figs 7.1 and 7.2).

Advantages

- Easy to use
- Cheap
- Dysphasic or comatose patients can be imaged safely
- Safe in patients with metallic implants and not claustrophobic
- The quality of the pictures is usually good when looking at the cerebral hemispheres or the skull vault. Many things that are eventually identified on MR will have been visible on the initial CT scan
- Blood is well visualized very soon after haemorrhage onset (see ➔ Figs 7.13 and 7.14).

Disadvantages

- It may miss subtle features of brain pathology
- Artefacts produced in the posterior fossa make it poor for examination of the brainstem and cerebellum
- May miss small infarcts, particularly lacunar ones
- It can be difficult to tell whether an old stroke is due to previous haemorrhage or infarct
- Not as sensitive as MRI for hyperacute ischaemia
- Involves ionizing radiation—a routine CT scan exposes the patient to the equivalent of 10 months of background radiation (2 days for chest X-ray).

Modern CT scanners

- These acquire data much quicker and with higher resolution than earlier generations
- Spiral scanners—these draw the subject into the scanner as the beam rotates around the subject. This allows continuous spiral acquisition
- Modern scanners can investigate a large block of tissue (rather than a single slice at a time). These scanners can do blocks of 32, 64 or even more slices during a single set of acquisitions.

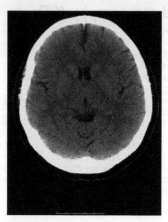

Fig. 7.1 CT scan of the brain. This is a normal section through the brain. The internal capsule and basal ganglia are clearly visible. © Anthony Pereira.

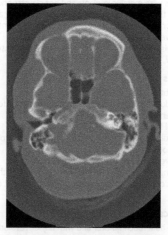

Fig. 7.2 This is a different slice through the brain with the CT windowing set to show the bones. This is used to seek fractures (e.g. after a fall and head injury). © Anthony Pereira.

CT in acute stroke

(See Figs 7.3–7.6.)
* Plain CT is not very sensitive for detecting early infarcts (<6 hours)
* However, ischaemic changes are often visible relatively early after stroke:
    * Loss of the grey–white matter interface
    * Loss of sulci
    * Loss of the insular ribbon
* Early mass effect and areas of hypodensity suggest irreversible injury and identify patients at higher risk of post-thrombolysis haemorrhage
* Significant hypodensity on the baseline scan if performed in the first few hours after stroke should prompt the physician to question the time of onset (see Fig. 7.5 and 7.6)
* A dense MCA sign suggests a clot in the MCA (see Fig. 7.4). Similar appearances can be seen in other intracerebral vessels due to clot, although differentiating this from a calcified vessel can be difficult.

CT is very sensitive to acute blood, which is visible soon after haemorrhage onset as high signal (white). One can see both:
* intracerebral haemorrhage (ICH)
* subarachnoid haemorrhage (SAH).

CT may demonstrate other causes of the patient's symptoms:
* Neoplasm
* Epidural and subdural haemorrhage
* Aneurysm
* Abscess
* Arteriovenous malformation
* Hydrocephalus.

Extra information is sometimes available by the addition of intravenous (IV) contrast:
* This identifies areas of high vascularity
* Also identifies regions where the blood–brain barrier is leaky
* Contrast-enhanced scans also highlight all major intracranial vessels
* However, contrast is not routinely used in cross-sectional imaging in acute stroke as it usually adds little extra information (see Fig. 7.3).

Images of early CT changes

When examining a CT, you should look for five findings:
* Look for evidence of thrombus in the MCA or other major intracerebral arteries (seen as white in the vessels)
* Look at the basal ganglia and internal capsule. Compare one side to the other. Are they distinct or hazy due to recent ischaemia? They have clearly been disrupted on the right in Fig. 7.3
* Look at the insular ribbon and see if it is still intact
* Look at the grey and white matter on the higher slices and see if detail in it has been lost
* Look at the sulci and gyri and see if the sulci have been compressed on one side (by cerebral oedema).

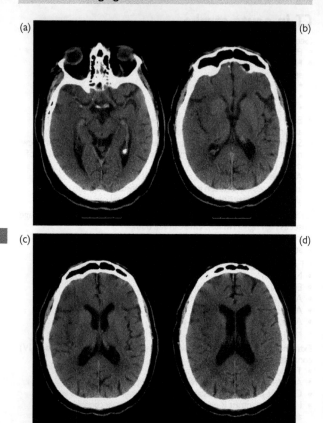

Fig. 7.3 Early CT appearances of a right middle cerebral artery infarct. Low density and loss of tissue definition is seen on all slices. There is loss of sulci and grey–white matter is not so easily distinguished.

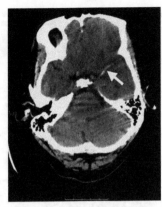

Fig. 7.4 The dense middle cerebral artery sign is seen on the left here. High-signal representing thrombus can be seen in the left middle cerebral artery (arrowed). © Anthony Pereira.

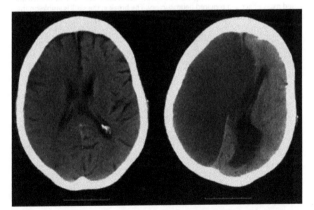

Fig. 7.5 Pair of CT images. The slice on the left shows subtle signs of an early large right carotid territory infarct. After 3 days, the infarct has swollen massively and is compressing the left hemisphere with midline shift and hydrocephalus. © Anthony Pereira.

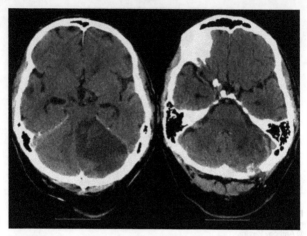

Fig. 7.6 Pair of images showing a left cerebellar hemisphere infarct. This swelled and caused mass effect and required neurosurgery. The break in the skull is visible on the left. © Anthony Pereira.

ASPECTS

The Alberta Stroke Programme Early CT Score (ASPECTS) (☞ http://www.aspectsinstroke.com/) has been devised to help structure the evaluation of acute CT scans and ensure the clinician looks at all aspects of the scan, although it only covers supratentorial regions and is primarily designed for MCA infarction. The territory of the MCA is allotted 10 points (Fig. 7.7). One point is subtracted for an area of early ischaemic change, such as focal swelling, or parenchymal hypoattenuation, for each of the defined regions. A normal CT scan has an ASPECTS value of 10 points. A score of 0 indicates diffuse ischaemia throughout the territory of the MCA.

In the initial evaluation, baseline (on pre-thrombolysis scans) ASPECTS score correlated inversely with stroke score on the NIH Stroke Scale and predicted functional outcome and symptomatic ICH following thrombolysis. Agreement between observers for ASPECTS, with knowledge of the affected hemisphere, was good (kappa 0.71–0.89). It was suggested that an ASPECTS of 7 might separate a group with a higher risk of post-thrombolysis haemorrhage. More recently, ASPECTS has been used in trials of thrombectomy as a surrogate for core infarct size in patient selection.

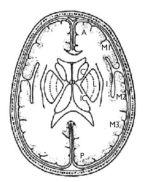
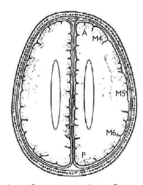

Fig. 7.7 The ASPECTS scale. A, anterior circulation; P, posterior circulation; C, caudate; L, lentiform; IC, internal capsule; I, insular ribbon; MCA, middle cerebral artery; M1, anterior MCA cortex; M2, MCA cortex lateral to insular ribbon; M3, posterior MCA cortex; M4, M5, and M6 are anterior, lateral, and posterior MCA territories immediately superior to M1, M2, and M3, rostral to basal ganglia. Subcortical structures are allotted 3 points (C, L, and IC), MCA cortex is allotted 7 points (insular cortex, M1, M2, M3, M4, M5, and M6).

Practising reading acute stroke CT scans

There are a number of interactive websites where you can review CT images of acute stroke patients online. This is a useful way to gain experience in this area. Here are some useful ones

Radiology Masterclass (🔗 https://www.radiologymasterclass.co.uk/) has useful training modules, including the two below:

How to read a normal CT brain scan

🔗 https://www.radiologymasterclass.co.uk/tutorials/ct/ct_brain_anatomy/ct_brain_anatomy_start

How to interpret acute changes on a CT brain scan

🔗 https://www.radiologymasterclass.co.uk/tutorials/ct/ct_acute_brain/ct_brain_start

The University of Edinburgh hosts a brain CT in stroke training course:

Acute Cerebral CT Evaluation of Stroke Study (ACCESS)

How to evaluate an acute stroke CT scan

🔗 https://www.ed.ac.uk/clinical-sciences/edinburgh-imaging/education-teaching/short-courses/training-tools/acute-cerebral-ct-evaluation-stroke-study-access

NeurovascularMedicine.com has a useful module on how to apply the ASPECTS score:

How to use the ASPECTS score

🔗 https://neurovascularmedicine.com/aspects.php

Magnetic resonance imaging (MRI)

- Nuclear MR signals have been used to study physics and chemistry since the 1940s
- In the 1970s it became possible to localize the signal and generate images
- For clinical applications, the 'nuclear' has been dropped
- The terms 'magnetic resonance (MR)' and 'magnetic resonance imaging (MRI)' are preferred
- The technique produces very high-quality images of brain parenchyma and individual structures. Small infarcts are well visualized
- In addition, different sequences can be tuned to identify very subtle brain pathology, such as early brain ischaemia, and to look at brain function (e.g. functional MRI, fMRI).

Advantages of MRI

- Images are more detailed than CT
- Small, including lacunar, infarcts are better detected than on CT
- Posterior fossa is better visualized (see Fig. 7.8)
- Best technique for imaging the spinal cord
- Sensitive to acute ischaemia within minutes/hours of ischaemia onset (diffusion-weighted imaging, DWI)
- Can detect evidence of old haemorrhage (haemosiderin seen as black holes on gradient-echo sequences—also called T2* imaging)
- It can also provide information on brain biochemistry (spectroscopy), brain function (fMRI), and white matter pathways (diffusion tensor imaging, DTI).

Limitations of MRI

- Relatively expensive
- Not as widely available as CT
- Longer scanning times than CT, although echo-planar MRI allows very rapid acquisition albeit with lower resolution
- Contraindications (e.g. pacemakers, metal in the eyes)
- Some patients are too claustrophobic in the 'tunnel'. Open magnets can overcome this but are not widely available. They also often have a lower magnetic field strength and may produce less clear images.

Recent advances in MRI

- Higher strength of magnetic field (3.0 Tesla field strength is now in routine clinical practice); provides higher resolution and better signal-to-noise ratio. 7T MRI has even higher resolution but is currently a research technique
- Open MRI for patients who are claustrophobic or overweight
- Intraoperative MRI scanner
- Low-field MRI scanners are being developed. These can be portable (e.g. MRI in outpatients or on ITU).

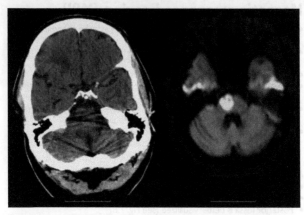

Fig. 7.8 A brainstem infarct on CT and MRI showing the much better sensitivity of MRI to lesions in the posterior fossa. The CT image on the left is very difficult to interpret. On the right is the DWI MR image, which clearly shows the abnormal area of infarction. The symmetrical areas of high signal in the temporal lobes on MRI are due to artefacts caused by nearby air cells in the bone. © Anthony Pereira.

Physics of MRI

- Atomic nuclei ^1H, ^{13}C, ^{19}F, and ^{31}P have a property called 'spin'
- The nucleus spins about its own axis
- Spinning creates a small magnetic field like a tiny bar magnet with its axis along the axis of rotation
- When an external magnetic field is applied (i.e. the MR scanner), the nuclei line up and spin at a given frequency
- When they are excited by a pulse of energy deliberately emitted from the MR scanner, two things happen:
  - They spin in a higher energy state and continue to do so until they give off that energy and return to their resting energy state
  - The energy pulse makes them all spin together in phase. However, they cannot maintain this and quickly spread out. They will still be in the high-energy state but no longer in phase.

T1

- The time it takes for the nuclei spins to return from the high-energy state to the resting energy state is the *T1 relaxation time*
- It depends on the actual structure of the brain
- Images based on this are called *T1-weighted images*
- T1 pictures tend to produce a good anatomical definition of the structure of the brain and are often used to estimate brain volume.

T2

- The time it takes for the spins to dephase is the *T2 relaxation time*
- It is very short
- Spins in solids dephase fast but spins in liquids are much slower
- Images based on this are called *T2-weighted images*
- Therefore, altered water content in tissues (e.g. brain oedema) is seen well
- T2-weighted images are good for looking at the pathological brain
- The scanner can be tuned to the spin frequency of different nuclei
- The main nucleus is ^1H (i.e. a proton)
- The commonest chemical containing this in the body is water
- Therefore, MR images often show the distribution of water molecules in different tissues in the body.

Commonly used MRI sequences

T1-weighted imaging

- Good for anatomical structure of normal tissue
- Used to measure whole brain volume or changes due to atrophy
- Sensitive to haemorrhage.

T2-weighted imaging

- Sensitive to oedema and increased water content (see Fig. 7.9)
- Good for showing most pathology
- Small lesions around the ventricles may be missed.

Fluid-attenuated inversion recovery (FLAIR)

- Essentially a T2 image with an added inversion recovery sequence. This suppresses signals from free water, i.e. in the ventricles and cerebrospinal fluid (CSF). This improves contrast and visualization, particularly of white matter hyperintensities (see Fig. 7.9)
- Lesions along the edges of the brain and ventricles are more clearly seen.

Gradient-echo imaging (T2*, pronounced 'T2 star')

- Sensitive to the presence of blood and blood products (i.e. haemorrhage), which are paramagnetic and degrades the image quality
- Haemorrhage appears as a large black 'hole' in the image
- Useful for looking at acute haemorrhage
- Can also detect old haemorrhage—blood is degraded to haemosiderin which is deposited and results in areas of signal loss (black). This also enables microhaemorrhages to be detected—they are particularly seen in small-vessel disease and cerebral amyloid.

Susceptibility-weighted imaging (SWI)

- Has similar clinical uses to gradient echo, and usually one or the other is used. More sensitive at detecting haemorrhage and microbleeds than T2*
- This is a neuroimaging technique, which uses tissue magnetic susceptibility differences to generate contrast
- Signals from substances with different magnetic susceptibilities go out of phase at long echo times (TEs)
- It is very good at differentiating blood products.

Diffusion-weighted imaging

- The most sensitive to detect acute ischaemic stroke; changes can appear within an hour of stroke onset.
- The infarct is bright on DWI and dark on apparent diffusion coefficient (ADC)
- In old stroke, the lesion will appear as a low signal on DWI—tissue breakdown results in increased diffusion.

Contrast can be added to MR sequences

- The contrast (gadolinium, a heavy metal) is paramagnetic
- It shortens the T1 signal and therefore appears bright

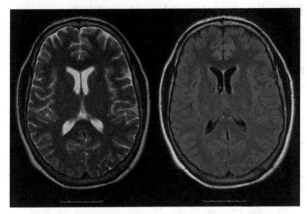

Fig. 7.9 T2 (left) and FLAIR (right) imaging. Both are good at detecting altered water content in brain tissue. In the FLAIR image, the free water in the CSF and ventricles is suppressed. © Anthony Pereira.

- It can be used to identify breakdown in the blood–brain barrier
- It is used to increase signal-to-noise ratio for angiographic imaging (contrast-enhanced MRA).

Perfusion imaging

- This can be performed either using a contrast injection (exogenous contrast) or using 'endogenous contrast'
- Exogenous contrast perfusion uses a very rapid gadolinium injection and echo-planar imaging to acquire very frequent images over the next 2–3 minutes. This allows the passage of the 'bolus' of contrast through the brain to be tracked and from this a perfusion map can be constructed. It is a good technique to detect perfusion deficits in acute stroke, and the signal changes seen are large. However, it is only semi-quantitative
- The following measures are commonly obtained—cerebral blood flow (CBF), cerebral blood volume (CBV), and mean transit time (MTT)
- Endogenous perfusion imaging creates 'contrast' in the tissue using a radiopulse. It is potentially quantitative but takes much longer to acquire and signal changes are much smaller. It is largely used as a research technique.

Diffusion-weighted imaging (DWI)

This sequence is very useful in early diagnosis of ischaemic stroke, and in differentiating recent stroke from old stroke and other pathologies.

It is an essential sequence to include in MRI in any acute stroke patient.

Physics

- Water molecules in the tissue are in a continuous state of Brownian motion
- Therefore, the ^1H (protons) in water are also in continuous motion
- When the protons in a selected slice are excited by the scanner radio frequency (RF) pulse, some of them will diffuse out of the slice
- Restriction of diffusion results in molecules rephasing in a more coherent fashion and giving off a stronger signal, whereas free diffusion results in them becoming out of phase and a weaker signal
- This phenomenon is used in DWI
- If diffusion of water molecules is impaired (after acute ischaemia), more stay in the slice and the signal acquired is altered
- This is called restricted diffusion. The mathematical value calculated is the ADC and it will be low because there is less diffusion. By convention, restricted diffusion is shown as dark as the ADC is low, whereas increased or free diffusion is shown as bright as the ADC is high
- In clinical practice, a DWI image is often used for interpretation. For this, the contrast is inverted so the dark areas of reduced ADC look bright—the light bulb sign of acute ischaemia.

DWI in acute stroke

- Restricted diffusion occurs rapidly (within an hour or two and can be in minutes) after stroke owing to cell swelling. This means DWI abnormalities are seen soon after stroke and it is the most sensitive technique to detect acute infarction (see Fig. 7.10)
- The reduced diffusion remains for 1–3 weeks on average. As tissue breakdown occurs, diffusion increases. Therefore, an old infarct is characterized by increased diffusion (dark on a DWI image). This makes DWI very useful in:
  - differentiating acute ischaemia from old infarcts—e.g. to determine if a new deficit is caused by a new stroke or a Todd's paresis (post-epileptic) in a patient with an old stroke
  - differentiating acute ischaemia from non-stroke pathology, e.g. migraine, non-organic, or functional weakness.
- High signal on DWI can occur if there is a high-signal lesion on T2, in the absence of acute ischaemia. This is called 'shine through'. One can differentiate this from acute ischaemia by looking at the ADC map—if it is acute ischaemia it will show a corresponding region of low signal. If it is 'shine through', ADC will not show a low signal, and instead usually also shows a high signal—a bright region
- High signal on DWI can also occasionally occur with acute haemorrhage—this can be differentiated by looking on the gradient-echo (T2*) sequence which will show low signal due to haemosiderin

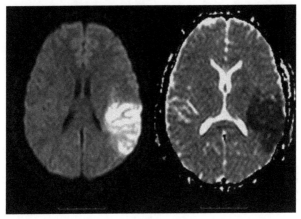

Fig. 7.10 DWI MRI in acute stroke. The left picture shows the DWI image of a slice through a left frontoparietal ischaemic infarct. It can be seen as high signal (white) on the DWI image. On the ADC map (right), the acute infarct is seen as a corresponding area of low signal. © Anthony Pereira.

- As well as the extent of diffusion, the directionality of diffusion can be determined using DTI. This is enabled by acquiring the diffusion data in multiple planes. Because diffusion is greater along white matter tracts, rather than across them, this allows visualization of white matter tract anatomy. It is very sensitive to white matter tract damage, although is largely used as a research tool.

Temporal profile of DWI in acute stroke

The mean diffusion of water molecules in the infarct changes over time. Fig. 7.11 shows how the ADC changes. Note that it is low for about 7–10 days and then increases.

There are a number of phases (see Fig. 7.12):
1. Initially restricted diffusion is seen—high signal on DWI
2. This DWI high signal persists for about 2 weeks
3. After this, diffusion increases as tissue breakdown occurs, allowing increased diffusion of water molecules—eventually the stroke appears dark on DWI. During the few days when the ADC is around normal, the image of the infarct may appear normal. But this will not be the case on structural sequences, so it is important not to use DWI alone except in special circumstances.

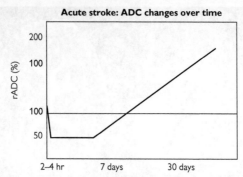

Fig. 7.11 ADC changes over time after acute ischaemic stroke. Remember that a reduction in ADC corresponds to an increase in signal on the DWI image. © Hugh Markus.

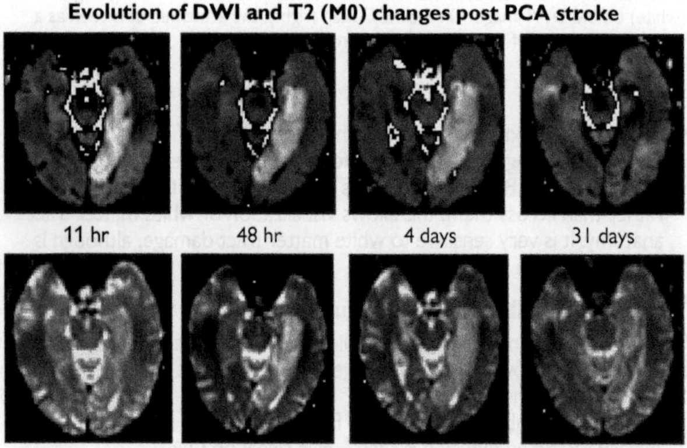

Evolution of DWI and T2 (M0) changes post PCA stroke

| 11 hr | 48 hr | 4 days | 31 days |

Fig. 7.12 DWI imaging of a posterior cerebral artery infarct at different time points after stroke. At 11 hours the infarct is clearly seen on DWI (top row) but is much less well seen on the T2 image (bottom row). By 48 hours it is visible on both DWI and T2. By 31 days the DWI image shows low signal (consistent with tissue breakdown and increased water diffusion). © Hugh Markus.

MRI in acute stroke

(See Table 7.1.)

Very early (0–24 hours)

- DWI detects ischaemia within minutes of onset. Reduced water diffusion is detected as decreased ADC/increased signal on DWI
- Early perfusion imaging detects reductions of CBF and CBV and increased MTT of blood. CBV may rise in non-infarcted ischaemic areas while tissue is still salvageable
- Matched diffusion- and perfusion-weighted abnormalities correlate with the region of infarction and are indicative of permanent neuronal death
- Mismatched diffusion and perfusion abnormalities with the perfusion abnormality larger than the diffusion abnormality may be indicative of a region of reversible ischaemic penumbra
- At 2–4 hours, T1-weighted image shows subtle effacement of the sulci owing to cytotoxic oedema
- At 8 hours, T2-weighted image shows hyperintense signal caused by both cytotoxic and vasogenic oedema
- At 16–24 hours, T1-weighted image shows hypointense signal caused by both cytotoxic and vasogenic oedema
- Contrast-enhanced images show arterial enhancement followed by parenchymal enhancement. The arterial enhancement can be very early and is caused by slow blood flow; it typically disappears after 1 week
- Although conventional MRI sequences most often do not show evidence of stroke in the hyperacute phase, conventional MRI may show signs of intravascular thrombus such as absence of flow void on T2-weighted sequences or vascular hyperintensity on FLAIR which can be an indication of patent vessels but altered flow.

MRI findings: 1–7 days

- Oedema increases at 48–72 hours and MRI abnormality becomes more prominent and well demarcated on the T2 images
- The ischaemic area appears hypointense on T1-weighted and hyperintense on T2-weighted images
- The mass effect can be appreciated in this phase
- Reperfusion occurs. Sometimes haemorrhage (petechial or larger accumulations of frank haemorrhage) can be observed, typically 24–48 hours after the onset of the stroke.

MRI findings: 7–21 days

- Mass effect becomes less marked
- The ischaemic area appears hypointense on T1-weighted and as a hyperintense area on T2-weighted images
- In contrast-enhanced images, the arterial enhancement usually improves but the parenchymal enhancement may persist
- DWI signal reduces in intensity, the infarct transiently becomes isointense, and then increased diffusion is seen (low signal on DWI)
- T2 high-signal lesions may normalize and not be visible before becoming identifiable again.

MRI findings: >21 days

- Oedema completely resolves
- The ischaemic area appears hypointense on T1-weighted and hyperintense on T2-weighted images
- There is usually some T1 hyperintensity as well by this stage (if not earlier) owing to haemorrhagic transformation. This can be gyriform or localized depending on the type of infarct and extent of transformation. The equivalent on T2 or T2* is hypointensity, which is usually visible to some degree, even on the spin-echo sequences
- Infarct becomes low intensity on DWI
- In contrast-enhanced images, parenchymal enhancement typically persists throughout this phase; it usually disappears after 3–4 months.

Table 7.1 MRI findings in acute ischaemic stroke

Time	MRI	Finding	Cause
2–3 minutes	PWI	Reduced CBF, CBV, MTT	Decreased CBF
2–3 minutes	DWI	Reduced ADC	Decreased motion of protons
0–2 hours	T2 FLAIR	Absent flow void signal most sensitively seen on FLAIR	Slow flow or occlusion
0–2 hours	T1	Arterial enhancement	Slow flow
2–4 hours	T1	Subtle sulcal effacement	Cytotoxic oedema
2–4 hours	T1	Parenchymal enhancement	Incomplete infarction
≈ hours	T2 FLAIR	Hyperintense signal— more sensitive on FLAIR	Vasogenic and cytotoxic oedema
16–24 hours	T1	Hypointense signal	Vasogenic and cytotoxic oedema
5–7 days		Parenchymal enhancement	Complete infarction

MRI and CT in cerebral haemorrhage

- MRI is as sensitive as CT for detecting acute haemorrhage. However, haemorrhage on MRI is more difficult to interpret than on CT for the inexperienced clinician (see Figs 7.13–7.15 and Table 7.2)
- Gradient-echo MRI is very useful in the diagnosis of haemorrhage and it is recommended to include it in any acute stroke MRI—blood appears as a 'black hole'
- Haemorrhage can appear bright on DWI (admittedly with a black ring round it but can be subtle), and therefore, acute stroke imaging cannot rely on DWI alone or you may thrombolyse bleeds in error. To avoid this, other MRI sequences, particularly T2*, must be performed with DWI
- Gradient-echo (GRE) MRI is the most sensitive sequence for detecting intraparenchymal haemorrhage (primary ICH and haemorrhagic transformation) in the hyperacute stages
- Conventional T1-weighted and T2-weighted sequences may show subacute and chronic bleeding
- T2* and FLAIR are the most sensitive MRI sequences for detecting acute SAH.

Table 7.2 Temporal sequence of appearances of cerebral haemorrhage on CT and MRI subject to variability depending on size and location of clot, haematocrit, sequences, etc.

	Immediate	Hours	Days	Weeks	Months
CT	Dense	Dense	Dense	Isodense >1 week	Hypodense
T1 MRI	Isodense		Bright	Bright	Dark eventually
T2 MRI	Bright	Bright	Dark around 2 days	Bright after about 2 weeks	Dark
GRE	Dark hole	Dark hole	Dark hole	Dark hole	Dark hole

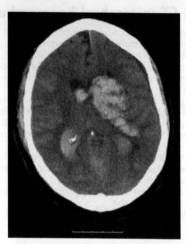

Fig. 7.13 CT in cerebral haemorrhage. A left subcortical haemorrhage can be seen with extension of blood into the ventricles and subarachnoid space. © Anthony Pereira.

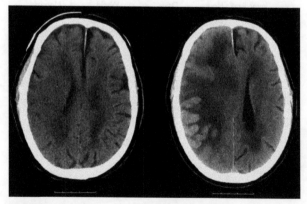

Fig. 7.14 Haemorrhagic transformation on CT. A pair of images show haemorrhagic transformation into a large infarct. The left-hand scan is in the first 24 hours. At this time no haemorrhage is present. The scan on the right is after a few days. © Anthony Pereira.

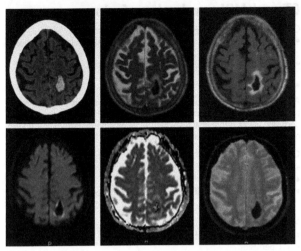

Fig. 7.15 CT and MRI images of an acute left parietal acute intracerebral haemorrhage. The top left-hand image is CT. The remaining images are all MRI sequences and are from left to right. Top row: T2-weighted, FLAIR; bottom row: DWI, ADC map, gradient echo. © Anthony Pereira.

CT and MRI cerebral perfusion

Cerebral perfusion imaging has a number of applications:
- Assessing the perfusion deficit in acute stroke and calculating perfusion–diffusion mismatch
- Assessing cerebral perfusion prior to revascularization for cerebral occlusive disease
- Research.

A number of techniques can be used. These differ in that some are quantitative and some are semi-quantitative. Some techniques measure tissue perfusion with a high spatial resolution while others estimate volume flow in major vessels (e.g. transcranial Doppler (TCD) and MRA methods).

Quantitative
- PET
- Xenon CT
- Endogenous contrast MRI arterial spin labelling (potentially quantitative).

Semi-quantitative
- Exogenous contrast perfusion MRI
- CT perfusion
- SPECT
- TCD—flow in major cerebral vessels.

The two most widely used in acute stroke are:
- CT perfusion
- MR Arterial spin labelling (ASL).

TCD ultrasound can also be used to assess relative changes in perfusion—it measures flow velocity rather than flow but if MCA diameter stays the same, changes in velocity are directly proportional to changes in flow.

CT perfusion

- CT perfusion measures brain parenchymal perfusion in a brain slice/block. Newer CT scanners offer whole brain coverage.
- Potentially, absolute quantification of CBF should be possible but, in practice, this is difficult and the technique is primarily semi-quantitative.
- During CT perfusion acquisition, the brain is repeatedly scanned during the intravenous infusion of iodinated contrast media.
- Contrast is followed as it passes through the brain.
- As the contrast flows through the region, the relative increase, peak, and then decrease in radiodensity, measured in Hounsfield units, allows an attenuation–time curve to be derived.
- These curves are calculated for an arterial input function and a venous outflow function, allowing a number of perfusion measures to be calculated for each voxel.
- Measures usually produced and displayed as colour-coded maps (Figs 7.16 and 7.17) are:
  - Cerebral blood volume is defined as the total volume of flowing blood in a given volume in the brain; low flow is considered a marker of already infarcted tissue.
  - Cerebral blood flow is defined as the volume of blood flowing through a given volume of brain per unit time. Low CBF values are associated with hypoperfused tissue, which could be salvageable; however, more severe CBF reductions are also considered a marker of infarction.
  - Time to peak is the time from the start of injection until the maximum peak of contrast enhancement.
  - Mean transit time (MTT) is the average time taken for contrast to flow through a brain region.
  - Tmax represents the time from the start of the scan until the maximum intensity of contrast material arrives at each voxel.
  - Time to drain is the time from maximum enhancement to a defined low cut-off.
- The ischaemic 'core' represents likely irreversibly damaged tissue and is identified by markedly reduced CBF and reduced CBV, with a marked delay in time to peak and MTT.
- The ischaemic penumbra, which represents potentially salvageable tissue, also has prolonged MTT or Tmax but in contrast has only moderately reduced CBF, and near normal or even increased CBV due to autoregulatory vasodilatation.
- Increased MTT is a sensitive indicator of ischaemic, but changes in MTT can also occur due to large artery stenosis/occlusion (e.g. carotid stenosis) in the absence of acute ischaemia.

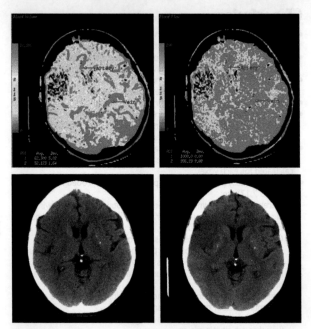

Fig. 7.16 CT perfusion in a patient presenting with a right frontal infarct. On the initial structural CT (bottom left), there are very early ischaemic changes. At this time a CT perfusion scan was performed. The cerebral blood volume and blood flow maps are shown on the upper left and right, respectively. There is a perfusion defect in the right frontal cortex with a matched reduction in cerebral blood volume, indicating the tissue is already damaged. On the follow-up CT scan (bottom right), there is an established infarct in this area. © Anthony Pereira.

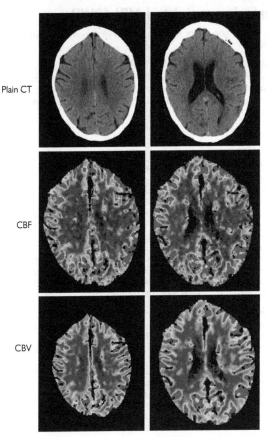

Plain CT

CBF

CBV

Fig. 7.17 Another patient in whom CT perfusion imaging suggests penumbral tissue. This patient with a left carotid stenosis presented with dysphasia. The CT perfusion showed a CBF deficit in the left frontal region but on CBV the blood volume was preserved consistent with salvageable tissue. The patient responded well to IV thrombolysis. © Hugh Markus.

Perfusion-weighted MRI (PWI)

This allows assessment of brain parenchymal perfusion. Two methods are used.

Endogenous contrast PWI (bolus tracking)

- Requires an IV infusion of an MRI contrast agent. Gadolinium is used
- Gadolinium is rapidly injected and images are acquired as it passes through the cerebral circulation. A bolus tracking technique is used to obtain maps of:
  - CBF
  - CBV
  - MTT
  - time to peak (TTP)
- CBF measurements require an input function to be obtained from a feeding artery
- Whole brain coverage can be obtained
- A robust technique with good signal-to-noise ratio
- The technique is claimed to provide quantitative CBF maps but in practice it is best thought of as semi-quantitative. Similar to CT perfusion, this may be very helpful in showing reduced perfusion in areas of acute stroke
- It is most often used clinically in acute stroke to determine the size of the perfusion deficit, and calculate diffusion–perfusion mismatch.
- It is less used now in acute stroke due to the need for a contrast injection; ASL (next) is preferred.

Endogenous perfusion MRI—arterial spin labelling (ASL)

- This uses flowing blood as the contrast agent—it is labelled using a spin labelling technique (see Fig. 7.18)
- The technique can potentially provide quantitative CBF values
- Signal-to-noise ratio is low
- Signal-to-noise ratio is higher with 3T scanners but still much lower than with exogenous contrast methods
- Can label individual arteries and potentially produce arterial territory maps.

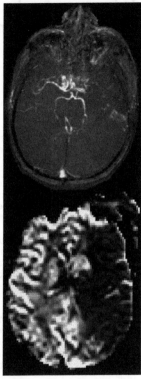

Fig. 7.18 An endogenous contrast MR perfusion study. On the upper image an MRA shows occlusion of the left MCA. On the perfusion image below, a large perfusion defect (low density) can be seen in the MCA territory. © Hugh Markus.

Positron emission tomography (PET) and single-photon emission computed tomography (SPECT)

PET

- This uses radionuclear isotopes that emit positrons
- As the isotopes decay they emit a positron
- As soon as the positron collides with an electron it will disintegrate
- The resulting disintegration produces two photons
- They travel in diametrically opposite directions
- These photons can be detected by gamma camera detectors
- These positron-emitting isotopes have a very short half-life; isotopes have to be made in a cyclotron and many have such a short half-life that the cyclotron has to be on site
- Multitracer 150 PET can be used in research studies to measure CBF, CBV, MTT, oxygen consumption, and then to derive oxygen extraction. The combination of CBF and oxygen consumption measurements allowed it to be used to perform seminal work investigating the ischaemic penumbra in man
- Pharmacological compounds can be labelled to investigate neuropharmacology. For example, fluorodopa is used to look at presynaptic integrity of the dopaminergic system in Parkinson's disease
- ^{11}C-flumazenil is a central benzodiazepine receptor labelled with ^{11}C. It detects neuronal damage in the cortex in the first few hours after acute stroke and is used in acute stroke research as a marker of tissue integrity
- ^{11}C-PK11195 has affinity for the translocator protein 18 kDa (TSPO) which is located in the mitochondrial membrane and is overexpressed in activated microglial cells. It is used as a marker of brain inflammation
- PET scanning is also a useful technique for detecting neoplastic malignant cells and may identify small tumours in the body
- PET is expensive.

SPECT

- This uses a gamma camera
- Drugs labelled with gamma-emitting ligands are injected. A variety of ligands can be used depending on the requirement. For example, ligands taken up across the blood–brain barrier where they are fixed in the tissues give pictures of CBF (e.g. HMPAO). Other ligands are taken up by dopaminergic receptors and are used in movement disorders to look at the basal ganglia
- Gamma radiation is emitted from the patient's brain
- The camera rotates around the patient and detects the gamma rays and their position in space from which it recreates a spatial map of the brain
- The resolution is much less than that of CT or MRI so images often need to be viewed with either CT or MRI scans to identify where the areas of high signal occur
- Measurements of CBF with HMPAO SPECT are relative (to a selected reference region) and do not give absolute quantitative values.

Cerebrovascular ultrasound

Ultrasound (US) is widely used in non-invasive imaging of the cerebral circulation. It has a number of applications:
- Identifying stenoses in both the extra- and intra-cranial circulation
- Imaging the arterial wall, primarily the carotid artery, to look both at intima–media thickness (IMT), a marker of cardiovascular risk, and at the morphology of established atherosclerotic plaque
- Studying haemodynamics: e.g. looking at reactivity or perfusion reserve in the MCA distal to a carotid stenosis or occlusion
- Monitoring circulating emboli.

Extracranial US (carotid and vertebral)

This is widely used to screen for carotid and vertebral stenosis.

It uses higher-frequency transducers (5–10 MHz) which allow higher spatial resolution. This is in contrast to TCD ultrasound where lower frequencies, with a corresponding reduction in resolution, are required to allow penetration through the skull.

It provides information on both structure (B-mode) and on flow (Doppler). The combination of the two is called Duplex ultrasound.

B-mode

A transducer (probe) is placed on the patient's neck over the artery being studied. It emits ultrasound waves. Every time the waves cross a boundary where the tissues have different densities, some of the waves are reflected back or back-scattered. The transducer also detects the reflected waves and their position and a computer image is generated. This image is continually updated, giving the real-time B-mode image. This is used to obtain anatomical data (e.g. identify the carotid or vertebral artery or measure the IMT).

Doppler

- The next stage is to use the Doppler principle to identify flowing blood.
- This relies on a shift in the frequency of the ultrasound waves as they are back-scattered and reflected back from the moving blood (red cells).
- From this frequency shift, combined with a knowledge of the angle between the ultrasound beam and the vessel, one can calculate the blood flow velocity.
- The Doppler information is conventionally colour-coded (red for arterial blood, blue for venous blood).
- Stenoses initially result in turbulence of blood flow and, as they become tighter, an increase in flow velocity.

Detection of stenoses on Duplex ultrasound

- A stenosis can be identified from visualization of plaque and also its effect on flow velocity. Measuring flow velocity is the most reliable way to determine the degree of stenosis
- Stenoses result in turbulent flow and loss of the spectral window. This reflects the fact that most blood flow is at a similar velocity with little flow at low velocities. With turbulence caused by stenosis, flow occurs

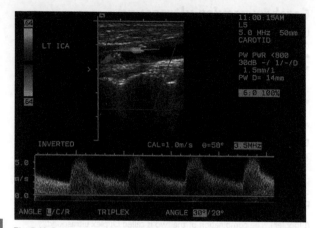

Fig. 7.19 Duplex ultrasound from a tight internal carotid stenosis. On the upper image the colour Doppler outlines the plaque and shows turbulent flow. On the lower image the peak systolic velocity is increased to above 5 m/s (normal up to 1.4 m/s). © Hugh Markus.

at all velocities, including low velocities, and therefore flow is seen at lower velocities. This change is seen before velocity starts to rise

- As stenosis increases above 50–60%, velocity increases (through the narrowed lumen). From the Doppler frequencies, the blood flow velocity and the degree of stenosis in the arterial lumen can be determined (see Fig. 7.19)
- The usual parameter recorded is the peak systolic velocity (PSV). Sometimes the ratio of the PSV over the end-diastolic velocity (EDV) is used. A conversion chart is used to convert this to stenosis; this may vary between laboratories
- If there is contralateral carotid occlusion, normal flow in the ipsilateral carotid will increase. In such cases, PSV measurements alone will overestimate stenosis and one should use the PSV:EDV ratio
- With very tight stenosis, velocities can fall. Sometimes differentiating tight stenosis from occlusion can be difficult. MRA or CTA is then useful
- Ultrasound contrast (which relies on the injection of minute air bubbles which are echogenic) can also help to differentiate tight stenosis from occlusion
- The degree of stenosis can also be determined from the B image. This gives a useful idea for lesser degrees of stenosis when velocities are not increased but is not as accurate as velocities for tighter stenoses.

Ultrasound plaque morphology

B-mode ultrasound also gives information on plaque morphology. There are three main types of plaque:

- Echolucent plaques (appear black) contain lipid and have highest stroke risk
- Echogenic plaques (appear white) are fibrous and have the lowest stroke risk
- Mixed.

Plaques may also be calcified, in which case the calcium casts an acoustic shadow, and the artery cannot be fully visualized.

Although plaque morphology relates to risk, it is observer-dependent and has not been widely adopted in risk prediction.

Advantages and disadvantages of carotid and vertebral Duplex

Advantages
- Quick
- Non-invasive
- Relatively inexpensive
- Widely available
- No radiation.

Disadvantages
- Experienced and skilled operator is required
- Inaccurate for stenoses below 50%
- Calcification of the artery may make it less accurate
- Distal carotid stenoses cannot be visualized (although abnormal flow patterns may give a clue to their presence)
- It is not very reliable at looking at the vertebral arteries—it can only visualize the vertebral origin well and sometimes even this is poorly seen; CTA or MRA are preferred as first line screening tests for posterior circulation stroke and TIA.

Carotid intima–media thickness

- The thickness of the intima–media complex is measured on the far wall of the common carotid artery using high-resolution B-mode ultrasound (see Figs 7.20 and 7.21)
- The IMT measured ultrasonically correlates well with the intima–media complex determined histologically
- Increased IMT is seen in patients with carotid stenosis, stroke, and ischaemic heart disease
- Increased IMT is an independent predictor of stroke and MI risk
- It is used as a screening test to assess vascular risk by some clinicians.

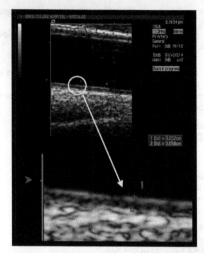

Fig. 7.20 Carotid artery intima–media thickness (IMT). On the posterior wall (lower wall) the intima–media complex can be seen. IMT is measured between the two interfaces as indicated on the lower magnified image by crosses. © Hugh Markus.

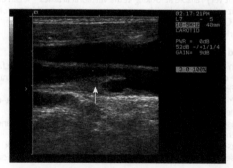

Fig. 7.21 Picture of an irregular plaque on B-mode ultrasound (arrowed). © Hugh Markus.

Transcranial Doppler (TCD) ultrasound

TCD allows detection of stenoses in the intracranial circulation (see Fig. 7.22).

Transmission of ultrasound through the skull is much less good than that through the skin:

- This means a lower-frequency ultrasound (2 MHz), which is better transmitted through the skull, has to be used
- This provides lower spatial resolution. Therefore, while limited information on structure can be obtained from the B-mode images, TCD primarily gives information on flow velocity
- Insonation has to be made through bone windows which are thinner and allow better transmission of ultrasound
- The most commonly used is the transtemporal window, which allows insonation of the MCA, distal ICA, and PCA
- In 10–20% of individuals, no signals can be detected through this window (described as an absent acoustic window). This absence of a TCD window is increased in older people and women
- A posterior window allows insonation of the basilar artery
- An orbital window allows insonation of the ophthalmic artery but insonating through the lens is associated with increased risk of cataracts.

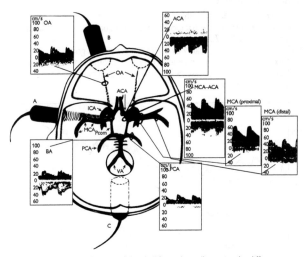

Fig. 7.22 A schematic diagram of the skull from above illustrating the different TCD windows and the appearance of the waveforms in the different vessels. ACA, anterior cerebral artery; BA, basilar artery; ICA, internal carotid artery; MCA, middle cerebral artery; OA, ophthalmic artery; PCA, posterior cerebral artery; Pcom, posterior communicating artery; VA, vertebral artery.

Advantages

- Non-invasive
- Suitable for repeated measurement of flow velocity and for continuous monitoring, e.g. during carotid endarterectomy
- High temporal resolution.

Disadvantages

- Operator dependent
- Poor spatial resolution
- Provides information on flow velocity, not absolute flow. Velocity correlates with flow if vessel diameter stays unaltered
- Does not allow visualization of all major intracerebral vessels
- Takes longer than CTA or MRA.

Clinical uses

- Screening for intracranial stenoses
- Monitoring for vasospasm in patients after SAH
- During carotid endarterectomy, monitoring flow in the ipsilateral MCA to determine whether shunting is necessary, and monitoring for emboli in the immediate postoperative phase.

Other uses of TCD

Assessment of cerebral reactivity

- This allows study of the haemodynamic consequences of stenosis or occlusion (see Fig. 7.23)
- If collateral supply, primarily by the circle of Willis, is good, a carotid stenosis may result in no haemodynamic compromise in the ipsilateral MCA. In contrast, if collateral supply is poor, then haemodynamics may be severely affected

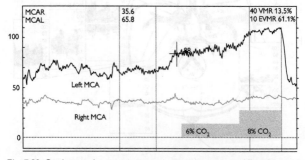

Fig. 7.23 Cerebrovascular reactivity measurement using transcranial Doppler. Increased inspired carbon dioxide (first 6% in air and then 8% in air) is given, which results in a marked increase in MCA flow in normal individuals. In a patient with a haemodynamically significant carotid stenosis this reactivity may be reduced or absent. In this patient with a right carotid occlusion, reactivity is normal in the left MCA but absent in the right MCA. Severely impaired reactivity has been associated with an increased future stroke risk, particularly in patients with carotid artery occlusion. © Hugh Markus.

- Only limited information can be obtained from resting MCA velocity measurements, owing to cerebral autoregulation preserving resting flow. Therefore, the circulation needs to be 'stressed'
- MCA flow velocity is measured at rest and then during a vasodilatory stimulus
- The commonly used vasodilatory stimuli are increased inspired CO_2 gas (5–8%) in air, or an IV injection of the carbonic anhydrase inhibitor acetazolamide
- In the presence of impaired haemodynamics, the vessels are already vasodilated to preserve flow. Therefore, they cannot vasodilate much further and reactivity (the percentage increase in flow velocity) is reduced
- If submaximal dilatory concentrations of CO_2 are used, the percentage increase in flow velocity needs to be divided by the increase in blood CO_2; this is estimated by the change in end-tidal CO_2
- In patients with carotid occlusion, a severely impaired reactivity predicts future stroke and TIA
- Reactivity is used by some clinicians to determine when to revascularize patients with carotid occlusion with extracranial–intracranial (EC–IC) bypass and when to treat asymptomatic carotid stenosis with carotid endarterectomy, although there are no trial data to support or contradict this approach.

Emboli detection

- TCD is the only technique which can detect circulating cerebral emboli
- Emboli reflect and back-scatter more ultrasound red blood cells and therefore result in high-intensity signals in the Doppler spectrum. As they are travelling rapidly through the insonated field, these increases are short duration. This is why they are called HITS (High InTensity short duration Signals) although most authorities use the simpler term 'embolic signals' (see Fig. 7.24)
- They have been detected in patients with a wide variety of potential embolic sources

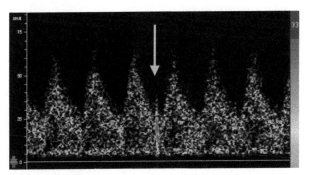

Fig. 7.24 An embolic signal (arrowed), seen as a short duration intensity increase, recorded from the MCA of a patient with carotid stenosis. © Hugh Markus.

- Most work has been done on carotid artery stenosis
- In recently symptomatic carotid stenosis they can be detected in about 40% of individuals during an hour-long recording from the ipsilateral MCA
- In this setting, they predict future stroke risk, and have been used to evaluate antiplatelet efficacy. For example, in the CARESS trial clopidogrel and aspirin were better than aspirin alone in preventing embolization in actively embolizing patients with symptomatic carotid stenosis
- The ACES study showed they predicted recurrent stroke risk in asymptomatic carotid stenosis
- Some surgeons use the technique to monitor for embolic signals in the immediate post-carotid endarterectomy period. A high embolic signal count predicts an early postoperative stroke rate. If this is detected, options are to check for technical problems with the operation and/or to give an additional antiplatelet agent (IV dextran has been commonly used).

CT angiography (CTA)

This uses CT and IV contrast to image the blood vessels in the neck and brain. The technique can be used to investigate the arteries (CTA, see Fig. 7.25) and the veins (CTV).

- Good-quality images require modern machines with spiral CT
- Here the patient is moved through the rotating X-ray beam
- This allows a faster scanning time and imaging while the bolus of contrast passes through the arteries
- The higher the number of slices (e.g. 16 versus 32 versus 64 versus 128), the quicker the acquisition, and the better the quality.

Advantages

- In contrast to ultrasound, CTA can visualize stenoses in the whole carotid and vertebral tree, and also the intracranial circulation. Therefore, it allows detection of vertebral and basilar stenosis and distal carotid stenoses
- Quick acquisition
- Can detect intracranial aneurysms
- Can show the collateral circulation present following acute large artery occlusion, which can be useful information in assessing patients for endovascular intervention.

Disadvantages

- Reconstructed images may be suboptimal if heavy calcification is present, as is often the case for carotid stenosis. However, examination of the axial source data at appropriate window settings usually enables estimation of the degree of carotid bifurcation stenosis. This is more difficult at the vertebral origins if they are very calcified
- Requires a contrast injection
- The contrast can exacerbate renal impairment in those with pre-existing kidney disease. Prior optimization of hydration and using appropriate contrast agents can help reduce the risk
- Involves ionizing radiation.

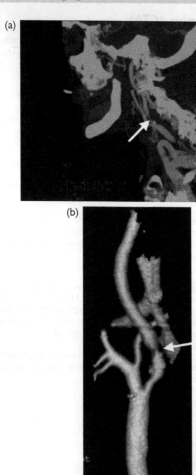

Fig. 7.25 CTA imaging of carotid stenosis. (a) On the upper image there is a proximal ICA stenosis with a speck of calcium visible in the plaque as high signal. (b) The lower image shows a reconstructed three-dimensional image from another patient with carotid stenosis. In both cases the stenosis is arrowed. © Hugh Markus.

Magnetic resonance angiography (MRA)

- This uses MR with or without IV contrast to image the blood vessels in the brain. The technique investigates:
  - the arteries (MRA)
  - the veins (MRV).
- MRA is very sensitive to flow and is based on the difference in signal between moving blood and stationary brain tissue
- MRA is particularly good for looking at the blood vessels in the carotid and vertebral circulation
- It is also very useful for looking at the intracranial circulation but is susceptible to small movements, so if a patient moves slightly it can severely degrade the quality of the images. CTA is equally susceptible to movement but the scan time is shorter so it is less likely to happen.

Methods

Non-contrast
- Time of flight
- Phase contrast.

Contrast
- Contrast-enhanced MRA.

Increasingly, contrast-enhanced MRI is used for the extracranial cerebral vessels because of the better signal-to-noise ratio.

Time of flight

- Depends on the relative contrast between flowing blood and stationary tissue
- Images correlate well with carotid angiography for analysing cervical bifurcation disease
- Flow signal dropout secondary to turbulent flow in tortuous and stenotic vascular segments makes interpretation of stenosis in these areas difficult (these are common predilection sites for atherosclerosis)
- In regions of slow flow, the spin saturation of the scan causes overestimation of stenosis
- MRA is flow dependent: absence of flow signal does not mean complete occlusion but rather that flow is below a critical value
- This means that stenosis is often overestimated and tight stenosis often appears as a flow gap. Such possible occlusions may then need further investigation to determine whether there is indeed stenosis or occlusion.

Phase contrast (PC-MRA)

- A technique that is helpful specifically in differentiating slow and absent flow from normal flow; it captures only truly patent vessels
- Other imaging sequences (e.g. spin-echo sequence or gradient-echo sequence) should be used with PC-MRA to avoid missing lesions such as perivascular haematomas, which are not captured by PC-MRA
- PC-MRA also has the disadvantage of signal loss because of turbulent flow in tortuous vessels
- Phase contrast is much less used now.

Contrast-enhanced MRA (CE-MRA)

- MRA can also be obtained by giving an IV contrast infusion: a paramagnetic contrast agent, based on gadolinium chelates, is given (see Fig. 7.26)
- Images are rapidly acquired as the bolus passes through the cerebral vessels
- The agent reduces the T1 relaxation times of the fluid in the blood vessels relative to surrounding tissues
- These images have a higher signal-to-noise ratio than non-contrast MRA methods
- The high quality of images from CE-MRA has made it the MRA modality of choice
- It overestimates degree of stenosis less than time of flight MRA. In particular, it is better at detecting vertebral origin stenosis, and at differentiating between tight stenosis and occlusion. However, it can still overestimate the degree of stenosis
- Rarely gadolinium is associated with nephrogenic systemic fibrosis (NSF) in patients with acute or chronic severe renal insufficiency (glomerular filtration rate <30 mL/min/1.73m²) and patients with renal dysfunction due to the hepatorenal syndrome or in the perioperative liver transplantation period. NSF leads to excessive formation of connective tissue in the skin and internal organs, including kidneys, and may be debilitating or fatal. Virtually every case has occurred following a high-dose gadolinium contrast MRI in a patient with pre-existing severe renal impairment. Dialysis is thought not to be protective. Therefore, gadolinium-based contrast media are avoided in all MRI scans in patients with significant renal impairment. Time of flight MRA or ultrasound should be used in these patients.

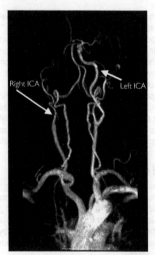

Fig. 7.26 A contrast-enhanced MRA showing a right carotid occlusion (arrowed). The right ICA is missing from its origin along its whole length. This can be appreciated when one looks at the normal left ICA (arrowed). © Hugh Markus.

Assessment of impaired cerebral haemodynamics

- When perfusion pressure falls, a series of compensatory events occur to try to preserve perfusion (see Fig. 7.27). These can be demonstrated by PET studies.
- Perfusion pressure can fall owing to a local occlusion or a systemic reduction (e.g. when the systemic blood pressure falls or after cardiac arrest).
- Initially, CBV rises to maintain CBF. This maintains adequate oxygen delivery. When this vasodilatory reserve is exhausted (i.e. the cerebral vessels are fully vasodilated), CBF starts to fall and oxygen extraction per unit volume of blood (the oxygen extraction fraction) rises to maintain adequate oxygenation. As CBF falls further, this compensatory mechanism fails and adequate oxygenation cannot occur, resulting in infarction.
- This compensatory mechanism, with vasodilatation and increased CBF, is also seen in patients with cerebral vessel occlusion (e.g. ICA occlusion) if they have inadequate collateral blood supply. The presence of this haemodynamic compromise can be assessed using a vasodilatory stimulus—see Fig. 7.23.

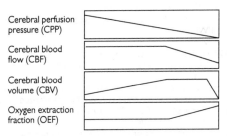

Fig. 7.27 Diagram showing how, as cerebral perfusion reserve falls, initially CBF is preserved owing to an increase in CBV until a critical point after which it falls. At this stage, oxygen extraction fraction starts to rise. © Hugh Markus.

Imaging the ischaemic penumbra in acute stroke

After an ischaemic stroke due to large artery occlusion there is a large area of hypoperfusion in the territory of the blocked artery, which can be imaged on CT perfusion or MR perfusion as reduced CBF. This progresses to infarction over a variable period of minutes to hours, depending primarily on the degree of collateral supply; this differs markedly between different people.

Studies using PET showed that after acute stroke due to middle cerebral artery occlusion there was an ischaemic penumbra (defined as tissue which is at risk due to reduced CBF but which is not yet infarcted). In some patients there is little penumbral or salvageable tissue at a couple of hours after stroke while in others penumbral tissue was still present as long as 16 hours after stroke. For further details, see ➋ Chapter 9.

This led to the hypothesis that reperfusion, even many hours after stroke, could improve outcome. However, this was only proven with the thrombectomy trials, which showed a benefit of the treatment in patients up to 24 hours after stroke onset if they had remaining penumbral tissue. In these trials CT and MR techniques were used to estimate the extent of the penumbra.

MRI perfusion–diffusion mismatch

- An estimate of the ischaemic penumbra can be obtained by combining DWI and PWI
- Simplistically:
  - the DWI deficit represents already infarcted tissue (core)
  - the PWI deficit represents tissue at risk (as well as the core) (i.e. hypoperfused)
- The mismatch between the two represents tissue which is not infarcted but hypoperfused, i.e. which could recover if revascularized but could die if not reperfused (see Figs 7.28 and 7.29)
- This concept is a bit simplistic:
  - DWI lesions can recover or reduce in size—they don't always represent irreversibly infarcted tissue
  - PWI deficits can represent oligaemia as well as critical hypoperfusion.
- Nevertheless, recent randomized clinical trials have shown that selecting patients with diffusion–perfusion mismatch can identify a group who will benefit from thrombolysis or thrombectomy at later time points
- An alternative MR method to identify the extent of salvageable DWI/FLAIR mismatch—this was successfully used in the WAKE-UP trial (see ➋ Chapter 9).

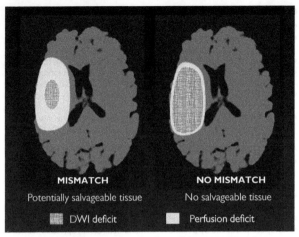

Fig. 7.28 Schematic diagram of the mismatch concept. © Hugh Markus.

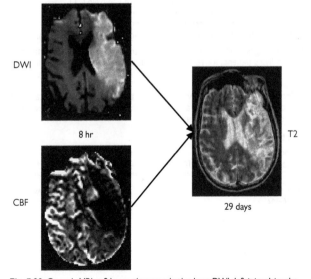

Fig. 7.29 On early MRI at 8 hours, there was both a large DWI deficit involving the whole of the left MCA territory and a similar sized perfusion deficit on the perfusion (CBF) map. As these two are matched, there is no mismatch. As predicted by the mismatch concept the final infarct size at 29 days was similar to the initial DWI deficit. © Hugh Markus.

CT ischaemic penumbra imaging

- CT perfusion can also be used to estimate mismatch.
- This is now widely used in acute stroke care due to its ease of use, wider availability, and lower costs.
- It provides maps of CBF, CBV, MTT, time to peak, and time to drain.
- Already damaged tissue (the ischaemic core) appears as markedly reduced CBF with delayed time to peak and MTT, and reduced CBV.
- Penumbral (potentially salvageable tissue) has moderately reduced CBF, but preserved CBV.
- Examples of CT scans showing mismatch, and not showing mismatch, are presented in ➔ Figs 7.16 and 7.17, respectively, pp. 172–173.

Automated AI packages to analyse acute stroke scans

- Artificial intelligence (AI) software has been developed to automatically analyse CT brain scans. Most packages provide analysis of non-contrast CT (NCCT), CT angiography (CTA) and CT perfusion (CTP) imaging
- They are now available on mobile phone apps, allowing easy review of data from remote sites
- Such packages are being increasingly used in routine clinical packages
- They are produced by a number of manufacturers. Proprietary names include RAPID-AI, Viz CTP, and Brainomix
- Uses include:
  - Detection of intracerebral haemorrhage (on plain CT)
  - Detection of ischaemic injury (e.g. using ASPECTS)
  - Detection of large vessel occlusion (on CTA)
  - Estimation of the extent of the ischaemic penumbra (on CTP).

Such packages can be very useful in the acute stroke pathways, particularly in identifying patients for reperfusion therapy and determining whether patient should be transferred for thrombectomy to a comprehensive stroke centre.

However they are not always accurate, particularly if the CT scan is of low quality or has artefacts, and the output should always be reviewed by an experienced human reader.

Further reading

CT perfusion

Chung CY, Hu R, Peterson RB, Allen JW (2021). Automated processing of head CT perfusion imaging for ischemic stroke triage: a practical guide to quality assurance and interpretation. *AJR Am J Roentgenol* **217**, 1401–1416.

Wing S, Markus HS (2019). How to do it: interpreting CT perfusion in stroke. *Pract Neurol* **19**, 136–142.

Chapter 8

Ischaemic stroke: common causes

Introduction

A large number of different pathologies can cause ischaemic stroke. This chapter covers the common causes. Rare causes of ischaemic stroke are covered in ➲ Chapter 11.

A full list of causes of ischaemic stroke is shown later in this topic.

The major mechanisms of ischaemic stroke are:

- thromboembolism from extracerebral and intracerebral arteries
- cardioembolism
- small-vessel disease or lacunar stroke.

List of causes of ischaemic stroke

Common

- Large-artery atherosclerosis:
  - extracranial atherosclerosis:
  - aorta
  - carotid artery
  - vertebral artery
  - intracranial atherosclerosis.
- Cardiac disease:
  - atrial fibrillation
  - valvular heart disease
  - left ventricular thrombus
  - other cardioembolic sources.
- Small-vessel disease.

Less common

- Carotid and vertebral artery dissection
- Connective tissue disorders and cerebral vasculitis
- Infections
- Trauma
- Drug related:
  - illicit drug abuse
  - oral contraceptives and hormone replacement therapy
  - other drug related.
- Moyamoya disease
- Haematological disorders, including prothrombotic states
- Migraine
- Genetic disorders.

Atheroma and large-vessel disease

- Atheroma is by far the most common disorder leading to narrowing of the larger arteries supplying the brain and subsequent stroke
- It affects mainly large and medium-sized arteries, especially at points of arterial bifurcation or curvature.

Extracranial atheroma causing stroke

- The most common sites are the:
  - aortic arch
  - carotid bifurcation
  - vertebral artery origin
  - proximal subclavian artery
- In addition, atheroma not infrequently affects more distal portions of the carotid and vertebral arteries.

Intracranial atheroma

- The intracranial arteries are structurally different from the extracranial arteries, having no elastic lamina, fewer elastic fibres in the media and adventitia, and a thinner intima
- Atheroma may occur at multiple intracranial sites, including:
  - carotid siphon
  - middle cerebral artery
  - anterior cerebral artery
  - distal vertebral artery
  - basilar artery.

Ethnic differences in distribution of atheroma

There are important ethnic differences in the distribution of atheroma. Knowledge of these differences can be useful when managing patients and deciding on optimal imaging approaches.

- In white individuals, extracranial atheroma, particularly of the carotid bifurcation and vertebral origin, is most common. Intracranial atheroma is much less common. Atheroma in the coronary arteries and aorta is also common
- In Black and East Asian individuals, intracranial atheroma is relatively more common, and extracranial carotid stenosis is less common
- The nature of these differences remains uncertain, including the relative contribution of genetic and environmental factors
- Table 8.1 shows comparative frequencies between ethnic groups.

Pathophysiology of atheroma

- The early stages of atherosclerosis begin in childhood or early adulthood.
- Fig. 8.1 shows a schematic diagram of the stages of atherosclerosis.
- A key early event is believed to be endothelial damage or dysfunction which is followed by deposition of fat (primarily LDL) within the arterial wall intima. resulting in a fatty streak.

Table 8.1 Comparative frequency of intracranial stenosis in patients presenting with stroke from different ethnic groups

Ethnic group	Frequency (%)
Chinese	33–50
Thai	47
Korean	56
South Asian	54
US white	1
UK white	3
US Black	6
UK Black	18
US Hispanic	11

Adapted from *Stroke*, 39(8), Gorelick PB, Wong KS, Bae HJ, Pandey DK, Large artery intracranial occlusive disease: a large worldwide burden but a relatively neglected frontier, pp. 2396–2399, Copyright (2008), with permission from Wolters Kluwer Health, Inc.; *Circulation*, 116(19), Markus HS, Khan U, Birns J, et al., Differences in stroke subtypes between black and white patients with stroke: the South London Ethnicity and Stroke Study, pp. 2157–2164, Copyright (2007), with permission from Wolters Kluwer Health, Inc.

- Hypertension can cause vessel wall stress and irritants such as cigarette smoking, high lipids, and high glucose can impair atheroprotective endothelial function.
- Wall stress causes smooth muscle cells to produce proteoglycans, which bind and trap LDL. Leucocytes migrate into the lesion attracted by chemoattractants and leucocyte adhesion molecules. Oxidized LDL induces tissue damage and stimulates angiogenesis, producing plaque vasa vasora.
- Circulating monocyte-derived macrophages invade the arterial wall. They scavenge modified LDL, eventually forming foam cells.
- Foam cells secrete platelet-derived growth factor and cytokines, which cause smooth muscle cells to migrate from the media to the intima and proliferate.
- Inflammation is a central process. There is an inflammatory response within the arterial wall with T-lymphocyte activation and cytokine production.
- Fibrosis occurs, and fibrous plaques are formed. These plaques have a lipid core and a fibrous cap and begin to encroach into the vessel lumen. Calcification in the vessel wall and plaque is common.
- For reasons not fully understood, these well-developed plaques may remain quiescent for many years but can become 'unstable' or 'active'.
- At some stage, this may lead to plaque ulceration and erosion and secondary thrombosis on the plaque surface. Platelet aggregation is believed to be particularly important in this process.

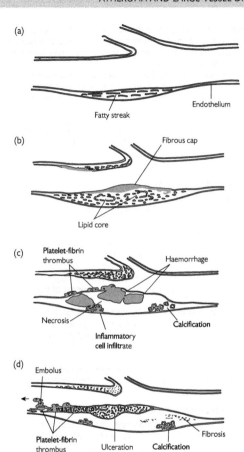

Fig. 8.1 Schematic diagram of the stages of carotid atherosclerosis. (a) Deposition of lipid in the vessel wall as a fatty streak; (b) increased deposition of lipid and formation of fibrous material occurs; (c) a more advanced plaque with inflammatory cell infiltration, calcification, necrosis, and new vessel formation; (d) ulceration occurring on the plaque surface with secondary platelet aggregation on the luminal wall. This final stage is called an unstable plaque and is associated with thromboembolism.

- Embolism can then occur from the adherent thrombus. Embolism is believed to be the primary mechanism by which atherosclerotic plaques cause stroke. It is much less common for them to cause stroke by haemodynamic compromise.
- Embolic and haemodynamic factors may interact, i.e. if perfusion pressure is lower, the effect of emboli may be greater because they may be less likely to fragment and break up, leading to less frequent vessel recanalization
- After becoming active, plaques can heal up. This has important clinical implications. Following a stroke or TIA secondary to a carotid stenosis, the risk of subsequent stroke is markedly increased for the next 2–3 years (particularly in the first month), after which it returns to that of an asymptomatic carotid stenosis.

Importance of embolism

- It was initially thought that large-artery stenosis usually caused stroke by haemodynamic compromise secondary to vessel obstruction
- We now know embolism is the predominant process. Evidence for this includes the following:
  - Emboli can be directly visualized in the retina
  - Embolic signals, representing circulating emboli, can be detected using TCD in the MCA of patients with carotid stenosis. They are more common in symptomatic stenosis, more frequent after a recent event, and predict future stroke risk independent of the degree of stenosis
  - Emboli occluding vessels can be seen on cerebral angiography
  - The risk of stroke is transiently, but markedly, increased after TIA or stroke in patients with carotid stenosis. This suggests the degree of stenosis, which does not change rapidly over time, is not the most important process
- Emboli may be platelet–thrombus aggregates, or less commonly cholesterol emboli. The latter can lodge in retinal vessels and be visible for a prolonged period.

The role of haemodynamic factors

- Although embolism is more important than haemodynamic compromise, haemodynamic factors can be important
- They can sometimes be a direct cause of stroke. During a reduction in perfusion pressure (e.g. severe hypotension), infarction may occur distal to the stenosis particularly in the watershed areas (see ➔ p. 85)
- Carotid occlusion is associated with an increased risk of stroke, although not as great as that seen in tight carotid stenosis
- Collateral supply, in particular the patency of the circle of Willis, plays a crucial role in determining the outcome of carotid stenosis and occlusion. For example, in a patient with a complete circle of Willis, internal carotid occlusion may be asymptomatic. In contrast, in a patient without either an anterior communicating artery or posterior communicating artery ipsilateral to the symptomatic carotid, carotid occlusion is likely to result in a large infarct.

Dolichoectasia

- This describes dilatation and tortuosity seen in the basal intracerebral vessels, particularly the basilar artery (see Fig. 8.2)
- Atheroma is the major cause, but other causes include congenital vessel wall defects, connective tissue disorders, and Fabry disease
- This appearance is particularly common in older people
- It is frequently an asymptomatic finding seen on structural MRI (as dilated signal voids in vessels, or on MRA)
- It most commonly causes symptoms in the basilar artery
- Symptoms may be caused by:
  - thromboembolism—thrombus within the dolichoectatic vessel
  - brainstem compression leading to cranial nerve and other brainstem dysfunction.

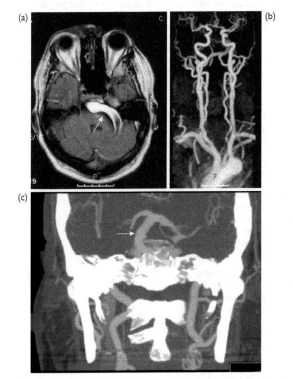

Fig. 8.2 Pictures of dolichoectatic basilar artery. (a) On the MRI there is a dilated and tortuous basilar artery. This is confirmed on the contrast-enhanced MRA (b) and on the CTA (c). The abnormality is arrowed.

Cardioembolism

- Embolism from the heart causes 20–25% of ischaemic stroke in most populations
- A large number of cardiac abnormalities can cause embolism
- Some of these are associated with a high risk of embolism. Therefore, if one of these is identified in a patient with stroke there is a high probability that they are related to the stroke
- Others are associated with a much lower risk of embolism. Therefore, their identification in a patient with stroke does not mean that they are necessarily the cause of stroke. An example of this is a patent foramen ovale (PFO)
- Atrial fibrillation (paroxysmal or sustained) is the most important cardioembolic source on a population basis. It accounts for about 20-30% of all strokes, with the highest proportion in older people
- Particularly in elderly patients, potential cardioembolic sources can coexist with other potential causes of stroke, and knowing which is the real cause of stroke may be impossible
- Thrombus emboli are believed to be particularly important in cardiac embolism. This is supported by the much greater reduction in stroke seen with warfarin, compared with antiplatelet agents, in conditions such as atrial fibrillation and valvular heart disease.

A list of cardioembolic sources is given here.

Left atrium
- Thrombus
- Atrial fibrillation
- Other atrial arrhythmias
- Atrial septal aneurysm
- Atrial myxoma.

Left ventricle
- Mural thrombus
- Post-acute myocardial infarction
- Left ventricular aneurysm/akinetic segment
- Cardiomyopathy
- Myxoma and other cardiac tumours.

Mitral valve disease
- Rheumatic mitral valve disease
- Prosthetic heart valve
- Infective endocarditis
- Marantic endocarditis
- Mitral valve prolapse (➜ p. 203).

Aortic valve
- Rheumatic aortic valve disease
- Prosthetic heart valve
- Infective endocarditis
- Marantic endocarditis

- Calcific stenosis
- Syphilis
- Other causes of aortic regurgitation, e.g. Marfan's disease.

Right-to-left shunt

- PFO
- Atrial septal defect
- Ventricular septal defect
- Pulmonary arteriovenous fistula
- Congenital heart disease.

Iatrogenic

- Cardiac surgery
- Cardiac catheterization
- Cardiac angioplasty and stenting
- Cardiac valvuloplasty.

Specific cardioembolic sources

Atrial fibrillation

- Non-rheumatic atrial fibrillation (AF) is by far the most common cause of cardioembolic stroke in developed countries
- Thrombus forms within the left atrium—particularly within the left atrial appendage, and embolizes to the brain
- AF secondary to rheumatic heart diseases is associated with a higher risk of embolism but is rare in developed countries
- In non-rheumatic AF, the absolute risk of stroke is 4% per annum, six times greater than for patients in sinus rhythm. This is an average
- Recent studies with long-term implantable cardiac monitors have suggested undiagnosed AF may be an important cause of apparently 'cryptogenic' stroke. In the CRYSTAL-AF study, it was found in 30% of cryptogenic patients when monitoring for 6 months. In many of these cases, the AF is likely to be the cause of stroke. However, whether occasional short bursts of AF detected on very long-term monitoring indicate that AF caused the original stroke is uncertain
- A number of factors are associated with higher or lower risk. Markers of increased risk include:
  - increasing age
  - previous embolic event
  - hypertension
  - diabetes
  - left ventricular dysfunction on echocardiography
  - enlarged left atrium on echocardiography.
- Lone AF—this describes AF in the absence of other cardiac disease and with normal echocardiography in younger individuals (<60 years). It is associated with a lower stroke risk of approximately 0.5% per annum
- Paroxysmal AF carries the same risk as persistent AF
- All patients with AF and previous stroke or TIAs should be considered for anticoagulation and not antiplatelet therapy. This is covered in detail on ➲ p. 289.

Infective endocarditis

- Bacterial or fungal infection occurs most commonly on already abnormal native valves, or in patients with prosthetic heart valves
- It is also common in intravenous drug abusers
- About 20% of patients with infective endocarditis have stroke or TIAs
- Stroke can be the presenting feature but more often it occurs in an already unwell patient. Mycotic aneurysms may occur which may bleed. Clues to diagnosis include fever, cardiac murmur, raised erythrocyte sedimentation rate (ESR), mild anaemia, raised white blood cell count (WBC), and vegetations on echocardiography. Blood cultures may not always be positive and repeated blood cultures are often required.

Prosthetic heart valves

- Mechanical heart valves are associated with a markedly increased risk of stroke
- Anticoagulation with warfarin is the standard treatment to prevent stroke in this group. With anticoagulation, the risk of embolism is approximately 2% per annum

- Bioprosthetic heart valves, including porcine valves, have a lower risk of embolism than metallic valves
- Patients with bioprosthetic valves are often treated with antiplatelet agents alone, although some authorities recommend anticoagulation, particularly in the first few months following valve insertion.

Rheumatic valve disease

- This is an important cause of stroke in developing countries
- Rheumatic fever earlier in life results in valvular damage and destruction
- Stroke is most common with mitral valve disease, particularly in patients who also develop AF.

Mitral valve prolapse

- This is a common clinical and echocardiographic finding
- It was thought to be associated with stroke but more recent data suggest this association is absent or very weak
- Therefore, it should not be thought of as the cause of stroke in an individual patient unless there are complicating features such as severe mitral regurgitation or infective endocarditis.

Patent foramen ovale and stroke

- PFO is a communication between the left and right atria. This is present in the foetus and persists into adult life in about 20% of individuals
- Case–control studies show PFO prevalence is higher in cryptogenic stroke patients under age 55 years compared with controls.
- Possible stroke mechanisms include:
  - paradoxical embolism from venous thrombosis
  - associated cardiac arrhythmias
  - the abnormality causing stroke is somehow structurally or pathophysiologically linked to PFO.
- Risk of stroke is higher with larger PFO and atrial septal aneurysm (ASA)
- PFO can be diagnosed on echocardiography (with contrast agent injection) or by TCD ultrasound of the MCA (also with contrast injection). Sensitivity of both tests is increased by a Valsalva manoeuvre which raises right atrial pressure
- TOE is more sensitive than TTE
- PFO can be closed percutaneously with a variety of umbrella and other devices with low complication rates (1%)
- For many years, although PFO was associated with stroke risk, no trials showed that closing a PFO reduced stroke risk. This lead people to question whether PFO was really a risk factor for stroke, and whether other features associated with PFO which would not be treated by PFO closure, such as the increased risk of arrythmias really accounted for the increased stroke risk.
- More recent randomized controlled trials (RCTs) and meta-analyses have shown that closing a PFO in someone who has had stroke does reduce recurrent stroke risk, as long as there are no other causes of stroke.
- This was shown to be because when other risk factors were present, these were much more important than the PFO itself. Only when

patients with no other risk factor apart from a PFO were treated were positive results obtained.
• PFO has also been associated with migraine with aura. Whether closing the PFO reduces migraine frequency remains controversial.

Atrial myxoma

• The most common primary cardiac tumour
• Portions of the tumour may embolize to the brain, resulting in stroke and TIA
• Occasionally, neoplastic cerebral aneurysms can form
• Clinical features include:
  • recurrent stroke
  • cardiac murmurs, which vary from day to day
  • mitral valve disease, either stenosis from mitral valve during diastole or regurgitation secondary to tumour-associated valve trauma
  • systemic symptoms and signs, including weight loss, malaise, fever, arthralgia, finger clubbing, anaemia, and raised ESR
• Diagnosis is made on echocardiography
• Cardiac catheterization may be necessary
• Surgical excision is the treatment of choice.

Small-vessel disease

This describes disease in the small perforating intracerebral arteries (<800 µm and, mostly, <400 µm).

Clinical importance

Small-vessel disease causes:
- lacunar stroke—the cause of 20% of ischaemic stroke
- vascular dementia—small-vessel disease is the most important cause of this
- lesser degree of cognitive impairment—vascular cognitive impairment (VCI)
- other cognitive symptoms, such as apathy
- gait disorders
- non-DOPA-responsive Parkinsonian syndrome (less commonly).

Pathology

Damage is seen both in the small arteries and in the brain parenchyma.

Arterial damage

A number of different pathologies may contribute, including:
- hyaline arteriosclerosis—hyaline wall thickening occurs with smooth muscle cells being replaced with collagen, presumably reducing the ability of the vessels to vasodilate normally
- lipohyalinosis
- fibrinoid necrosis—with more aggressive vessel destruction
- atheroma at or near the origin of the small perforating vessels.

Parenchymal lesions

- Small, discrete lacunar infarcts (referred to as 'lacunes' or 'small lakes')
- Diffuse ischaemic injury without frank infarction seen radiologically as leukoaraiosis (low signal on CT), or confluent white matter hyperintensities (WMH, high signal on T2 or FLAIR MRI, see Fig. 8.3). Pathologically, axonal loss, ischaemic demyelination, and gliosis are found.

Two types of small-vessel disease

C. Miller Fisher first suggested that the arterial pathology underlying lacunar infarcts is heterogeneous and proposed that there may be two main patho-logical patterns causing different sorts of lesions. This is now supported by radiological and risk factor data.

Type 1: isolated lacunar infarction

Microatheroma in the larger vessels from which the perforating arteries arise, or in the larger proximal perforating arteries (200–800 µm diameter), causes larger, often isolated, lacunar infarcts in the absence of leukoaraiosis (see Fig. 8.4).

Type 2: lacunar infarcts with leukoaraiosis

Lipohyalinosis or other similar pathologies in the smaller perforating ar-teries (<400 µm diameter) cause multiple smaller lacunar infarcts and often also leukoaraiosis (see Fig. 8.4).

(a)

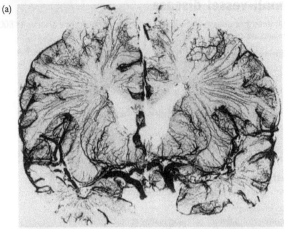

(b)

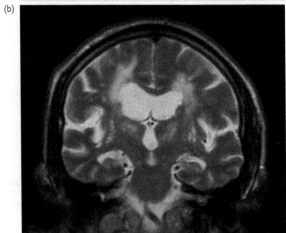

Fig. 8.3 Leukoaraiosis first occurs in the regions at the distal end of the perforating arterial supply. (a) This is illustrated by the microinjection radiological plate showing the arteriolar supply of the periventricular region. (b) An MRI scan of a similar coronal view is also shown. The high signal on MRI (leukoaraiosis) first develops in those areas furthest from the origin of the perforating arteries, i.e. those which have the lowest perfusion pressure.

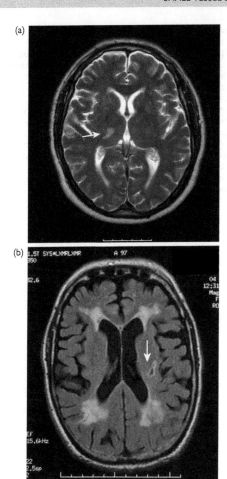

Fig. 8.4 MRI scans from patients with cerebral small-vessel disease. Both have presented with lacunar stroke. (a) A single larger lacunar infarct (arrowed) and no leukoaraiosis is seen; (b) image shows the combination of lacunar infarcts (arrowed) and extensive confluent leukoaraiosis. © Hugh Markus.

- These two patterns can be distinguished radiologically, particularly on MRI
- There appear to be risk factor differences between these two subtypes. Hypertension is a particularly strong risk factor for lacunar infarcts with leukoaraiosis (present in 90% of cases). The classical atherosclerotic risk factors (smoking, atherosclerosis in other parts of the body) are commoner for the isolated lacunar infarct subtype
- How the small-vessel disease pathology causes the type 2 subtype is uncertain. An important factor may be impaired vessel reactivity and autoregulation, leading to hypoperfusion and inability to cope with fluctuations in blood pressure. It has also been suggested that increased blood–brain barrier permeability may occur, resulting in exudation of plasma constituents into the vessel wall and parenchyma
- Embolism is not thought to play a major role in either subtype of small-vessel disease, although there is no doubt that emboli can occasionally cause small, deep lesions.

Embolic stroke of undetermined source

- Cryptogenic (of unknown cause) ischaemic strokes are now thought to comprise about 25% of all ischaemic strokes. Advances in imaging techniques and an improved understanding of stroke pathophysiology prompted a reassessment of cryptogenic stroke.
- The term embolic stroke of undetermined source (ESUS) patients was introduced to describe a group of patients with an embolic pattern of infarction on brain imaging but no obvious source of embolism—defined by a process of exclusion after echocardiography, ECG telemetry, and imaging of the large arteries.
- ESUS is a conceptual entity without a definite pathological correlate.
- It was hypothesized that emboli could arise from a number of causes, including undetected atrial fibrillation and other cardiac disease, and minor non-stenotic atheroma plaques.
- The risk of recurrent stroke is about 4.5% per year.
- As many emboli may come from cardioembolic sources, it was suggested that ESUS patients may be better treated with anticoagulants than with antiplatelets.
- This led to interest in a number of RCTs comparing anticoagulation to antiplatelets in ESUS patients.
- All trials to date have shown no benefit of direct oral anticoagulants (DOACs) over antiplatelets. (see Chapter 10).
- The reasons for these negative RCTs are unclear. It may be that many ESUS strokes are caused not by cardioembolism, but by other causes such as non-stenotic atheroma plaques, which respond better to antiplatelets.

Further reading

Atherosclerosis

Delewi R, Yang H, Kastelein J (2024). Atherosclerosis. *Textbook of cardiology.org*. Available online at: https://www.textbookofcardiology.org/wiki/Atherosclerosis

Evans NR, Bhakta S, Chowdhury MM, Markus H, Warburton E (2024). Management of carotid atherosclerosis in stroke. *Pract Neurol* **24**, 382–386.

Specific cardioembolic sources

Atrial fibrillation

Chao, TF, Potpara, TS, Lip, GYH (2024). Atrial fibrillation: stroke prevention. *Lancet* **37**, 100797.

Patent foramen ovale and stroke

Alakbarzade V, *et al.* (2020). Patent foramen ovale. *Pract Neurol* **20**, 225–233.

Embolic stroke of undetermined source

Ntaios G, *et al.* (2024). Embolic strokes of undetermined source: a clinical consensus statement of the ESC Council on Stroke, the European Association of Cardiovascular Imaging and the European Heart Rhythm Association of the ESC. *Eur Heart J* **45**, 1701–1715.

Intracranial stenosis

Hoh BL, Chimowitz MI (2024). Focused update on intracranial atherosclerosis: introduction, highlights, and knowledge gaps. *Stroke* **55**, 305–310.

Hurford R, Rothwell PM (2021). Prevalence, prognosis, and treatment of atherosclerotic intracranial stenosis in Caucasians. *Int J Stroke* **16**, 248–264.

Chapter 9

Acute stroke treatment

Acute treatment of stroke

This chapter deals mainly with ischaemic stroke, although many of the principles also apply to haemorrhagic stroke; details specific for cerebral haemorrhage are given in ➔ Chapter 13. Following stroke, a series of damaging consequences occur, each of which requires appropriate action to treat and/or prevent:

- Initial ischaemic damage
- Subsequent extension of brain damage into the ischaemic penumbra
- Early recurrent stroke
- Secondary deterioration owing to a number of causes, including:
  - brain oedema
  - raised intracranial pressure
  - epilepsy
  - secondary complications
  - decompensation of pre-existing medical conditions
- Secondary complications, including:
  - aspiration and pneumonia
  - epilepsy
  - DVT and pulmonary embolus
  - Other infections (e.g. cellulitis related intravenous cannula insertion, urinary tract infection related to urethral catheter insertion)
- Organ systems may fail:
  - heart failure, arrhythmia, myocardial infarction
  - respiratory distress
  - renal failure
  - liver compromise from drug treatment
  - skin breakdown
  - muscle and bone changes
  - dehydration
  - decreased nutrition but increased catabolism
  - psychological difficulties
- Physiological variables may become deranged:
  - blood pressure
  - diabetes
  - fever.

In addition, most stroke patients are elderly and commonly have other comorbidities. Therefore, acute treatment of the stroke patient requires consideration of many different aspects.

Key principles of stroke care

Care of the acute stroke patient requires:
- a systematic approach
- attention to detail
- concentration on doing the simple things well.

This is greatly aided by having agreed protocols and, for some areas (e.g. thrombolysis), having standard proformas.

Scheme of treatment

Treatment of acute stroke may be split into several components:
- General emergency treatment of the patient
- Acute treatment of the cerebral ischaemia/haemorrhage itself:
  - Thrombolysis or other reperfusion strategies
  - For haemorrhage, reversing coagulation disorders
- Treatment of specific causes of stroke
- Treatment of physiological variables
- Prevention and treatment of complications
- Early secondary prevention.

General emergency treatment

These are the steps taken when any seriously ill patient arrives in hospital:
- Check and protect the airway. Intubate if necessary
- Check breathing:
  - Suction the patient if necessary
  - Use a bedside saturation monitor to check the capillary oxygen
- Check the circulation:
  - Good pulse?
  - Is there an arrhythmia?
  - Is the blood pressure adequate, or too high or too low?
- Is there fever?
- Check BM/blood glucose in all patients on arrival: occasionally hypoglycaemia will masquerade as stroke
- Set up IV access
- Give IV fluids if drowsy or unsafe swallow
- Treat seizures if needed. Seizures that occur during the first week of stroke are called acute symptomatic seizures. We treat them with anticonvulsants for 14 days and then wean and stop the medication.

Key points in acute treatment of stroke

- Consider thrombolysis/thrombectomy or acute treatment of haemorrhage
- Treat physiological variables
- Identify and treat problems with systemic organ systems
- Start secondary prevention as soon as possible
- Anticipate and treat complications
- Manage patients on a specialized stroke unit

Pathophysiology of stroke

Treatment of the vascular event

The primary problem in ischaemic stroke is an occlusion of a cerebral artery. This needs to be unblocked as soon as possible if ischaemic neurons are to be saved. Spontaneous reperfusion occurs in a proportion of cases, but this can be increased by reperfusion therapies.

There are several methods of achieving this, including:

- IV thrombolysis
- intra-arterial thrombolysis
- mechanical retrieval of the embolus (thrombectomy).

In cerebral haemorrhage, haematoma (see ➔ Chapter 13 on cerebral haemorrhage) expansion occurs over the first few hours, worsening the clinical outcome. Therefore, here the specific treatment must be aimed at:

- stopping the haematoma growth, e.g. acute lowering of BP
- reversing any coagulopathy
- removing the haematoma in selected cases.

The rationale for reperfusion: the ischaemic penumbra

- If recovery is to occur, successful reperfusion must take place before neuronal death.
- As perfusion pressure in the brain falls, different cerebral blood flow (CBF) thresholds which relate to the possibility of recovery of function are passed (see Fig. 9.1).
- Recovery depends on the concept of the ischaemic penumbra, i.e. that there is tissue which is critically hypoperfused but not yet infarcted (see Fig. 9.2).
- After an acute ischaemic stroke, there is:
  - a central core of irreversibly damaged tissue
  - surrounding this is an ischaemic penumbra
  - surrounding this is an area of hypoperfusion.
- Studies in primates have shown that tissue in the ischaemic penumbra can survive if reperfusion occurs early enough, but will die if no reperfusion occurs.
- Duration of ischaemia is important. The longer the ischaemia, the less likely penumbral tissue will survive. The rate of progression to core infarction varies widely between different patients and is dependent on collateral blood supply.
- Studies with PET demonstrated the existence of penumbral tissue in humans (identified as tissue with increased oxygen extraction which may progress to recovery or infarction). The extent of this 'penumbral' tissue was very variable: none at 3 hours in some stroke patients, whereas in exceptional patients penumbral tissue existed as late as 18 hours. For more details on PET and imaging of penumbral tissue see ➔ Chapter 7. More recent studies with MRI and CT perfusion have confirmed that the amount of salvageable tissue varies greatly between different patients in the early hours after stroke, reflecting differing degrees of collateral supply.

>50	Normal
>21	Oligaemia: normal neuronal activity, reduced CBF
11–20	Ischaemic penumbra: functionally silent but viable
6–10	Irreversibly damaged tissue

Fig. 9.1 The relationship between blood flow levels and ischaemic injury, illustrating levels at which the ischaemic penumbra occurs. The data are derived from animal models. CBF, cerebral blood flow, measured in mL/100 mg/min.

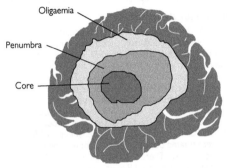

Oligaemia

Penumbra

Core

Fig. 9.2 Diagram of the ischaemic penumbra, which surrounds an inner core of irreversibly damaged tissue.

Thrombolysis

Thrombolysis is the first treatment that was shown to be effective in acute stroke. A lytic agent, most commonly recombinant tissue plasminogen activator (rtPA; generic name alteplase) is administered either intravenously (most commonly) or intra-arterially to break down the clot.

- The *in vivo* target is the enzyme plasmin which breaks down the crosslinked fibrin of the clot and disrupts the thrombus
- Plasmin circulates in inactive form as plasminogen but is activated by thrombolytic agents
- There is trial evidence for alteplase, urokinase, and tenecteplase
- In randomized clinical trials, streptokinase given within 6 hours of stroke onset increased haemorrhage and death rates and is not used in stroke.

The evidence for thrombolysis

The pivotal stroke thrombolysis trial was the National Institute for Neurological Disorders and Stroke (NINDS) trial published in December 1995. This was the first to demonstrate a treatment benefit with stroke thrombolysis using alteplase, which when administered within 3 hours of stroke onset improved patient outcome by about one-third on average. This was offset against a small but significant increase in the risk of cerebral haemorrhage (6%).

- No other individual trials of IV thrombolysis given within 3 hours have shown a statistical benefit, but meta-analysis of available trials shows a consistent benefit for IV alteplase given within 3 hours.
- In 2008, the ECASS 3 trial confirmed a benefit up to 4.5 hours—patients were treated between 3 and 4.5 hours (mean 3 hours 59 minutes) post-stroke. There was a significant 1.3–1.4 times increase in excellent outcomes (modified Rankin score 0 or 1).
- In IST3, 3035 patients were enrolled within 6 hours of stroke onset to receive alteplase or placebo. 1617 (53%) were older than 80 years of age. Although the overall trial results were neutral, indicating that the time window for IV thrombolysis should remain up to 4.5 hours, IST 3 did indicate that age, presence of AF, pre-treatment with antiplatelet agents, presence of subtle changes on the admission CT scan, and diabetes should not be barriers to administering thrombolysis.
- The benefit is much greater when alteplase is given earlier within the initial 4.5-hour period. The chance of a good outcome is better if the patient is thrombolysed at say 60 minutes than at 90 minutes. Therefore, although patients must be treated within 4.5 hours, *do not wait to treat; treat as quickly as possible* (see Fig. 9.3).
- An individual patient data meta-analysis of 6756 patients in the alteplase trials showed treatment within 3 hours resulted in good outcomes in 32.9% of treatment vs. 23.1% who received control. From 3 to 4.5 hours, the outcomes were 35.3% and 30.1%, respectively. Beyond 4.5 hours, the figures were 32.6% vs. 30.6%, respectively, and no longer significant. 90-day mortality was 17.9% with alteplase vs. 16.5% with control. Therefore, despite an increased risk of fatal intracranial haemorrhage during the first few days after treatment, this risk was offset by an average absolute increase in disability-free survival of about 10% for patients treated within 3 hours and about 5% for patients treated from 3 to 4.5 hours (see Fig. 9.4).

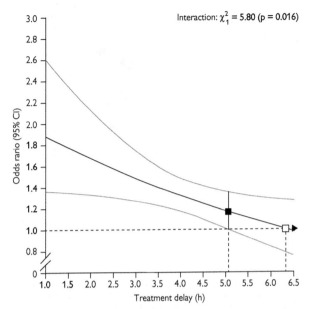

Fig. 9.3 Effect of timing of alteplase treatment on good stroke outcome (modified Rankin Scale score 0–1) showing the marked reduction of benefit as time passes after stroke onset. The solid line is the best linear fit between the log odds ratio for a good stroke outcome for patients given alteplase compared with those given control (vertical axis) and treatment delay and gives a clinically useful estimate of the benefit of treating a patient at different time points post-stroke. Estimates are derived from a regression model in which alteplase, time to treatment, age, and stroke severity are included as main effects but the only treatment interaction included is with time to treatment. The white box shows the point at which the estimated treatment effect crosses 1. The black box shows the point at which the lower 95% CI for the estimated treatment effect first crosses 1.0.

Reproduced from *Lancet*, 384(9958), Emberson J, et al., Effect of treatment delay, age, and stroke severity on the effects of intravenous thrombolysis with alteplase for acute ischaemic stroke: a meta-analysis of individual patient data from randomised trials, pp. 1929–1935, Copyright (2014), with permission from Elsevier.

- For thrombolysis given within 3 hours for every 10 patients treated, one returns to normal (Rankin 0) or almost to normal (Rankin 1). The benefit is higher if thrombolysis is given earlier (in the first 90 minutes) but lower if given between 3 and 4.5 hours (1 in 19).

Thrombolysis outside the 0–4.5-hour window

- Initially IV thrombolysis was shown to benefit patients only when given within the first 4.5 hours.

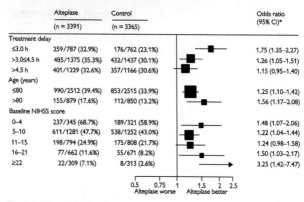

	Alteplase (n = 3391)	Control (n = 3365)		Odds ratio (95% CI)*
Treatment delay				
≤3.0 h	259/787 (32.9%)	176/762 (23.1%)		1.75 (1.35–2.27)
>3.0≤4.5 h	485/1375 (35.3%)	432/1437 (30.1%)		1.26 (1.05–1.51)
>4.5 h	401/1229 (32.6%)	357/1166 (30.6%)		1.15 (0.95–1.40)
Age (years)				
≤80	990/2512 (39.4%)	853/2515 (33.9%)		1.25 (1.10–1.42)
>80	155/879 (17.6%)	112/850 (13.2%)		1.56 (1.17–2.08)
Baseline NIHSS score				
0–4	237/345 (68.7%)	189/321 (58.9%)		1.48 (1.07–2.06)
5–10	611/1281 (47.7%)	538/1252 (43.0%)		1.22 (1.04–1.44)
11–15	198/794 (24.9%)	175/808 (21.7%)		1.24 (0.98–1.58)
16–21	77/662 (11.6%)	55/671 (8.2%)		1.50 (1.03–2.17)
≥22	22/309 (7.1%)	8/313 (2.6%)		3.25 (1.42–7.47)

0.5   0.75   1   1.5   2   2.5
Alteplase worse   Alteplase better

Fig. 9.4 Effect of alteplase on good stroke outcome (modified Rankin Scale score 0–1), by treatment delay, age, and stroke severity from a meta-analysis of individual patient data from randomized trials.

* For each of the three baseline characteristics, estimates were derived from a single logistic regression model stratified by trial, which enables separate estimation of the OR for each subgroup after adjustment for the other two baseline characteristics (but not for possible interactions with those characteristics).

Reproduced from *Lancet*, 384(9958), Emberson J, et al., Effect of treatment delay, age, and stroke severity on the effects of intravenous thrombolysis with alteplase for acute ischaemic stroke: a meta-analysis of individual patient data from randomised trials, pp. 1929–1935, Copyright (2014), with permission from Elsevier.

- With better understanding of the pathophysiology of stroke and progression to infarction, it has allowed thrombolysis to be given to carefully selected patients well outside the previous time constraints.
- The main improvements in understanding the pathophysiology, which have made this possible are
- The total area of ischaemia is the perfusion lesion. This can be separated into core and surrounding penumbra. The penumbra may survive for several hours. Provided the core is very small, thrombolytic agents may rescue the penumbra without increasing the risk of haemorrhage in the core.
- Penumbra tissue may survive for several hours because there may be some perfusion from the pial collateral circulation.
- Irreversibly infarcted brain can be detected almost straightaway by MRI using DWI. It takes on average 4 hours for the blood–brain barrier to break down and vasogenic oedema to occur. This can be seen on FLAIR imaging.
- Therefore, if you can see an abnormality on DWI but no abnormality on FLAIR, this acts as a tissue clock making the onset of stroke within the last four hours. One can then give thrombolysis.
- DWI/FLAIR is an MRI tissue clock and must not be confused with perfusion mismatch between the core and penumbra.

- PET imaging suggests that some patients have remaining ischaemic penumbra beyond 4.5 hours while others do not. The implication is that the former group may benefit from thrombolysis beyond 4.5 hours while the latter group will not (but may get side effects). Selecting these patients with PET is not practical, but MRI and CT offer methods by which the 'ischaemic penumbra' may be estimated.
- CT perfusion is being used in a similar way (see → Chapter 7). The core defined by the cerebral blood volume threshold matches DWI lesion volume and penumbral plus core on CT perfusion matches the PWI lesion volume.
- An alternative approach is to use CT angiography with extra delayed imaging phases to identify patients who have a persistent intracerebral artery occlusion and to assess the collateral supply.

Thrombolysis guided by MRI: Wake-Up stroke

- In the Wake-Up trial, MRI-guided thrombolysis was used.
- 503 patients with an unknown time of stroke onset were selected with DWI/FLAIR mismatch on their MRI scans, suggesting that stroke onset was within 4.5 hours.
- 254 were randomized to alteplase and 249 to placebo.
- Thrombectomy patients were excluded.
- 53.3% in the alteplase group and 41.8% in the placebo group had an mRS of 0–1 at 90 days (adjusted OR 1.62; 95% CI, 1.17 to 2.23; $P = 0.003$)
- The rate of symptomatic intracranial haemorrhage was 2.0% in the alteplase group and 0.4% in the placebo group (odds ratio, 4.95; 95% CI, 0.57 to 42.87; $P = 0.15$)
- The mean age was about 65 years and the median NIHSS score was 6 (IQR 6–9). Therefore, these were younger patients with smaller syndromes.
- However, the number needed to treat for 1 extra patient to have an excellent outcome was 8.7.

Thrombolysis guided by perfusion imaging: EXTEND

- EXTEND randomized patients 4.5 and 9.0 hours after the onset of stroke or on awakening with stroke (if within 9 hours from the midpoint of sleep) between intravenous alteplase or placebo.
- The mismatch between the perfusion lesion and the core was obtained using CT perfusion or MRI DWI/perfusion mismatch.
- The ratio between perfusion lesion and core had to be at least 1.2 and there had to be at least 10 mL of tissue to save.
- Cores up to 70 mL were allowed.
- 13 patients were randomly assigned to alteplase and 112 to placebo.
- The mean age of patients was about 72 years and median NIHSS was about 11.
- Most importantly, the median volume of irreversibly injured ischaemic-core tissue at initial imaging was 4.6 mL (IQR 0–23.2) in the alteplase group and 2.4 (0–19.5) in controls.
- 35.4% who received alteplase group and 29.5% in the placebo group had an mRS 0–1 at 90 days (adjusted risk ratio, 1.44; 95% confidence interval [CI], 1.01 to 2.06; $P = 0.04$).

- Symptomatic intracerebral haemorrhage occurred in 6.2% receiving alteplase vs. 0.9% in the placebo group ($P = 0.05$).
- It is important to note that while patients could be recruited with an infarct core of up to 70 mL, in fact 75% of all recruits had a core of less than 23.2 mL.
- A meta-analysis that included EXTEND but also ECASS4-EXTEND, and EPITHET studied individual patient data from 414 patients.
- 36% of patients in the alteplase group and 29% in the placebo group had excellent functional outcome at 90 days ($P = 0.011$), with 5% vs. <1% respectively suffering a symptomatic ICH ($P = 0.031$).
- Using the meta-analysis, the NNT for 1 extra patient to have an excellent outcome was 14 but remember that these patients generally actually had very small core infarcts.

Thrombolysis in mild stroke

- There is still controversy about whether or not to thrombolyse patients suffering mild stroke symptoms.
- PRISMS randomized 313 stroke patients with NIHSS 0–5 presenting with 4.5 hours of either alteplase or aspirin.
- 78.2% treated with alteplase and 81.5% treated with placebo achieved favourable outcome (mRS 0–1) at 90 days (non-significant), while 3.2% vs. 0% respectively suffered symptomatic ICH.
- ARAMIS was a non-inferiority trial comparing DAPT to alteplase in 760 patients with acute minor nondisabling stroke (NIHSS 0–5) treated within 4.5 hours of symptom in China. DAPT was 100 mg of aspirin on the first day, followed by 100 mg daily for up to two weeks and 300 mg of clopidogrel on the first day followed by 75 mg daily.
- At 90 days, 93.8% of DAPT patients and 91.4% of alteplase patients had an excellent functional outcome (mRS 0–1). P for non-inferiority was <0.001. Symptomatic intracerebral haemorrhage at 90 days occurred in 0.3% DAPT patients and 0.9% in the alteplase group.
- TEMPO-2 looked at the benefit of treating patients with *non-disabling* mild stroke (NIHSS 0–5) with evidence of a large vessel occlusion (LVO) or focal perfusion deficit within 12 hours of symptom onset, with TNK or standard of care therapy (typically DAPT with aspirin and clopidogrel). The trial was stopped early due to futility and a signal of harm due to excessive ICH and increased death in the TNK arm
- The Pro-Urokinase in Mild IsChemic strokE (PUMICE) trial randomized almost 1500 patients in China with mild ischaemic stroke (NIHSS <5) within 4.5 hours to pro-urokinase or standard medical therapy. The was no benefit from thrombolysis.
- Our practice is to thrombolyse patients low on NIHSS (<5) if we consider their symptoms disabling (e.g. an isolated severe aphasia) but to treat others with DAPT.

Tenecteplase (TNK)

- Tenecteplase, a genetically engineered mutant tissue plasminogen activator, can be given as a single bolus. It has less specificity for circulating fibrinogen compared to alteplase, which in effect leads to more Tenecteplase being available to act on plasmoinogen held to fibrin at the clot surface.

- Tenecteplase is also more resistant (around 80 times) to plasminogen activator inhibitor-1 (PAI-1) and due to different pharmacokinetics and dynamics has a longer half-life than alteplase
- Tenecteplase is licensed for the treatment of myocardial infarction. It has similar efficacy to alteplase but fewer bleeding side effects.
- In stroke, the 0.25 mg/kg dose of Tenecteplase has the best risk/benefit profile.
- Trials have used a higher 0.4 mg/kg dose but this resulted in an excess of bleeding complications.
- A number of large, randomized trials (AcT, TRACE2, and ATTEST-2) have demonstrated that Tenecteplase 0.25 mg/kg is non-inferior to alteplase for good clinical outcome when delivered within 4.5 hours of stroke onset (Menon et al., 2022; Wang et al., 2023).
- AcT compared Tenecteplase with alteplase for acute ischaemic stroke in Canada. 1600 patients were randomized to Tenecteplase (n = 816) or alteplase (n = 784); 36.9% of Tenecteplase patients vs. 34.8% in the alteplase group had an mRS score of 0–1 at about 3 months meeting the prespecified non-inferiority threshold. In safety analyses, 3.4% patients in the Tenecteplase group and 3.2% in the alteplase group had symptomatic intracerebral haemorrhage at 24 hours.
- TRACE 2 in China recruited 1430 patients randomized to Tenecteplase (716) or alteplase (714). 62% of the Tenecteplase group versus 58% in the alteplase group had a mRS score of 0–1 at 90 days. Symptomatic intracranial haemorrhage within 36 hours was observed in 2% patients in each group. Tenecteplase was non-inferior to alteplase.
- In ATTEST-2, 885 patients were allocated Tenecteplase and 892 allocated alteplase, within 4.5 hours of stroke onset. Tenecteplase was non-inferior to alteplase for mRS score distribution at 90 days, but was not superior (odds ratio 1.07; 95% CI, 0.90–1.27; P value for non-inferiority <0.0001; P = 0.43 for superiority). There was no difference in haemorrhage rates.
- TASTE Participants identified patients within 4.5 h of ischaemic stroke onset or last known well, who were not being considered for endovascular thrombectomy, and met target mismatch criteria on CT brain perfusion imaging. 680 patients were randomized between Tenecteplase and alteplase. There was no difference between the two treatments. In the intention-to-treat analysis, the primary outcome (mRS score of 0–1 at 3 months) occurred in 191 (57%) of 335 participants allocated to Tenecteplase and 188 (55%) of 340 allocated to alteplase.
- TRACE-3 studied Tenecteplase administered beyond 4.5 hours (from 4.5 to 24 hours). Patients with MCA or ICA occlusion with salvageable brain tissue on perfusion imaging were randomized to Tenecteplase or standard medical treatment without thrombolysis. (These were patients who did not undergo thrombectomy.) 516 patients were recruited. 33.0% vs. 24.2% receiving Tenecteplase were mRS0-1 at 90 days (P = 0.03). Mortality was not significantly affected. Symptomatic intracranial haemorrhage within 36 hours after treatment was higher with Tenecteplase (3.0% and 0.8%) but this difference was not significant.

- Tenecteplase trials have shown that it is noninferior to alteplase.
- Tenecteplase has clear practical work-flow advantages over alteplase given its relative ease of preparation and administration.

Lower dose alteplase and other thrombolysis agents

- The ENCHANTED trial compared low-dose alteplase (0.6 mg/kg) with the standard dose (0.9 mg/kg); in 3310 patients (63% Asian). The primary outcome (death or Rankin score >2) occurred in 53.2% in the low-dose group and 51.1% in the standard-dose group (odds ratio, 1.09; 95% confidence interval, 0.95–1.25). Major symptomatic intracerebral haemorrhage occurred in 1.0% in the low-dose group and 2.1% in the standard-dose group (P=0.01). The results suggest the lower dose may be a treatment option for patients at higher risk of bleeding, or possibly for patients already taking aspirin..
- The PROST-2 study compared pro-urokinase with alteplase in patients with ischaemic stroke presenting within 4.5 hours. The primary endpoint, a modified Rankin of 0 to 1 at 90 days, was equivalent in the two groups, demonstrating noninferiority for pro-urokinase. The rate of major haemorrhage was significantly lower in the pro-urokinase group (2.1% versus 0.5%). Pro-urokinase is currently licensed for thrombolysis in China.
- Reteplase is a recombinant plasminogen activator that is characterized by a double-bolus approach where the boluses are separated by 30 minutes. Reteplase versus Alteplase for Acute Ischaemic Stroke (RAISE, 2024) was a trial comparing reteplase at a double-bolus dose of 18

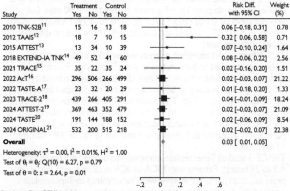

Study	Treatment Yes	Treatment No	Control Yes	Control No	Risk Diff. with 95% CI	Weight (%)
2010 TNK-S2B[11]	15	16	13	18	0.06 [−0.18, 0.31]	0.78
2012 TAAIS[12]	18	7	10	15	0.32 [0.06, 0.58]	0.71
2015 ATTEST[13]	13	34	10	39	0.07 [−0.10, 0.24]	1.64
2018 EXTEND-IA TNK[14]	49	52	41	60	0.08 [−0.06, 0.22]	2.56
2021 TRACE[15]	35	22	35	24	0.02 [−0.16, 0.20]	1.51
2022 AcT[16]	296	506	266	499	0.02 [−0.03, 0.07]	21.22
2022 TASTE-A[17]	23	32	20	29	0.01 [−0.18, 0.20]	1.33
2023 TRACE-2[18]	439	266	405	291	0.04 [−0.01, 0.09]	18.24
2024 ATTEST-2[19]	369	463	352	479	0.02 [−0.03, 0.07]	21.09
2024 TASTE[20]	191	144	188	152	0.02 [−0.06, 0.09]	8.54
2024 ORIGINAL[21]	532	200	515	218	0.02 [−0.02, 0.07]	22.38
Overall					0.03 [0.01, 0.05]	

Heterogeneity: $\tau^2 = 0.00$, $I^2 = 0.01\%$, $H^2 = 1.00$
Test of $\theta_i = \theta_j$: Q(10) = 6.27, p = 0.79
Test of $\theta = 0$: z = 2.64, p = 0.01

Random-effects REML model

Fig. 9.5. The figure below shows a meta-analysis of trials comparing Tenecteplase 0.25 mg versus alteplase 0-4.5 hours after stroke onset for the outcome of mRS 0-1 at 90 days. (Campbell 2024).

From Campbell BC. Hyperacute ischaemic stroke care-Current treatment and future directions. Int J Stroke. 2024;19:718-726. Copyright © 2024 World Stroke Organization. Reprinted by Permission of Sage Publications.

mg plus 18 mg (with a 30-minute interval) to standard alteplase. 1412 patients were randomized. 79.5% in the reteplase group vs. 70.4% in the alteplase group were mRS 0–1 at 90 days (P <0.001 for noninferiority and P = 0.002 for superiority). Any intracranial haemorrhage at 90 days was higher with reteplase than alteplase (7.7% vs. 4.9%) (P = NS) and symptomatic intracranial haemorrhage was 2.4% with reteplase vs. 2.0% with alteplase (P = NS).

- Argatroban is a short-acting direct thrombin inhibitor. Combined with IV alteplase, it was shown to be safe in patients with moderate to severe ischaemic stroke due to proximal intracranial arterial occlusion in the ARTSS-2 study but did not improve clinical outcome in the larger Chinese conducted ARAIS RCT. Argatroban, given as an infusion over 7 days, however, has shown to have a beneficial role in a recent RCT of 628 Chinese patients with AIS, which demonstrated early neurological deterioration (increase of >1 in NIHSS 48 hours after symptom onset. Further studies are required to reproduce this.

Sonothrombolysis
- *In vitro* data suggest ultrasound itself may cause clot lysis
- It may act synergistically with alteplase
- One phase 2 trial, CLOTBUST, found increased recanalization rates in patients undergoing IV thrombolysis
- The addition of an ultrasound contrast agent (such as microbubbles) may increase recanalization rates further
- However the phase 3 CLOTBUST-ER trial of TCD in acute ischaemic stroke was stopped early due to futility.

Thrombolysis in clinical practice
There has been concern that the results of thrombolysis might be worse in clinical practice than in clinical trials but this does not seem to be the case.
- A very large European audit (The Safe Implementation Thrombolysis Stroke-Monitoring Study; SITS-MOST) looked at the safety of thrombolysis with IV alteplase when given within 3 hours of stroke onset in 6483 patients (see Fig. 9.6)
- Results suggested that outcomes were as good, if not better, than those reported in clinical trials and better than pooled data from placebo-treated patients in the clinical trials
- Other aspects of stroke care have improved during that time since the trials and this may explain why SITS-MOST patients appeared to do better than those patients treated with alteplase in the clinical trials.

Administering thrombolysis—the practicalities
- The patient must be seen by a clinician who is competent in diagnosing stroke and is able to distinguish stroke mimics
- The patient must have a clinical diagnosis of a stroke syndrome
- The time of onset of stroke should be known or be deducible.
- A collateral history from relatives, carers, or others is often very helpful in assessing time of onset
- The patient needs a brain scan to exclude contraindications
- Most often, the first scan will be a plain CT scan

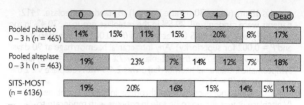

Fig. 9.6 Results from the SITS-MOST register. The figure shows the outcome at 3 months according to Rankin score. Numbers at the top are the Rankin scores. 0 means excellent recovery. The results suggest that 5% more people are Rankin 0 (cured) after thrombolysis and 5% more patients are Rankin 1 (minor symptoms but no disability) after thrombolysis.

Reproduced from *Lancet*, 369(9558), Wahlgren W, Ahmed N, Dávalos A, *et al.*, Thrombolysis with alteplase for acute ischaemic stroke in the Safe Implementation of Thrombolysis in Stroke-Monitoring Study (SITS-MOST): an observational study, pp. 275–282, Copyright (2007), with permission from Elsevier.

- It is very important to remember that you do not need to see the infarct or the subtle signs suggesting infarction
- On the scan, check that there is no:
  - haemorrhage
  - cause for the symptoms other than stroke, e.g. brain tumour
  - well-established infarct—suggesting the time period is longer than 4.5 hours
- The patient must have no standard contraindication to being given thrombolysis such as a bleeding diathesis or being on anticoagulants
- As long as these rules are obeyed, thrombolysis may be given safely to most patients and will improve outcomes overall
- A proforma is very useful in ensuring the protocol is adhered to, and contraindications are identified, and it can be used as a checklist when seeing the patient

Thrombolysis-related intracerebral haemorrhage

- This is the major complication of thrombolysis
- The haemorrhage is usually within the area of infarction—haemorrhage at a remote site is rare
- To screen for haemorrhage, all patients who have been treated with thrombolysis should have repeat brain imaging at 24 hours
- A systematic review of the published literature sought to identify the risk factors for ICH. 55 studies were identified, including a total of 3953 ICH cases in 65 264 acute ischaemic stroke patients. Almost all studies used alteplase at the currently recommended dose of 0.9 mg/kg. A range of definitions of ICH were used (see Table 9.1) and according to which one was used, the incidence of ICH varied from 4.1% (parenchymal haemorrhage with significant neurological deterioration) to 12.2% (any parenchymal haemorrhage, with or without neurological deterioration)

- Fatal intracranial haemorrhage within 7 days was 2.7% in alteplase-treated patients vs. 0.4% in non-treated patients (OR 7.14, *P* <0.0001).
- Type 2 parenchymal haemorrhage definition was 6.8% vs. 1.3% of 3365, OR 5.55, *P* <0.0001.

Factors which have been related to an increased risk of haemorrhage include:
- Larger infarcts
- higher stroke severity (higher NIHSS)
- higher glucose
- AF
- congestive heart failure
- renal impairment
- previous antiplatelet agents
- leukoaraiosis
- visible acute cerebral ischaemic lesion on pre-treatment brain imaging
- renal impairment
- previous antiplatelet agents.

There is no definitive RCT evidence as to whether blood pressure should be brought down to permit thrombolysis
- Some patients' BP settles spontaneously once the initial peak in fear of coming to hospital abates
- Some physicians use pharmacological means to reduce BP to the 'safe' range after which thrombolysis is given. If this is done, it is important to ensure the BP is maintained at the lower level
- The Dutch TRUTH study suggested lowering BP actively to facilitate thrombolysis increased thrombolysis rates, was safe but did not improve patient outcome
- One option in this setting is to use IV labetalol and a regimen is given as follows.

Labetalol to treat hypertension during/after infusion of alteplase

- Diastolic BP >140 mmHg: IV labetalol 40 mg over 2 minutes, then infuse 2–8 mg/min
- If BP is 230/(121–140): IV labetalol 20 mg over 2 minutes, then infuse 2–8 mg/min
- If systolic BP (185–230)/(110–120): IV labetalol 10 mg over 2 minutes, then 2–8 mg/min
- If the patient needs antihypertensive medication, monitor BP every 15 minutes.

Immediate post-thrombolysis care

- After thrombolysis, the current guidelines are that patients should not be given anticoagulants or antiplatelet agents for approximately 24 hours
- By 24 hours, the patient may be given antiplatelet agents for secondary prevention

- BP should be monitored closely over the first 24 hours and aggressively managed if excessive (e.g. systolic BP >185 mmHg, diastolic BP >110 mmHg)
- If haemorrhage occurs, neurosurgical consultation is not indicated. However, agents to reverse bleeding (e.g. cryoprecipitate should be readily available).

Avoiding and treating complications

- A number of studies show that if the protocol is not adhered to, the risk of complications increases and possibly efficacy decreases
- The major complication is cerebral haemorrhage within the infarcted region. If one should try to identify signs of early ischaemia and not thrombolyse if they are present and extensive is controversial:
  - The NINDS trial did not use any such CT cut-off
  - However, later trials used extensive early CT changes as an exclusion criterion: if greater than one-third of the MCA territory has ischaemic changes, then thrombolysis was not administered. Many units still use this
  - Identifying early CT changes may be difficult and requires training. This is covered in → Chapter 7. A standardized scoring system (e.g. the ASPECTS scale, described on → p. 155) may be helpful to ensure that all brain regions are inspected methodically.

Angio-oedema and anaphylaxis

- This is a rare complication of alteplase; it is more common in patients on ACE inhibitors.
- It is life-threatening but reversible if managed promptly.
- Symptoms include bronchospasm, hypotension, laryngeal and facial oedema, and urticaria.
- tPA activates plasminogen to plasmin. In addition to its therapeutic 'clot-busting' action, plasmin also causes bradykinin to be released. Bradykinin is the main cause of orolingual angioedema.
- tPA-related hypersensitivity is seldom allergic (i.e. due to mast cell degranulation). However, plasmin may also activate the complement cascade, which can produce histamine.
- Most reactions are minor and will stop after discontinuation of treatment and treatment of the histamine component with H1 antihistamines (e.g. Chlorpheniramine) and steroids.
- If the airway is threatened, ITU should be involved immediately.
- Agents which treat the bradykinin component include icatibant, a selective bradykinin B2 receptor antagonist approved to manage hereditary angioedema in which bradykinin accumulates owing to a genetic deficiency in C1 inhibitor activity.

Combination of alteplase and aspirin

Aspirin is normally delayed until 24 hours after thrombolysis. However, hypothetically co-administration or aspirin with IV alteplase might reduce the risk of reocclusion and improve outcome. In the multicentre, open-label, ARTIS trial, 642 patients were randomized to receive early addition of IV aspirin (300 mg) to alteplase versus alteplase alone. The trial was terminated prematurely because of an excess of symptomatic intracranial haemorrhage and no evidence of benefit in the aspirin group. At 3 months, 174 (54.0%) patients in the aspirin group versus 183 (57.2%) patients in the standard treatment group had a favourable outcome (P = NS). Intracerebral haemorrhage occurred more often in the aspirin group (14 (4.3%) patients) than in the standard treatment group (five (1.6%); P = 0.04). Therefore, it is still recommended to wait 24 hours before starting an antiplatelet agent.

Thrombectomy

This has transformed the care of acute ischaemic stroke and is one of the most effective treatments for acute medical conditions.

Older clot retrieval devices

A number of devices were developed to mechanically disrupt or re-trieve the clot. The most studied was the Mechanical Embolus Removal in Cerebral Ischaemia (MERCI) retrieval device. This is a catheter with a cork-screw on the end, which is inserted into the artery, then corkscrewed into the clot and pulled out, taking the clot with it.

- The recanalization rates are about 40–50%
- The results may be dramatic
- Initial results were encouraging, and the US Food and Drug Administration licensed the device
- In 2013, three trials (Interventional Management of Stroke (IMS) III, MR RESCUE, and SYNTHESIS Expansion) were published simultaneously in *The New England Journal of Medicine*. Disappointingly, they reported non-superiority of clot retrieval over IV alteplase alone
- A number of reasons for the lack of success were suggested including:
  - length of time to endovascular recanalization
  - use of older devices or less effective devices such as MERCI retriever were used in the majority of patients
  - only one of the three (MR RESCUE) routinely identified LVO of an artery on either CTA or MRA; in IMS III 20% of patients had no LVO or an inaccessible distally located thrombus, while in SYNTHESIS approximately 10% did not have an LVO.

Next-generation thrombectomy studies

- Newer thrombectomy devices, such as retrievable stents and the Penumbra system, were shown to result in better recanalization rates and faster reperfusion times than older devices such as the MERCI retriever
- In late 2014 and early 2015, a series of studies using these devices demonstrated impressive results. They showed that, when implemented rapidly, thrombectomy was more effective than IV thrombolysis alone for patients with occlusion of large intracranial arteries
- The landmark MR CLEAN study was presented at the World Stroke Congress in Istanbul in 2014 to a standing ovation. Following this presentation multiple ongoing studies were halted for efficacy after review by their data and safety monitoring committees. These studies included ESCAPE, EXTEND, EXTEND-IA, SWIFT PRIME, REVASCAT, THERAPY, and THRACE
- MR CLEAN enrolled 500 patients from 16 medical centres in the Netherlands (233 assigned to thrombectomy and 267 to usual care alone). Eligible patients had a proximal arterial occlusion in the anterior cerebral circulation that was confirmed on vessel imaging and that could be treated intra-arterially within 6 hours after symptom onset. Mean age was 65 years and 89% were treated with IV alteplase before randomization. Retrievable stents were used in 81.5% assigned to intra-arterial treatment. There was an absolute difference of 13.5 percentage

points (95% CI, 5.9–21.2) in the rate of functional independence (modified Rankin score, 0 to 2) in favour of the intervention (32.6% vs. 19.1%). There were no significant differences in mortality or the occurrence of symptomatic intracerebral haemorrhage

- The different trials varied in their inclusion criteria, including time to randomization and methods used to select patients suitable for thrombectomy. The key features and findings of each study are summarized in Table 9.1

- MR CLEAN had the least restrictive inclusion criteria. ESCAPE, SWIFT PRIME, and REVASCAT used the ASPECTS score and EXTEND-IA used perfusion imaging to exclude patients with large core infarcts. THERAPY was the only study to use clot length to screen patients (minimum 8 mm for inclusion)

- The allowable time between stroke onset and intervention varied from 4.5 hours in THERAPY to 12 hours in ESCAPE

- Stent retriever devices were used in 82% and 86% of the interventional arms of MR CLEAN and ESCAPE, respectively, and in 100% of the interventional arms of EXTEND-IA, SWIFT PRIME, and REVASCAT. The rates of recanalization rates were higher than those in the earlier studies (IMS III, MR RESCUE, and SYNTHESIS Expansion)

- All studies, with the exception of THERAPY, showed a significant improvement in the rate of functional independence (modified Rankin Scale score 0 to 2) at 90 days, with an absolute difference of 8%-31%. THERAPY was halted before a significant benefit was observed in functional independence, but ordinal analysis showed significantly greater improvement in modified Rankin Scale score for the interventional arm

- Although every study, except REVASCAT, reported a decrease in mortality with endovascular treatment, the difference was only statistically significant in ESCAPE (absolute difference, 8.6%)

- Taken together, the studies, which had many similarities in design, produced results that were strikingly consistent and favourable for endovascular treatment
  - All relied on referral to experienced endovascular centres, required documentation of intracranial occlusion,
  - most patients (82–96%) had M1 or distal ICA occlusions documented by CTA
  - aimed at recanalization usually within 6 hours
  - using stent-retriever technology (82–100% overall).
  - Patients included were similar in NIHSS severity,
  - most patients received alteplase,
  - patients older than 80 years were included in most trials,

- Furthermore, and perhaps most reassuringly, despite differences in the timing and amount of recanalization achieved, there was a consistent difference across all studies in good outcome between the interventional and control arms favouring thrombectomy

- The best way to appreciate the overall results of all the trials and the benefit of thrombectomy is from the HERMES meta-analysis. This reported that 46% of thrombectomy patients compared to 26% of controls were independent at 3 months. This gives a NNT of 5.

Table 9.1 A historical summary of the initial major thrombectomy trials of stent retrieval approaches in treating acute ischaemic stroke

Trial	MR CLEAN	ESCAPE	EXTEND-IA	SWIFT PRIME	REVASCAT	THERAPY	THRACE
Key inclusion criteria	NIHSS ≥2, age ≥18	NIHSS>5, ASPECTS>5, moderate/good collaterals (CTA)	Eligible for IV alteplase <4.5 hours from stroke onset ischaemic core <70 cm³, mismatch†	Eligible for IV alteplase <4.5 hours from stroke onset, age 18–80, NIHSS 8–29, ASPECTS ≥6	*Age 18–80, NIHSS ≥6, ASPECTS ≥7	Eligible for IV alteplase <4.5 hours from stroke onset, age 18–85, NIHSS≥8, Clot lenght≥8 mm	Eligible for IV alteplase <4.5 hours from stroke onset, age 18–80, NIHSS 10–25
Interventional arm	Intra-arterial therapy	Intra-arterial therapy	Endovascular thrombectomy with Solitaire FR stentriever	Endovascular thrombectomy with Solitaire FR stentriever	Endovascular thrombectomy with Penumbra aspiration system	Endovascular thrombectomy with Penumbra aspiration system	Endovascular mechanical thrombectomy
Control arm	Best medical management (± IV alteplase)	Best medical management (± IV alteplase)	IV alteplase only	IV alteplase only	Best medical management (± IV alteplase)	IV alteplase only	IV alteplase only
Time window for intervention	<6 hours from onset	<12 hours from onset	<6 hours from onset	<6 hours from onset	<8 hours from onset	<4.5 hours from onset	<5 hours from onset
Number of patients	500 (I: 233, C: 65.7)	315 (I: 165, C: 70)	70 (I: 35, C: 35)	196 (I: 98, C: 98)	206 (I: 103, C: 103)	108 (I: 54, C: 54)	385 (I: 190, C: 195)
Mean/median age (year)	I: 65.8, C: 65.7	I: 71, C: 70.2	I: 68.6, C: 70.2	I: 66.3, C: 65.0	I: 65.7, C: 67.2	NR	I: 62, C: 62
Median NIHSS	I: 17, C: 18	I: 16, C: 17	I: 17, C: 13	I: 17, C: 17	I: 17, C: 17	NR	I: 17, C: 17
Median ASPECTS	I: 9, C: 9	I: 9, C: 9	NR	I: 9, C: 9	I: 7, C: 8	NR	NR

Received IV alteplase	I: 87.1%, C: 90.6%	I: 72.7%, C: 78.7%	I: 100%, C: 100%	I: 100%, C: 100%	I: 68.0%, C: 100%	I: 77.7%, C: 100%	I: 100%, C: 100%
Median time from stroke onset to groin puncture (minute)	260	241‡	210	224	269	226	255‡
Intervention with stentriever device	8.15%	86.1%	100%	100%	100%	0%§	NR
Improvement in mRS 0-2 at 90 days	13.5%* (I: 32.6, C: 19.1%)	23.7%* (I: 50.0, C: 29.3%)	31.4%* (I: 71.4, C: 40.0%)	24.7%* (I: 60.2, C: 35.5%)	15.5%* (I: 43.7, C: 28.2%)	7.6% (I: 38.0, C: 30.4%)	12.1% (I: 54.2, C: 42.1%)
Decrease in mortality at 90 days	1.1% (I: 21.0%, C: 22.1%)	8.6* (I: 10.4%, C: 19.0%)	11.4% (I: 8.6%, C: 20.0%)	3.2% (I: 9.2%, C: 12.4%)	−2.9% (I: 18.4%, C: 15.5%)	11.9% (I: 12.0%, C: 23.9%)	0.6% (I: 12.5%, C: 13.1%)
TICI grade 2b/3 recanalization	58.70%	72.40%	86.20%	88.00%	65.70%	NR	NR
Symptomatic ICh	I: 7.7%, C: 6.4%	I: 3.6%, C: 2.7%	I: 0%, C: 5.7%	I: 0%, C: 3.1%	I: 1.9%, C: 1.9%	I: 10.9%, C: 11.3%	NR

*Statistically significant (P <0.05); †Mismatch defined, based on CT perfusion imaging, as a match ratio >1.2 and absolute mismatch volume >10 cm³; ‡Time from stroke onset to first reperfusion (time to groin puncture not reported); §All patients in THERAPY were treated with the Penumbra System; ¶Results from presentation at the 2015 European Stroke Organization Conference (Glasgow, UK) based on available data from 385 of 414 enrolled patients (93%) with 90 day follow-up; ¶After enrolment of 160 patients, the inclusion criteria were modified to include patients with age 81–85 who had an ASPECTS >9.

ASPECTS = Alberta stroke programme early computed tomography score, C = control, CTA = computed tomography angiography, FR = flow restoration; I = intracranial haemorrhage, IV alteplase = intravenous alteplase, mRS = modified Rankin Scale, NIHSS = National Institutes of Health Stroke Scale, NR = not reported, TICI = thrombolysis in cerebral ischaemia.

Reproduced from J Stroke, 17(2), Ding D, Endovascular mechanical thrombectomy for acute ischaemic stroke: a new standard of care, pp. 123–126, Copyright (2015) Korean Stroke Society, reproduced under the Creative Commons Attribution License 3.0.

- Also reassuringly, the likelihood of good outcomes increased with a greater amount of recanalization.

Talking all the results together, it is reasonable to consider thrombectomy in the following patients:
- mRS 0–2. Almost all patients had a pre-stroke mRS 0 with a small group having mRS 1
- Any age
- Definite anterior circulation occlusion (middle cerebral artery M1 69%, Carotid-T 21%, M2 8%)
- Within 6 hours of stroke
- Use a stentriever

Thrombectomy for medium sized vessels

- Endovascular Treatment to Improve Outcomes for Medium Vessel Occlusions (ESCAPE-MeVO) randomized 530 patients within 12 hours from onset of acute stroke caused by a medium vessel occlusion (M2 or M3 segments).
- 255 patients randomized to thrombectomy and 275 to usual care.
- Median mRS at 90 days was 2 in each group; not significant.
- Mortality at 90 days: 13.3% thrombectomy group vs. 8.4% in controls.
- Endovascular Therapy plus Best Medical Treatment (BMT) versus BMT Alone for Medium Vessel Occlusion Stroke—A Pragmatic, International, Multicentre, Randomized Trial (DISTAL) randomized 543 patients with occlusion of medium or distal vessels within 24 hours of suspected stroke onset.
- 271 randomized to thrombectomy vs. 272 BMT.
- The predominant occlusion locations were the M2 segment (44.0%), M3 (26.9%), P2 (13.4%), P1 (5.5%).
- No significant difference in mRS at 90 days between the two groups.
- Mortality at 90 days was 15.5% in the thrombectomy group and 14.0% in controls.
- These well-conducted and rigorous trials do not support the routine use of thrombectomy for medium vessel occlusions.
- The NIHSS scores of randomized patients in both trials were rather low (7–8 in ESCAPE-MeVO and 6 in DISTAL), suggesting potential bias recruiting patients with, say, an M2 occlusion and a large clinical syndrome. Further, rigorous studies are needed to identify whether there is a subgroup of patients with MeVO stroke who may benefit from thrombectomy.

Thrombectomy at later time windows up to 24 hours

- The DAWN and DEFUSE-3 Trials demonstrated that selecting patients using advanced imaging could allow patients to be treated up to 24 hours after stroke onset.
- Both trials used a measure of the perfusion lesion and a measure of the infarct core to identify patients with salvageable penumbra who might benefit from thrombectomy.
- In DAWN, the perfusion lesion was estimated using the NIHSS and the core was identified on DWI.

- 206 patients with a mean age of 70 years were randomized.
- Patients could be recruited from 6 to 24 hours.
- The median NIHSS was 17 in both groups (i.e. big stroke syndromes and by inference large perfusion lesions).
- Most patients had an M1 (78%) or carotid-T (20%) occlusion.
- Infarct core volumes were small: 7.6 mL in the thrombectomy groups vs. 8.9 mL in controls.
- In the thrombectomy group, 49% were independent at 90 days compared to 13% in controls. The NNT was 2.7.
- In DEFUSE-3, the perfusion lesion and core were identified using perfusion imaging
- 182 patients were randomized, with a mean age of 70 years.
- Patients could be recruited from 6 to 16 hours.
- The median NIHSS was 16 in both groups (reflecting severe strokes)
- This was reflected in the large median perfusion lesion volumes: 114.7 mL in the thrombectomy group vs. 116.1 in controls.
- The median ASPECTS was 8 in both groups
- Most patients had an M1 (60–65%) or carotid-T occlusion (35–40%)
- Infarct core volumes were small: 9.4 mL in the thrombectomy group vs. 10.1 mL in controls
- In the thrombectomy group, 45% were independent at 90 days compared to 17% in controls. The NNT was 3.5.

Therefore, using modern imaging techniques to identify the core and sometimes the perfusion lesion, if there was a large area of threatened ischaemic tissue and as yet only a small core, intervention with thrombectomy is indicated.

Thrombectomy in older people and the frail

- The elderly have been underrepresented in many stroke trials.
- The MR CLEAN registry reported 1526 patients, of whom 25% were over 80
- Mortality after thrombectomy is higher in older patients. 51% of ≥80 years of age died compared to 22% of younger patients.
- Median mRS at 90 days was 6 in ≥80 compared to 3 in younger patients
- However, 20.3% pf ≥80 were independent at 90 days compared to 45.6% of younger patients.
- Therefore older people should not be denied thrombectomy.
- Frailty has also been shown to reduce the benefit of thrombectomy.
- In one study, poor outcome, defined as an mRS 4–6 at three months, was observed in 52.4% of non-frail and 79.4% of those defined as frail (Clinical Frailty Scale ≥5)

Should thrombolysis be given in thrombectomy patients?

- The main thrombectomy trials randomized patients to thrombolysis and thrombectomy versus control. However, it has been questioned whether thrombolysis is necessary in patients with thrombectomy, particularly as it might increase intracerebral haemorrhage risk.

- SWIFT-DIRECT recruited patients with stroke to receive stent-retriever thrombectomy alone or intravenous alteplase plus stent-retriever thrombectomy. This was a non-inferiority trial.
- 423 were randomized to thrombectomy alone or intravenous alteplase plus thrombectomy.
- 57% of thrombectomy vs. 65% of 207 alteplase plus thrombectomy were independent at 3 months.
- Symptomatic intracranial haemorrhage occurred in 2% thrombectomy vs. 3% alteplase plus thrombectomy.
- Successful reperfusion was less common in patients assigned to thrombectomy alone 91% vs. 96% alteplase plus thrombectomy $P = 0.047$).
- Thrombectomy alone was not non-inferior to intravenous alteplase plus thrombectomy and resulted in decreased reperfusion.
- In SKIP, 204 patients with acute ischaemic stroke due to LVO were randomly assigned to mechanical thrombectomy alone (n = 101) or combined intravenous thrombolysis (alteplase at a 0.6-mg/kg dose) plus mechanical thrombectomy (n = 103).
- Favourable outcomes occurred in 59.4% in the mechanical thrombectomy alone group and 57.3% in the combined intravenous thrombolysis plus mechanical thrombectomy group (P = NS).

Therefore, unless there is a contraindication, patients should receive thrombolysis (where eligible) and thrombectomy.

Is penumbral imaging necessary for thrombectomy after 6 hours?

There remains controversy about the need for advanced imaging to facilitate thrombectomy. The argument is that if one cannot see an infarct on the plain CT and the clinical diagnosis and CTA agree that there is a symptomatic LVO, one should just pull out the clot. Previous trials (e.g. **Dawn and Defuse-3**) relied on multimodal brain imaging, whereas non-contrast CT is mostly used in clinical practice. The counter-argument is that one can make better-informed patient selection when one can evaluate the underlying pathophysiology.

- TENSION studied this.
- It was a multicentre, open-label, randomized trial in 253 patients, where patients with acute ischaemic stroke due to LVO in the anterior circulation and a large established infarct (ASPECTS of 3–5) were randomized to thrombectomy or usual care up to 12 h from stroke onset.
- The trial was stopped early for efficacy.
- At 90 days, thrombectomy was associated with a shift in mRS scores (P = 0.0001) and with lower mortality (P = 0.038).
- However, reviewing plain CT scans is difficult particularly in the ED acute setting.
- When the core lab re-evaluated the randomization scans, only about 80% were deemed accurately assessed.
- If such practice is to be implemented, training in reading plain CT scans is essential.

- After 12 months' follow-up, the median mRS in the endovascular group was 5 while it was 6 in the medical treatment group.

Does thrombectomy work in patients with large cores?

Trials had already shown that restrictive patient selection produced excellent outcomes after thrombectomy. The next question was whether less restrictive selection using plain CT alone would also be successful.

- Angel-ASPECTS was a large trial in China involving patients with acute anterior circulation LVO and ASPECTS of 3–5 or an infarct core volume of 70–100 mL.
- Patients were randomized within 24 hours of onset.
- 456 patients were enrolled with average age was about 67 years.
- Median NIHSS was about 16.
- Occlusion sites were M1 (63%) or carotid-T (36%).
- Median infarct volume was 60.5 mL thrombectomy vs. 63 mL control.
- At 90 days, 30% thrombectomy and 11.6% control were independent.
- Symptomatic intracranial haemorrhage occurred in 6.1% thrombectomy 2.7% control.
- SELECT-2 was a randomized, controlled trial of patients with a large core ASPECTS 3–5 or a core volume of at least 50 mL on CT perfusion or DWI within 24 hours after onset.
- 352 patients were randomized with mean age was about 66 years.
- Median NIHSS was 19.
- LVO was M1 (51.1–57.5%) or carotid-T (37.9–44.9%).
- Core volume was about 80 mL.
- Perfusion lesion volume was about 170 mL.
- 20% in thrombectomy group 7% in control had functional independence at 90 days.
- Mortality was similar in the two groups.
- Symptomatic ICH occurred in 1 thrombectomy patient and in 2 in control

These trials show that broadening the selection criteria for thrombectomy is appropriate. Substantially fewer patients have excellent outcomes. Part of the explanation for the improvement seen comes from data in SELECT-2, which shows that while patients may have very large core volumes, they also have very large penumbras.

In our practices, we have adopted the results of these two trials but still individualize our treatment decision, taking into account the plain CT, data from perfusion imaging, as well as the clinical state and relevant comorbidity of each patient.

Does thrombectomy work in patients where the infarct is large and unrestricted in size?

- LASTE examined whether thrombectomy was beneficial where there was a large infarct. It randomized patients with a large LVO infarct core and ASPECTS ≤5 within 6.5 hours after symptom onset to undergo thrombectomy or BMT alone.
- 333 patients were recruited, with a mean age of about 73 years.
- Median NIHSS was 21.

- Median infarct volume was 132 mL thrombectomy vs. 137 mL control.
- The median mRS 0–2 at 90 days was 4 in the thrombectomy arm versus 6 in controls.
- Mortality was 36.1% thrombectomy vs. 55.5% control.
- Symptomatic ICH was 9.6% with thrombectomy and 5.7% in controls.
- The trials shows that even patients with a large infarct benefit from thrombectomy, although most are still left with severe disability, and there was a higher ICH rate.

Thrombectomy for basilar artery occlusion

- Early trials (e.g. BASICS) showed no benefit for thrombectomy for basilar artery occlusion compared with thrombolysis alone, although this was contrary to many stroke physicians' clinical experience. However, the recent ATTENTION and BAOCHE trials, both performed in China, have shown that it is as effective for basilar artery occlusion as it is for anterior circulation stroke.
- ATTENTION recruited 340 patients of mean age 66 years who were within 12 hours after the estimated time of onset; median time to onset was about 5 hours in each group.
- Intravenous thrombolysis was used in 31% thrombectomy and 34% control.
- Median NIHSS was 24.
- Median PC-ASPECTS (based on CT imaging) was 9–10 (i.e. little evidence of infarction).
- At 90 days, 46% of thrombectomy vs. 23% of controls had an mRS 0–3.
- Independent at 90 days was 33% thrombectomy vs. 11% controls.
- Mortality at 90 days was 37% with thrombectomy and 55% in the control.
- These patients were younger, and randomized early without much evidence of infarction in the basilar territory.

BAOCHE recruited patients who presented between 6 to 24 hours after symptom onset to thrombectomy or control
- The median time to randomization was 11 hours for each group
- 217 patients (110 thrombectomy and 107 control) were recruited
- Mean age was 64
- Median NIHSS was 19–20
- Median PC-ASPECTS was 8 in each group
- Median Pons-midbrain index was 1 in each group
- Thrombolysis was used in 14% thrombectomy and 21% control
- At 90 days 46% thrombectomy and 24% controls had an mRS of 0–3 (P <0.001)
- mRS 0–2 (i.e. independent) was 39% thrombectomy vs.14% control
- Symptomatic ICH occurred in 6% thrombectomy and 1% control
- Mortality at 90 days was 31% thrombectomy and 42% control
- Procedural complications occurred in 11% of the patients who underwent thrombectomy.

Neuroprotection

Following brain ischaemia, a sequence of events occurs that results in brain damage (see Fig. 9.7):

- Brain ischaemia rapidly depletes intracellular ATP
- This leads to the failure of membrane-bound ion channels
- This metabolic aberration results in the accumulation of intracellular ions (especially calcium) and water by osmosis: cytotoxic oedema
- The falling blood flow means the cells cannot maintain their ionic balance and depolarize
- Calcium floods into the cells, triggering cell death mechanisms.

Several hours after the onset of ischaemia, the blood–brain barrier starts to break down and becomes permeable, allowing large plasma proteins to enter the extracellular space. Water follows when reperfusion occurs, causing vasogenic oedema. This process starts within a few hours of stroke and peaks at 5 days. It may result in leakage of blood into the brain tissues and haemorrhagic transformation.

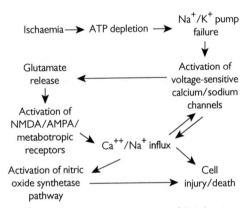

Fig. 9.7 A simplified diagram of events in the early part of the ischaemic cascade.

Trials of neuroprotection in stroke

It has been hoped that drug therapy can intervene in this ischaemic cascade and this is the rationale behind neuroprotection. Many agents have worked in animal models, but none have had replicable positive results in humans.

Drugs have been developed that target many aspects of the ischaemic cascade. Agents tested include the following:
- Calcium channel antagonists: after SAH, nimodipine reduces vasospasm and therefore subsequent stroke but it has no effect in acute ischaemic stroke
- Potassium channel openers
- Glutamate antagonists
- Anti-adhesion molecules
- N-methyl-D-aspartate (NMDA) receptor antagonists and modulators:
  - NMDA receptors control the entrance of calcium into cells
  - They are therefore a logical therapeutic target
  - Unfortunately, no drug has been shown to be effective
  - The simplest agent, magnesium, which is a voltage-dependent channel blocker, showed some initial promise but a large trial (IMAGES) failed to confirm this
- Alpha-amino-3-hydroxy-5-methyl-4-isoxazolepropionic acid (AMPA) receptor antagonists
- Membrane stabilizers:
  - Citicoline is a compound involving the synthesis of cell membranes
  - A small study showed that it may help stroke patients recover
  - However, no large-scale trials have confirmed this
- Growth factors: experiments have been done on fibroblast growth factor and transforming growth factor and these have not been successful
- Glycine-site antagonists
- Free radical scavengers: the free radical scavenger NXY-059 appeared to show benefit in The Stroke Acute Ischaemic NXY-059 Treatment (SAINT-I) study but this was not replicated in the SAINT-2 trial

Possible reasons for negative neuroprotection trials despite positive animal studies include the following:
- They really don't work
- Poor experimental methods in animal studies
- Animal models are not representative for human stroke
- Treating one aspect of the ischaemic cascade is too simplistic and cocktails of a number of drugs may be more effective
- They were tested in animal models when given before or just after stroke; in human stroke, they are given later.

There is current interest in combining neuroprotective agents with thromb-ectomy to protect recently re-perfused tissue from reperfusion injury

Antiplatelet therapy

Aspirin

- Most trials of antiplatelet agents in stroke have been in long-term secondary prevention rather than the acute phase.
- In this setting, aspirin, clopidogrel, the combination of aspirin and dipyridamole and the combination of aspirin and ticagrelor have been shown to be effective.
- The risk:benefit ratio could be different in acute stroke due to the potential risk of promoting haemorrhagic transformation within an infarct.
- The International Stroke Trial (IST) and Chinese Aspirin Stroke Trial (CAST) showed in 40 000 patients that aspirin, given within 48 hours of stroke onset, has a small benefit in improving acute stroke outcome (see Table 9.2).
- Both trials showed a small but significant reduction in recurrent ischaemic stroke risk of about 1 in 100 patients treated.
- This was not accompanied by a significant risk of haemorrhagic stroke.
- In each trial individually, there was no significant reduction in death or dependency, but when both trials were combined in a meta-analysis there was a significant reduction in both end points.
- Therefore as soon as haemorrhage has been excluded on brain imaging, aspirin should be started. A loading dose of 300 mg is usually given. 300 mg daily may be continued for 2 weeks and then replaced by clopidogrel 75 mg once daily. During the transition, a 300 mg loading dose of clopidogrel is usually given to achieve therapeutic levels rapidly. If the patient cannot swallow, aspirin may be given rectally.
- The benefit of aspirin is that it reduces the risk of recurrent stroke by about one-third.
- A meta-analysis of aspirin use in patients with minor stroke and TIA found that aspirin vs. control reduced the risk of recurrent ischaemic stroke by about 60%. The reduction in risk exceeded 50% by 36–48 hours after the aspirin was started.

Table 9.2 Summary of results of the IST and CAST trials. Outcomes were assessed at 28 days in CAST and at 14 days and 6 months in IST

	CAST		IST	
	Aspirin	No aspirin	Aspirin	No aspirin
Number randomized	10335	10320	9719	9714
Early death (%)	3.3[a]	3.9[a]	9.0	9.4
Recurrent ischaemic stroke (%)	1.6[b]	2.1[b]	2.8[c]	3.9[c]
Haemorrhagic stroke (%)	1.1	9	9	8
Recurrent stroke or death (%)	5.3[a]	5.9[a]	11.3[a]	12.4[a]
Dead or dependent at 28 days/ 6 months (%)	30.5	31.6	61.2	63.5

Alternative antiplatelet agents in acute stroke

Dipyridamole

- The combination of dipyridamole and aspirin has been shown to be more effective than aspirin alone, and of similar effectiveness to clopidogrel alone, in the long-term secondary prevention of stroke (see ➔ Chapter 10)
- However, there is no trial data supporting the use of dipyridamole in acute stroke (i.e. being given within the first 48 hours).

Clopidogrel

- Clopidogrel has been shown to be slightly more effective than aspirin alone, and to have similar efficacy to the combination of aspirin and dipyridamole in the long-term secondary prevention of stroke (see ➔ Antiplatelet agents, p. 239).
- Nevertheless, if patients cannot tolerate aspirin we give clopidogrel during the acute phase.
- If clopidogrel is given acutely, a loading dose of 300 mg is recommended to achieve therapeutic plasma levels rapidly.
- In patients with TIA and minor stroke, there is a high early risk of recurrent stroke, which is much higher than previously appreciated. This is as high as 10–12% in the first week.
- Large RCTs suggest the combination of dual antiplatelet therapy DAPT given for a period of a few weeks over this high-risk period reduced recurrent stroke risk.
- DAPT with aspirin and clopidogrel reduced the rate of asymptomatic embolization monitored on TCD, compared with aspirin alone in patients with acute carotid stenosis and stroke/TIA (CARESS study) and also in patients with acute symptomatic intracranial stenosis (CLAIR).
- In the randomized, double-blind, placebo-controlled CHANCE trial conducted in China, 5170 patients within 24 hours after the onset of minor ischaemic stroke or high-risk TIA were randomized to clopidogrel and aspirin or placebo plus aspirin. Stroke occurred in 8.2% of patients in the clopidogrel–aspirin group compared to 11.7% of those in the aspirin group (P <0.001). The rate of severe haemorrhage or haemorrhagic stroke was 0.3% in each group.
- In POINT 4881 patients were enrolled to receive either clopidogrel plus aspirin or aspirin alone for 3 months. Major ischaemic events occurred in 121 of 2432 patients (5.0%) receiving clopidogrel plus aspirin and in 160 of 2449 patients (6.5%) receiving aspirin plus placebo (HR 0.75; P = 0.02), with most events occurring during the first week. Major haemorrhage occurred in 0.9% DAPT and 0.4% aspirin.
- A meta-analysis suggested an optional period of DAPT, balancing the risk of recurrent stroke versus the risk of bleeding, was three weeks.
- A reasonable option in patients with TIA and minor stroke, and particularly those with large artery stroke who represent the highest risk group, is to give DAPT for about a month and then switch to clopidogrel alone.
- The early risk of recurrent stroke is risk appears to be particularly high in large artery disease (carotid, vertebral, or intracranial stenosis).

- Ticagrelor is an alternative to clopidogrel. THALES 11 016 patients were randomized either receive a 30-day regimen of either ticagrelor plus aspirin or aspirin alone. Stroke or death occurred in 303 patients (5.5%) in the ticagrelor–aspirin group and in 362 patients (6.6%) in the aspirin group (HR 0.83; $P = 0.02$). Severe bleeding occurred in 28 patients (0.5%) in the ticagrelor–aspirin group and in 7 patients (0.1%) in the aspirin group ($P = 0.001$).

Anticoagulation

Anticoagulation can be used in a number of settings in acute stroke:
1. At full dose for all patients with ischaemic stroke
2. In patients with cardioembolic sources, particularly AF
3. As prophylaxis for DVT.

Full-dose anticoagulation in acute stroke

- Trial data have shown no benefit for full-dose anticoagulation in the acute phase
- The largest trial, the International Stroke Trial (IST), showed no overall benefit of subcutaneous heparin, with virtually identical death and dependency rates at 6 months (see Table 9.3)
- There was a reduction in recurrent stroke risk of about 1 in 100 (similar to that seen with aspirin), but this was countered by a similar increase in the risk of haemorrhagic stroke (which was not seen with aspirin)
- An early trial of low-molecular-weight heparin (LMWH) in Hong Kong showed a benefit, but this could not be confirmed in a subsequent trial
- Therefore, heparin at therapeutic doses should not be routinely used in acute stroke.

Table 9.3 Results from the IST showing that subcutaneous heparin reduced recurrent stroke risk, but increased haemorrhagic stroke risk

	IST	
	Heparin	No heparin
Number randomized	9717	9718
Death within 28 days (%)	9.0	9.3
Recurrent ischaemic stroke (%)	2.9[a]	3.8[a]
Haemorrhagic stroke (%)	1.2[b]	0.4[b]
Recurrent stroke or death (%)	11.7	12.0
Dead or dependent at 6 months (%)	62.9	62.9

All the figures except the numbers randomized are percentages. [a]$P < 0.01$; [b]$P < 0.00001$.

Reproduced from *Lancet*, 349(9065), International Stroke Trial Collaborative Group, The International Stroke Trial (IST): a randomised trial of aspirin, subcutaneous heparin, both, or neither among 19 435 patients with acute ischaemic stroke, pp. 1569–15681, Copyright (1997), with permission from Elsevier.

Anticoagulation in acute cardioembolic stroke

- Anticoagulation is a proven treatment for secondary prevention of cardioembolic stroke, primarily with AF (see ➋ p. 289).
- When to start anticoagulation in patients with acute stroke and AF is controversial. The concern is that it may result in haemorrhagic transformation, particularly for larger infarcts
- A common approach has been to wait for 2 weeks in patients with larger infarcts, but to start straight away in cases of TIA and minor

stroke. However, there are now data from a number of RCTs suggesting early initiation as good, and possibly more effective, than waiting.

- In the Early versus Later Anticoagulation for Stroke with Atrial Fibrillation (ELAN) trial, patients were randomized
  - within 48 hours after a minor stroke to start anticoagulation on day 3 or 4.
  - within 48 hours after a moderate stroke to start anticoagulation on day 6 or 7
  - day 6 or 7 after a major stroke to start anticoagulation on days 12–14.
- The primary outcome was a composite of recurrent ischaemic stroke, systemic embolism, major extracranial bleeding, symptomatic intracranial haemorrhage, or vascular death within 30 days after randomization.
- 2013 patients were recruited (37% minor, 40% moderate, and 23% major stroke).
- A primary outcome event occurred in 29 (2.9%) in the early-treatment group and 41 (4.1%) in the later-treatment group (P = NS) by 30 days.
- Recurrent ischaemic stroke occurred in 14 (1.4%) in the early treatment group and 25 (2.5%) in the later treatment group (P = NS) by 30 days.
- Symptomatic intracranial haemorrhage occurred in 2 (0.2%) in both groups by 30 days.
- OPTIMAS (Optimal timing of anticoagulation after acute ischaemic stroke with atrial fibrillation) randomized 3648 patients (1:1) to early (i.e. ≤4 days from stroke symptom onset) or delayed (i.e. 7–14 days) anticoagulation initiation with any DOAC.
- The primary outcome was a composite of recurrent ischaemic stroke, symptomatic intracranial haemorrhage, unclassifiable stroke, or systemic embolism incidence at 90 days. There was no difference in the primary outcome, which occurred in 3.3% in each group.
- Some patients in OPTIMAS had severe strokes, and some had minor haemorrhagic transformation.
- Symptomatic intracranial haemorrhage occurred in 0.6% early anticoagulated patients vs. 0.7% allocated to delayed initiation (P = NS).
- The catalyst meta-analysis used individual patient data of all the other early versus late anticoagulation trials (ELAN, TIMING, START), as well as OPTIMAS.
- In 5411 participants, it suggested that early anticoagulation may be associated with a lower risk of stroke at 30 days.
- We now have results from many thousands of patients, which tell us that, even in patients with mild haemorrhagic transformation, early anticoagulation is as safe as late anticoagulation, and may be beneficial.
- We will be starting anticoagulation early in our patients from now on.

Prophylaxis for DVT and pulmonary embolus

- DVT is very common after stroke, particularly in patients with hemiparesis and may result in pulmonary embolus.
- In our experience many unexpected deaths in acute stroke patients turn out to have pulmonary embolus as a contributing cause at postmortem.

- There is evidence that low-dose heparin reduces pulmonary embolus risk in other settings, such as the postoperative period.
- However, in acute stroke there is no trial evidence that the routine use of subcutaneous heparin improves outcome when given to all stroke patients.
- In the PREVAIL trial, patients with ischaemic stroke with leg weakness of at least 2 on the NIHSS were randomized to receive either 5000 units unfractionated heparin twice daily or 40 mg of the LMWH enoxaparin daily starting within 48 hours of stroke and continued for 10 days. Treatment allocation was not blinded, but the end points were objectively defined by routine venography (in 82% of subjects) and/or compression ultrasound in all subjects.
- Enoxaparin was associated with a reduced risk of venous thromboembolic events of 43%, representing eight fewer events per 100 patients treated (number needed to treat for benefit: 13). Bleeding complications were rare.
- Therefore, if pharmacological DVT prophylaxis has to be used, LMWH is the agent of choice.
- Intermittent pneumatic compression stockings are a proven method for preventing DVT after stroke. CLOTS 3 was a multicentre, parallel group, randomized trial assessing intermittent pneumatic compression (IPC) versus no IPC in immobile stroke patients. 2876 patients were enrolled. A compression duplex ultrasound (CDU) of both legs at 7–10 days was performed and, wherever practical, at 25–30 days after enrolment. The primary outcome was a DVT in the proximal veins detected on a screening CDU or any symptomatic DVT in the proximal veins, confirmed on imaging, within 30 days of randomization. The primary outcome occurred in 8.5%of patients allocated IPC and 12.1%) of those allocated no IPC; an absolute reduction in risk of 3.6%. There was a significant reduction in asymptomatic DVTs and a just significant reduction in symptomatic DVTs but no reduction in pulmonary emboli or 30-day mortality.
- Patients with proven pulmonary embolus should receive full anticoagulation with heparin followed by a DOAC, which is usually given for 3–6 months.
- A not uncommon situation is the stroke patient with cerebral haemorrhage or other haemorrhagic complication (e.g. GI bleed) who develops pulmonary embolus. A 'bridging' inferior venous cava filter is an option in such cases until anticoagulation can be reasonably started.
- Thigh-length graduated compression stockings have been shown not to prevent DVT in acute stroke patients (CLOTS trial).

Acute stroke unit care

Considerable evidence from randomized trials has shown care on a stroke unit reduces mortality. Much of this is from subacute and rehabilitation units (see ➔ Chapter 16) but there is also evidence for acute stroke units.

A large study comparing acute stroke unit care versus conventional care across many hospitals in Italy confirmed this finding. The results are shown in Table 9.4.

Therefore, all stroke patients should be managed in a specialized unit. Patients with intracerebral haemorrhage also benefit from stroke unit care.

Exactly what components of acute stroke unit care improve outcome is uncertain, but important factors include the following:
• Improved control of physiological parameters:
• Glucose
• Pyrexia
• Hypoxia
• Blood pressure
• Prevention of complications:
• DVT and pulmonary embolus
• Infection
• Hydration and feeding
• Reduced early recurrence
• Attention to detail and standard management protocols
• Thrombolysis is an important aspect of acute stroke care but does not account for the benefit seen in the trials as very few patients were thrombolysed in these studies and most were before widespread alteplase use
• Reorganization of care with rapid admission to a stroke unit can have a major impact on outcomes. In London, UK, a major change in stroke organization was implemented using a 'hub and spoke' model for acute stroke care. Patients are admitted directly via ambulance triage to the hub for evaluation and acute treatment and then moved to the spoke hospitals on day 3 for rehabilitation. There was a significant decline in risk-adjusted mortality at 3, 30, and 90 days after admission. At 90 days, the absolute reduction was −1.1% (relative reduction 5%). There was also a significant decline in risk-adjusted length of hospital stay: −1.4 days. Therefore, there is evidence that a centralized hyperacute service results in lower mortality and reduced overall length of stay

Table 9.4 Two-year outcome in patients admitted to acute stroke units compared with non-stroke unit/specialized stroke care

	Stroke unit (n = 4936)	Control (n = 6636)
Follow-up (months)	19.7 (6.9)	20.4 (7.2)
Lost to follow-up	172 (3%)	175 (3%)
In-hospital case fatality	542 (11%)	1034 (16%)
Death after discharge	821 (17%)	1348 (20%)
Alive at follow-up	3401 (69%)	4079 (61%)
Rankin score = 0[a]	735 (22%)	804 (20%)
Rankin score = 1[a]	871 (26%)	941 (23%)
Rankin score = 2[a]	547 (16%)	604 (15%)
Rankin score = 3[a]	590 (17%)	740 (18%)
Rankin score = 4[a]	471 (14%)	713 (17%)
Rankin score = 5[a]	187 (5%)	277 (7%)
Stroke recurrence	195 (4%)	265 (4%)
Rehabilitation programme	1089 (22%)	1381 (21%)
New hospital admissions	835 (17%)	992 (15%)

Data were acquired from a large number of Italian hospitals although the study was observational rather than randomized. Data are mean (SD) or number (%). [a] Data are numbers (percentage of those alive at follow-up).

Controlling physiological parameters

There is only limited evidence from randomized trials as to how intensively to control physiological and biochemical variables in the acute phase of stroke.

Studies comparing stroke outcome between countries have suggested that those units with better outcome control these variables more intensively.

Blood pressure in ischaemic stroke

- Approximately 80% of stroke patients are hypertensive on admission, partly owing to pre-existing hypertension and also as an acute stress response to the stroke itself.
- A higher BP after stroke could be:
  - a good thing by increasing cerebral perfusion.
  - a bad thing if it extended infarction, and increased the risk of both haemorrhagic transformation and recurrent stroke.
- Considerable epidemiological evidence suggests that high BP after acute stroke is associated with worse outcome.
- However, a number of large trials of BP lowering have failed to change outcome whether treatment was started prehospital, in the community, or in hospital.
- Therefore we do not know whether, and how much, to reduce elevated blood pressure in ischaemic stroke.
- In the acute phase of stroke, cerebral autoregulation can be impaired and therefore an excessive drop in BP could reduce CBF.
- Collateral blood vessels may take time to open after stroke.
- Several trials investigated treating hypertension pre-hospital in patients with suspected stroke. None showed this was effective for clinical outcome.
- RIGHT (Rapid Intervention With Glyceryl Trinitrate in Hypertensive Stroke Trial) and the subsequent, larger RIGHT 2 used GTN patches as the pre-hospital antihypertensive agent. Overall, they did not demonstrate an improvement in clinical outcome. However, GTN was associated with worse outcome in intracerebral haemorrhage.
- Acute hospital trials have also not demonstrated an early clinical benefit of acute BP-lowering treatment.
- The Scandinavian Candesartan Acute Stroke Trial (SCAST) recruited 2029 patients presenting within 30 hours of acute stroke. There was no benefit of candesartan in acute stroke.
- In the ENOS trial, 4011 patients with an acute ischaemic or haemorrhagic stroke and raised SBP (140–220 mmHg) were randomized to 7 days of transdermal glyceryl trinitrate (5 mg per day), started within 48 hours of stroke onset, or to no glyceryl trinitrate (control). Functional outcome at day 90 did not differ in either group.
- BP lowering in the context of thrombolysis was studied in ENCHANTED (Enhanced Control of Hypertension and Thrombolysis Stroke Study). It showed a lower rate of intracerebral haemorrhage in the intensive BP lowering arm (target SBP, 130–140 mmHg) versus

patients with looser BP control (<180 mmHg). However, there was no difference in clinical outcome at 90 days.

- In the context of Thrombectomy, a meta-analysis of 25 studies comprising 6474 patients showed that higher post-thrombectomy systolic BP was associated with higher 3-month mortality and symptomatic intracranial haemorrhage and lower odds of 3-month functional independence.
- A reasonable approach is:
  - avoid more than a 10% reduction in SBP within the first 24 hours unless BP exceeds a high threshold value.
  - start treatment if SBP exceeds 180 mmHg or diastolic BP exceeds 100 mmHg or there is clinical evidence of malignant hypertension (e.g. papilloedema)
  - if BP is below these limits, then wait 48 hours before deciding on treatment
  - As a rule of thumb, during the acute phase of stroke where hypertension or hypotension need to be avoided, a blood pressure of about 150/90 should keep the intercranial CBF within the limits of cerebral autoregulation
- In most cases, BP can be lowered using oral agents (for choice, see ➋ Chapter 10)
- If more rapid reduction is required this can be achieved with transdermal glyceryl trinitrate, IV agents such as labetalol or nicardipine. If less severe, oral calcium channel blockers such as nifedipine can be used. Sublingual nifedipine administration is not recommended as this may cause the BP to drop excessively
- If rapid reduction of BP is performed it should not be lowered at a rate >15 mmHg/hour, and precipitous falls should be avoided
- In patients with carotid occlusive disease, or other large artery stenoses/occlusions, lowering BP may induce ischaemia and should be done more cautiously.

Blood pressure in intracerebral haemorrhage

While lowering BP too aggressively in infarction has not been proven effective, it may be more effective in ICH.

- INTERACT 3 assessed whether a care bundle could improve outcomes acute ICH. The study was conducted in low- and middle-income countries and included patients who presented within 6 h of the onset of symptoms.
- The care bundle included early intensive lowering of systolic blood pressure (target <140 mm Hg), strict glucose control (target 6.1–7.8 mmol/L in those without diabetes and 7.8–10.0 mmol/L in those with diabetes), anti-pyrexia treatment (target body temperature ≤37.5°C), and rapid reversal of warfarin-related anticoagulation (target INR <1.5) within 1 h of treatment.
- 7036 patients were enrolled at 121 hospitals, with 3221 assigned to the care bundle group and 3815 to usual care.
- The likelihood of a poor functional outcome was lower in the care bundle group (odds ratio 0.86; 95% CI, 0.76–0.97; P = 0.015).

- Patients in the care bundle group had fewer serious adverse events versus those with usual care (16.0% vs. 20.1%; $P = 0.0098$).
- Therefore it seems reasonable to reduce BP to <140mmHg systolic in acute ICH

Hypotension

Hypotension episodes in the acute stroke setting may lead to hypoperfusion of the collateral supply to the penumbra, and stroke extension.

Therefore, BP and heart rate should be closely monitored in the first few days post-stroke.

The causes of hypotension are:
- bleeding (e.g. GI haemorrhage on aspirin)
- MI
- cardiac arrhythmia
- heart failure
- dehydration
- sepsis
- massive pulmonary embolus.

Treatment includes:
- treatment of the underlying cause
- fluid replacement
- raising the foot of the bed
- stopping hypotensive drugs
- sometimes cardiac pressor drugs (e.g. noradrenaline) are necessary.

Hyperglycaemia

- An acute elevation of blood glucose often occurs in stroke
- This may represent:
  - underlying diabetes mellitus in a known diabetic
  - underlying diabetes mellitus in a newly diagnosed diabetic
  - a stress response in non-diabetics
- In animal models, elevated glucose is associated with increased infarct size and worse outcome
- Epidemiological data have associated elevated glucose in the acute phase following stroke with poor outcome. However, whether this is a consequence of the elevated glucose, or the elevated glucose is merely associated with some other parameter that worsens outcome, is not known
- It makes sense that better glycaemic control might improve outcome after stroke. However, this hypothesis as yet is unproven
- Two large randomized trials (GIST and SHINE) failed to show a benefit of intensive glycaemic control using insulin infusions, with a signal of harm—predominantly due to symptomatic hypoglycaemia
- The GLP-1 agonist exenatide was recently trialled in acute ischaemic stroke hyperglycaemia in the TEXAIS trial and achieved improved glycaemic control without significant hypoglycaemia but did not reduce neurological impairment as measured by NIHSS at 7 days

Table 9.5 Sliding scale protocol for insulin administration post stroke

Blood glucose (mmol/L)	Units of insulin/ hour	IV fluid
<3.0	0	40 mL 10% glucose STAT, then 40 mL/hour
3.1–4.0	0	Glucose 10% 40 mL/hour
If, after 2 hours, blood glucose is still <3 mmol/L call diabetic team		
4.1–6.9	1	Glucose 10% 40 mL/hour
7–8.9	2	Glucose 10% 40 mL/hour
9–11.9	3	Glucose 10% 40 mL/hour
12–14.9	4	Glucose 10% 40 mL/hour
15–17	6	Normal saline (0.9%) 40 mL/hour
>17	8	Normal saline (0.9%) 40 mL/hour and seek urgent advice from diabetes team

• While it is still reasonable to treat excessively raised glucose immediately after stroke, the cut-off at which treatment should be instituted remains controversial
• Avoid giving IV fluids high in glucose
• In our units, we try to keep blood sugar below between 5–15 mmol/L (not as strict as in SHINE and GIST) and use insulin to treat higher blood sugar concentrations. Our protocol is shown in Table 9.5.

Fever

• Pyrexia is associated with worse outcome following stroke in animal models
• Pyrexia appears to be associated with worse outcome in stroke in males. However, whether this is a causal relationship is uncertain
• Fever may be central in origin but is often indicative of infection somewhere
• Common sites are:
  • pneumonia
  • urinary tract infection (especially if catheterized)
• And, less commonly:
  • biliary
  • large bowel diverticuli
  • cellulitis
  • joints
• Stroke itself may be associated with mild pyrexia.

Any patient with a fever should be carefully evaluated to identify a source of infection.
Appropriate other investigations may help, such as:
• FBC looking at the white cell count
• C-reactive protein

- chest X-ray
- urinalysis and culture
- blood culture.

It has been suggested that fever should be treated with antipyretics (e.g. paracetamol). In 2008, the Paracetamol in Stroke study (PAIS) randomized stroke patients to high-dose paracetamol (6 g/day) or placebo started in the first 12 hours after symptom onset and continued for 3 days. Patients were included if they had a body temperature of between 36°C and 39°C at baseline. The planned sample size was 2500, but the trial was stopped after the inclusion of 1368 patients for 'logistical reasons'. The primary analysis showed that 37% (260/697) of patients improved beyond expectation in the paracetamol group, and 33% (232/703) improved beyond expectation in the placebo, a difference that was not statistically significant (OR 1.21, 95% CI, 0.97–1.51, $P = 0.09$). There was a suggestion that there might be a benefit in patients with a higher baseline temperature (>37°C) (OR 1.43, 95% CI, 1.02–1.97).

Do not forget other causes of fever, such as DVT or comorbidities, e.g. inflammation owing to flare-ups of arthritis (crystal arthropathy or other forms of acute but non-infective arthritis can cause fever and be simply treated by joint aspiration and injection).

Hypothermia as a treatment

- Hypothermia is effective in stroke treatment in animal models
- A 2–3°C drop in temperature may be associated with a reduction in infarct volume of as much as 80%
- Cooling appears to delay a number of deleterious phenomena, including intracerebral acidosis, changes in blood–brain barrier permeability, impaired cerebral energy metabolism, and changes in the release of excitotoxic amino acids
- In humans it has been shown to improve outcome in the treatment of cardiac arrest
- There have been several small phase 2 randomized trials of cooling in stroke (COOL AID, ICTuS-L, EuroHYP-1) which found variable difficulties in recruitment and achieving target levels of hypothermia. More recently, the feasibility and safety of cooling thrombectomy patients has been demonstrated in The ReCCLAIM 2 study from the US (66 thrombectomy patients cooled to a core temp of <34°C with intravascular cooling). This selective approach to therapeutic cooling seems the most promising.

Hypoxia

The Stroke Oxygen Study (SO_2S) found no benefit from oxygen supplementation in acute stroke when 8000 patients were randomized within 72 hours of stroke onset. However the mean time to randomization was about 20 hours and therefore it cannot exclude a benefit during the very early period after stroke.

Complications of stroke

Avoiding and treating complications is an important part of acute stroke care.
   Common complications include:
- the deteriorating patient
- cerebral oedema
- aspiration and pneumonia
- DVT and pulmonary embolus
- haemorrhagic transformation of an infarct
- hydrocephalus (with cerebral haemorrhage)
- epilepsy.

The deteriorating patient

Deterioration occurs in about 40% of patients during the first week after stroke and may present as:
- worsening neurological scores: GCS or NIHSS
- new neurological signs
- reduced conscious level.

   Causes include:
- extension of initial stroke
- recurrent stroke
- haemorrhagic transformation
- cerebral oedema
- hyponatraemia
- secondary complications:
  - epilepsy
  - pneumonia and aspiration
  - pulmonary embolus.

Risk factors include:
- infarct already visible on CT
- large infarct
- high BP
- high glucose.

Management should include:
- correction of physiological and metabolic derangements (see
   ➜ p. 247)
- treatment of secondary infections
- treatment of dehydration
- treatment of hypoxia, which may result from aspiration, pneumonia, or pulmonary embolism
- brain imaging to exclude haemorrhagic transformation, cerebral oedema, or recurrent stroke.

Cerebral oedema

- Cerebral oedema is an important cause of deterioration after a large stroke. It is a greater problem in younger stroke. In older individuals, atrophy may have created space into which the swollen brain may expand (see Fig. 9.8)
- Transtentorial herniation occurs mainly within 24–48 hours of cerebral haemorrhage and at 4–5 days after cerebral infarction

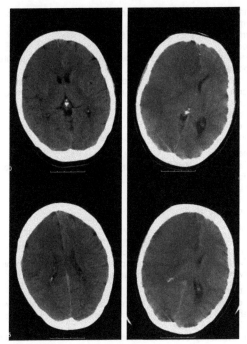

Fig. 9.8 CT scans showing massive right hemisphere swelling. The two images on the left are from a scan at 4 hours post stroke and show early ischaemic changes in the right carotid (both MCA and ACA) territory. The corresponding images on the right are from a scan the following day and show an established infarct with brain swelling into the left hemisphere. © Hugh Markus.

- The principal cause is supratentorial cerebral oedema resulting in secondary brainstem compression
- It may cause:
  - drowsiness and reduced conscious level
  - pupil asymmetry
  - breathing abnormalities
- There is often a stable period followed by a deterioration with progressive impairment of consciousness, coma, and respiratory failure.

Treatment of cerebral oedema

General measures:
- Elevate the head and upper body 20–30°
- Position the patient to avoid compression of jugular veins

- Avoid glucose-containing IV solutions and/or hypotonic solutions
- Normothermia
- Normovolaemia and mean arterial BP >110 mmHg
- Intubation
- Hyperventilation can be used as a supportive measure prior to surgery
- Barbiturates
- Steroids have little or no benefit—they are effective in vasogenic oedema (e.g. associated with brain tumours) but not in the cytotoxic oedema associated with infarction.
- Osmotherapy—see the following subsection
- Hemicraniectomy is used in cases where massive MCA infarction and secondary oedema lead to brain compression.

Osmotherapy
- These agents are often used, although this is not supported by trial data
- Options used include:
  - mannitol
  - glycerol
  - hypertonic saline.

Mannitol
- Start with 0.5–1.0 g/kg
- Then give 0.25–0.5 g/kg every 4 hours
- It is best used as a temporary holding measure before more definitive interventions such as surgical intervention.

Hemicraniectomy
- First described in 1935, there have now been 9 RCTs including over 500 patients and it is now a well-established lifesaving operation in patients with large MCA stroke.
- A large bone flap is removed on the side of the infarction site and the dura opened to reduce the pressure (see Fig. 9.9).
- A meta-analysis of data from 129 younger patients from three small RCTs showed a highly significant reduction in mortality from 71% to 22%.
- There has been concern that the operation merely saves disabled patients.
- Results are less good in older patients (>50 years). The Decompressive Surgery for the Treatment of Malignant Infarction of the Middle Cerebral Artery II (DESTINY II) evaluated hemicraniectomy in 112 patients 61 years of age or older (median, 70 years; range, 61–82) within 48 hours after the onset of symptoms.
  - There was a lower mortality in the surgery group (33% vs. 70%) but in either group who had a good outcome, no patients had a modified Rankin Scale score of 0 to 2 (survival with no disability or slight disability) while only 7% of patients in the surgery group and 3% of patients in the control group had a score of 3 (moderate disability). The remainder were more disabled (Rankin 4; moderately severe disability—requirement for assistance with most bodily needs) (see Fig. 9.10).
- If it is to be performed, patients with early signs of large MCA infarcts should be identified early and operated upon within 24–48 hours.

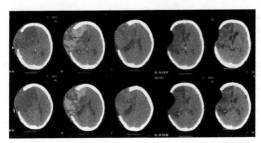

Fig. 9.9 A series of scans from a patient in their 40s with a right MCA infarct who had a hemicraniectomy. On the day 17 scan (second from left), a secondary haemorrhage into the infarct can be seen. Over time, the swelling resolves and has completely resolved by the day 50 scan (far right). © Geoffrey Cloud.

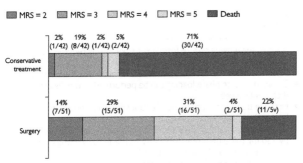

Fig. 9.10 Results of meta-analysis of the DECIMAL, DESTINY, and HAMLET studies showing improved outcomes (measured by modified Rankin Scale) in operated versus non-operated patients.

Reproduced from *Lancet Neurol* 6(3), Katayoun Vahedi K, Hofmeijer J, Juettler E et al., Early decompressive surgery in malignant infarction of the middle cerebral artery: a pooled analysis of three randomised controlled trials, pp. 215–222, Copyright (2007), with permission of Elsevier.

All the figures except the numbers randomized are percentages. [a]P <0.05; [b]P <0.01; [c]P <0.001.

Adapted from *Lancet*, 349(9065), International Stroke Trial Collaborative Group, The International Stroke Trial (IST): a randomised trial of aspirin, subcutaneous heparin, both, or neither among 19 435 patients with acute ischaemic stroke, pp. 1569–1581, Copyright (1997), with permission from Elsevier; *Lancet*, 349(9066), Zheng-Ming C and CAST (Chinese Acute Stroke Trial) Collaborative Group, CAST: randomised placebo-controlled trial of early aspirin use in 20 000 patients with acute ischaemic stroke, pp. 1641–1649, Copyright (1997), with permission from Elsevier.

- Some clinicians only operate if the stroke affects the non-dominant hemisphere on the premise that quality of life will be poor if the speech areas are affected.
- It is important to discuss what the patient would have wished with his family, and to look at any advance directives. Some people would like to live despite a major disability, while others would not.

Seizures after stroke

- Seizures complicate about 10% of strokes and are more common if there is cortical involvement.
- About a third occur within the first week, and most of these within the first 24 hours. These are acute symptomatic seizures and have a 33% 10-year recurrence risk for unprovoked seizures.
- Late-onset seizures, occurring 2 weeks after the acute event, peak within 6–12 months after the stroke; they have a higher recurrence rate than early-onset seizures.
- Single, acute symptomatic seizures post-stroke (within the first 7 days normally do not need treatment).
- Check physiological parameters.
  - Fever and markers of infection
  - Hypoxia
  - Sodium
  - Calcium
  - Magnesium
  - Glucose
  - Renal function
  - Remember alcohol withdrawal
- A single self-limiting seizure following stroke usually requires no treatment.
- If there is more than one seizure, we start anticonvulsant medication.
- During the acute phase loading can be performed to rapidly achieve therapeutic levels.
- First-line treatment options include lamotrigine, levetiracetam or lacosamide
- Levetiracetam, can be given with oral, NG, or IV loading at 1 g followed by 250 mg twice daily oral, NG, or IV increasing by 250 mg every 2 days up to a maximum of 500 mg twice daily.
- Seizures developing 1 week after stroke represent the development of post-stroke epilepsy. These have a recurrence rate of 72% over 10 years.
- The principle for all AEDs is to use the lowest dose at which seizures are controlled. If rapid titration is needed (recurrent seizures), levetiracetam is the better option.
- Outside the acute phase when loading is not required, Lamotrigine should be started at 25 mg once daily oral or NG for 2 weeks, increased by 25 mg every 2 weeks until on 50 mg twice daily, and thereafter if needed by no more than 50 mg increments every 2 weeks. Most patients respond between 150–300 mg/day and the maximum daily dose is 400 mg/day.
- Lacosamide can be started at 50 mg twice daily, increased to 100 mg twice daily after one week, and then slowly (in steps of 50 mg twice daily) to a maximum dose of 300 mg twice daily.
- If seizures only occur during the acute phase (e.g. first 48 hours) they often do not recur, and we tail off medication after 1–2 weeks.
- For patients receiving short-term (7-day) treatment for acute symptomatic seizures, document clearly on the discharge summary

how to withdraw the AED with instructions to refer to local epilepsy or neurology services if seizures recur.
- If seizures are recurrent, standard anticonvulsants should be used.
- Seizures developing more than 1 week after stroke represent the development of post-stroke epilepsy. These have a recurrence rate of 72% over 10 years.
- IV benzodiazepines should not be used after a single seizure in the acute phase. They are associated with respiratory depression and are sometimes used inappropriately, particularly in emergency departments. These seizures are usually self-terminating.
- Status epilepticus complicating acute stroke is very uncommon but must be treated aggressively according to local protocols including admission to ITU if deemed appropriate.

Dysphagia, swallowing, and aspiration

Dysphagia is common following stroke, particularly in patients with hemiparesis and/or brainstem stroke.
- The dysphagic patient is unable to protect their airway and may develop aspiration pneumonia or choke on food.
- They cannot take medication and sufficient nutrition orally.
- Therefore, it is imperative that swallowing is assessed early in all stroke patients.
- The gag reflex is not a good determinant of the competence of swallowing.
- The only way to test swallowing is to get the patient to swallow something (e.g. a small amount of water) and watch them do it.
- Patients who cannot swallow should have a NG tube placed to facilitate the administration of their medication, oral nutrition, and hydration.
- There is some debate as to the best timing for this; there is no strong evidence for guidance.
- The FOOD trial randomized patients within 7 days of admission between early tube feeding and no tube feeding. A total of 859 patients were enrolled on the early versus avoid trial. Early tube feeding was associated with a non-significant reduction in risk of death of 5.8% (95% CI, –0.8 to 12.5, $P = 0.09$) and a reduction in death or poor outcome of 1.2% (–4.2 to 6.6, $P = 0.7$).
- In most patients with dysphagia, we tend to insert a NG tube soon after stroke (within 48 hours) both to make the patient more comfortable with adequate hydration and to allow medication administration. It also allows IV fluids to be avoided, which have the risk of precipitating cardiac failure in the predominantly elderly stroke population who often have cardiac comorbidity.
- RCTs have found no improvement in outcome with prophylactic antibiotics given to reduce the risk of infection following aspiration.

Swallowing assessment

Clues to difficulty swallowing include:
- impaired conscious level
- difficulty managing secretions
- a 'wet' sounding voice
- choking or coughing while eating and/or drinking.

To assess swallowing, we use the following approach:
1. With the patient sitting in upright position, place your index and middle fingers over the patient's thyroid cartilage
2. Give the patient 60 mL of water in a cup
3. Instruct the patient to first take a small sip of water
4. If a problem is detected, *stop!*
5. If no problem occurs, proceed
6. Ask the patient to drink the remaining water as quickly and comfortably as possible
7. Allow 5 seconds to drink the water
8. Ask the patient to count out loud from 1 to 10.

If the patient fails the swallowing assessment or is too drowsy to swallow, then refer to speech therapy for further expert assessment and consider inserting a NG tube to facilitate the administration of usual medication, nutrition, and hydration on an individualized patient basis.

It is important to remember that swallowing may be normal soon after stroke but become unsafe. This is particularly common in larger infarcts that develop cerebral oedema, and swallowing may deteriorate a few days after stroke. Therefore, swallowing needs monitoring with repeated assessment over the first few days.

Acute psychiatric problems

Acute psychotic states may develop unexpectedly in acute stroke patients. Causes include:
- acute organic reactions
- severe depression
- acute paranoid psychosis
- exacerbation of pre-existing schizophrenia or mania.

Clues to the cause and management may be obtained from the history including:
- neurological and endocrine symptoms
- past psychiatric problems
- suicide attempts
- medication history (cimetidine, anticholinergics)
- drug history, including alcohol, cannabis, cocaine
- drug withdrawal (e.g. benzodiazepines, barbiturates)
- underlying systemic disease (cardiac, renal, hepatic, or respiratory failure)
- dementia
- infection.

Management
- It is important to try to manage patients using a calm approach in a well-lit, quiet place.
- Remember that an apparent psychiatric illness may be mimicked by delirium, so look for comorbidity that may be provoking the symptoms.
- Management involves treatment of the underlying cause and withdrawal or reduction of as many psychotropic drugs as possible.
- Avoid hypnotics.

- If sedation is required, small doses of lorazepam (1–2 mg) or risperidone (250–500 micrograms or haloperidol 500–1000 micrograms) may be given orally.

Alcohol withdrawal

This is not uncommon. It may need treatment.

A benzodiazepine in reducing doses can be given to cover the withdrawal period.

Withdrawal can be monitored using the Clinical Institute Withdrawal Assessment of Alcohol Scale–Revised (CIWA-Ar Score, Sullivan JT 1989).

Patients with possible severe thiamine depletion or Wernicke's should have IV administration of B vitamins (e.g. Pabrinex®) for 5 days, followed by oral administration. If in doubt, give this.

If oral intake is good and one can give vitamin B₁ (thiamine), then give 100 mg orally two or three times daily for 3 weeks.

Early secondary prevention of stroke

- Data have suggested that the risk of recurrent stroke after TIA and minor stroke is higher than was previously appreciated.
- In the prospective OXVASC study, the risk of recurrent stroke following TIA was 8.0% (95% CI, 2.3–13.7) at 7 days and 11.5% (4.8–18.2) at 1 month. Following minor stroke, the 7-day and 1-month risks were 11.5% (4.8–11.2) and 15.0% (7.5–22.5). The risk is highest very soon (within a couple of days) after the initial event.
- The risk seems to be highest in patients with large artery disease (carotid and vertebral stenosis).
- This means that patients should be assessed urgently for secondary prevention measures.
- The CHANCE and POINT trials have shown that clopidogrel and aspirin are more effective than aspirin alone when given within 24 hours of onset of minor stroke or TIA. See ➋ p. 240 for more detail on this topic.
- More intensive antiplatelet regimens may be useful, particularly for patients with large artery stroke (ICA, intracranial or vertebral stenosis).
- Carotid endarterectomy should be performed as soon as possible in patients with TIA and minor stroke (see ➋ p. 297)

Further reading

Pathophysiology of stroke

Ermine CM, Bivard A, Parsons MW, Baron JC (2021). The ischemic penumbra: from concept to reality. *Int J Stroke* **16**, 497–509.

Hyperacute stroke care

Campbell BC (2024). Hyperacute ischemic stroke care—current treatment and future directions. *Int J Stroke* **19**, 718–726. *A useful overview of acute ischaemic stroke in 2024.*

Thrombolysis

Emberson J, Lees KR, Lyden P, *et al*. (2014). Effect of treatment delay, age, and stroke severity on the effects of intravenous thrombolysis with alteplase for acute ischaemic stroke: a meta-analysis of individual patient data from randomised trials. *Lancet* **384**, 1929–1935.

Hacke W, Kaste M, Bluhmki E, *et al*. (2008). Thrombolysis with alteplase 3 to 4.5 hours after acute ischemic stroke. *N Engl J Med* **359**, 1317–1329.

IST-3 collaborative group (2012). The benefits and harms of intravenous thrombolysis with recombinant tissue plasminogen activator within 6 h of acute ischaemic stroke (the Third International Stroke Trial [IST-3]): a randomised controlled trial. *Lancet* **379**, 2352–2363.

Ma H, Parsons M, Campbell B, *et al*. (2019). Thrombolysis guided by perfusion imaging up to 9 hours after onset of stroke. *New Eng J Med*. **380**, 1795–1803. The EXTEND trial.

The National Institute of Neurological Disorders and Stroke rt-PA Stroke Study Group (1995). Tissue plasminogen activator for acute ischemic stroke. *N Engl J Med* **333**, 1581–1587.

Thomalla G, Simonsen CZ, Boutitie F, *et al*. (2018). MRI-guided thrombolysis for stroke with unknown time of onset. *New Eng J Med*. **379**, 611–622. The Wake-UP Trial.

Tenecteplase

Menon BK, Buck BH, Singh N, *et al*. (2022). Intravenous tenecteplase compared with alteplase for acute ischaemic stroke in Canada (AcT): a pragmatic, multicentre, open-label, registry-linked, randomised, controlled, non-inferiority trial. *Lancet* **400**, 161–169.

Muir KW, Ford GA, Ford I, *et al*. (2024). ATTEST-2 Investigators. Tenecteplase versus alteplase for acute stroke within 4.5 h of onset (ATTEST-2): a randomised, parallel group, open-label trial. *Lancet Neurol* **23**, 1087–1096.

Muir KW (2025). Should we switch to tenecteplase for all ischemic strokes? Evidence and logistics. *Int J Stroke* **20**(3), 261–267.

Palaiodimou L, Katsanos AH, Turc G, et al. (2024). Tenecteplase vs alteplase in acute ischemic stroke within 4.5 hours: a systematic review and meta-analysis of randomized trials. *Neurology* **103**, e209903.

Parsons MW, Yogendrakumar V, Churilov L, et al. (2024). TASTE investigators. Tenecteplase versus alteplase for thrombolysis in patients selected by use of perfusion imaging within 4.5 h of onset of ischaemic stroke (TASTE): a multicentre, randomised, controlled, phase 3 non-inferiority trial. *Lancet Neurol* **23**, 775–786.

Xiong Y, Campbell BCV, Schwamm LH, et al. (2024). Tenecteplase for ischemic stroke at 4.5 to 24 hours without thrombectomy. *New Eng J Med* **391**, 203–212. TRACE 3.

Thrombectomy

Albers GW, Marks MP, Christensen KS. et al. (2018). Thrombectomy for stroke at 6 to 16 hours with selection by perfusion imaging, *New Eng J Med* **378**, 708–718. DEFUSE-3.

Berkhemer OA, Fransen PSS, Beumer D, et al. (2015). A randomised trial of intraarterial treatment for acute ischemic stroke. *N Engl J Med* **372**, 11–20.

Bendszus, M, Fiehler J, Subtil F, et al. (2023). Endovascular thrombectomy for acute ischaemic stroke with established large infarct: multicentre, open-label, randomised trial. *Lancet* **402**, 1753–1763. TENSION.

Costalat V, JOvin TG, Albucher JK, et al. (2024). Trial of thrombectomy for stroke with a large infarct of unrestricted size. *New Eng J Med* **390**, 1677–1689. LASTE.

Goyal M, Menon BK, van Zwam WH, et al. (2016). Endovascular thrombectomy after large-vessel ischaemic stroke: a meta-analysis of individual patient data from five randomised trials. *Lancet* **387**, 1723–1731.

Huo X, Ma G, Tong X, et al. (2023). Trial of endovascular therapy for acute ischemic stroke with large infarct. *New Eng J Med* **388**, 1272–1283. ANGEL-ASPECTS.

Nogueira RG, Jadhav AP, Haussen DC. et al. (2018). Thrombectomy 6 to 24 hours after stroke with a mismatch between deficit and infarct. *New Eng J Med*, **378**, 1–21. DAWN Trial.

Sarraj A, Hassan AE, Abraham MG. et al. (2023). Trial of endovascular thrombectomy for large ischemic strokes, *New Eng J Med* **388**, 1259–71. SELECT-2.

Thrombectomy for basilar artery occlusion

Goyal M, Ospel JM, Ganesh A, et al. (2025). Endovascular treatment of stroke due to medium-vessel occlusion. *New Eng J Med.* doi: 10.1056/NEJMoa2411668.

Jovin TG, Li C, Wu C, et al. (2022). Trial of thrombectomy 6 to 24 hours after stroke due to basilar-artery occlusion. *New Eng J Med* **387**, 1373–1384. BAOCHE.

Psychogios M, Brehm A, Ribo M, et al for the DISTAL Investigators (2025). Endovascular treatment for stroke due to occlusion of medium or distal vessels. *New Eng J Med.* doi: 10.1056/NEJMoa2408954.

Tao C, Nogueira RG, Zhu Y, et al. (2022). Trial of endovascular treatment of acute basilar-artery occlusion. *New Eng J Med*, **387**, 1361–1372. ATTENTION.

Neuroprotection

Pérez-Mato M, López-Arias E, Bugallo-Casal A, et al. (2024). New perspectives in neuroprotection for ischemic stroke. *Neuroscience* **550**, 30–42.

Antiplatelet therapy

Chen H-S, Cui Y, Zhou Z-H, et al. (2023). Dual antiplatelet therapy vs alteplase for patients with minor nondisabling acute ischemic stroke: the ARAMIS randomized clinical trial. *JAMA* **329**(24), 2135.

Johnston SC, Amarenco P, Denison H, et al. (2020). Ticagrelor and aspirin or aspirin alone in acute ischemic stroke or TIA. *New Eng J Med* **383**(3), 207–217. THALES.

Johnston SC, Easton JD, Farrant M, et al. (2018). Clopidogrel and aspirin in acute ischemic stroke and high-risk TIA. *New Eng J Med* **379**(3), 215–225. POINT.

Pan Y, Elm JJ, Li H, et al. (2019). Outcomes associated with clopidogrel-aspirin use in minor stroke or transient ischemic attack: a pooled analysis of clopidogrel in high-risk patients with acute non-disabling cerebrovascular events (CHANCE) and platelet-oriented inhibition in new TIA and minor ischemic stroke (POINT) trials. *JAMA Neurol* **76**, 1466–1473.

Rothwell PM, Algra A, Chen Z, *et al.* (2016). Effects of aspirin on risk and severity of early recurrent stroke after transient ischaemic attack and ischaemic stroke: time-course analysis of randomised trials. *Lancet* **388**, 365–375.

Wang Y, Wang Y, Zhao X, *et al.* (2013). CHANCE Investigators. Clopidogrel with aspirin in acute minor stroke or transient ischemic attack. *N Engl J Med* **369**, 11–19.

Prevention of VTE

CLOTS (Clots in Legs Or sTockings after Stroke) Trials Collaboration (2013). Effectiveness of intermittent pneumatic compression in reduction of risk of deep vein thrombosis in patients who have had a stroke (CLOTS 3): a multicentre randomised controlled trial. *Lancet* **382**, 516–524.

Acute stroke unit care

Candelise L, Gattinoni M, Bersano A, *et al.* (2007). Stroke-unit care for acute stroke patients: an observational follow-up study. *Lancet* **369**, 299–305.

Morris S, Hunter RM, Ramsay AIG, *et al.* (2014). Impact of centralising acute stroke services in English metropolitan areas on mortality and length of hospital stay: difference-in-differences analysis. *BMJ* **349**; g4757.

Controlling physiological parameters

Treating blood pressure

Bath PM, Somn L, Silva GS, *et al.* (2022). Blood pressure management for ischemic stroke in the first 24 hours. *Stroke* **53**, 1074–1084.

The ENOS Trial Investigators (2015). Efficacy of nitric oxide, with or without continuing antihypertensive treatment, for management of high blood pressure in acute stroke (ENOS): a partial-factorial randomised controlled trial. *Lancet* **385**, 617–628.

Zonneveld TP, Vermeer SE, van Zwet EW, *et al.* (2024). Safety and efficacy of active blood-pressure reduction to the recommended thresholds for intravenous thrombolysis in patients with acute ischaemic stroke in the Netherlands (TRUTH): a prospective, observational, cluster-based, parallel-group study. *Lancet Neurol* **23**, 807–815.

Hyperglycaemia

Sacco S, Foschi M, Ornello R, *et al.* (2024). Prevention and treatment of ischaemic and haemorrhagic stroke in people with diabetes mellitus: a focus on glucose control and comorbidities. *Diabetologia* **67**, 1192–1205.

Complications of stroke

Alakbarzade V, O'Kane D, Pereira AC (2020). Hypersensitivity reactions to recombinant tissue plasminogen activator. *Pract Neurol* **20**, 75–79.

Dennis MS, Lewis SC, Warlow C; FOOD Trial Collaboration (2005). Effect of timing and method of enteral tube feeding for dysphagic stroke patients (FOOD): a multicentre randomised controlled trial. *Lancet* **365**, 764–772.

Galovic M, Ferreira-Atuesta C, Abraira L, *et al.* (2021). Seizures and epilepsy after stroke: epidemiology, biomarkers and management. *Drugs & Aging* **38**, 285–299.

Kneihsl M, Berger N, Sumerauer S, *et al.* (2024). Management of delirium in acute stroke patients: a position paper by the Austrian Stroke Society on prevention, diagnosis, and treatment. *Ther Adv Neurol Disord* **17**, 1–19.

Lin J, Frontera JA (2021). Decompressive hemicraniectomy for large hemispheric strokes. *Stroke* **52**, 1500–1510.

Sullivan JT, Sykora K, Schneiderman J, *et al.* (1989). Assessment of alcohol withdrawal: the revised clinical institute withdrawal assessment for alcohol scale (CIWA-Ar). *Br J Addict* **84**, 1353–1357.

Early secondary prevention of stroke

Fischer U, Koga M, Strbian D, *et al.* (2023). Early versus later anticoagulation for stroke with atrial fibrillation. *N Engl J Med* **388**, 2411–2421. ELAN.

Werring DJ, Dehbi H-M, Ahmed N, *et al.* (2024). Optimal timing of anticoagulation after acute ischaemic stroke with atrial fibrillation (OPTIMAS): a multicentre, blinded-endpoint, phase 4, randomised controlled trial. *Lancet* **404**, 1731–1741.

Secondary prevention of stroke

Introducing stroke prevention

Types of stroke prevention

- Primary—in people who have never suffered stroke or TIA
- Secondary—in patients who have suffered stroke or TIA.

Secondary prevention can be usefully considered in two phases:

- Early secondary prevention.
- Long-term secondary prevention.
- The early risk of stroke after minor stroke and TIA is high—about 10–12% in the first week.
- The recurrent stroke risk appears highest in stroke due to large-artery stenosis, both in extracranial and intracranial arteries.
- In this setting, a higher risk of treatment-related complications may be acceptable because of the greater potential benefit: for example, more intensive combination antiplatelet regimens might have a benefit owing to the very high risk of stroke (compared to the slightly increased risk of bleeding) over a short period of time. More intensive antiplatelet and other preventative regimens may well be appropriate in this setting and are being tested
- Early carotid endarterectomy (CEA) is important in appropriate cases
- For guidance on early secondary prevention see ➔ p. 260.

Most data on secondary prevention are on long-term secondary prevention. Most of these studies have included few patients within the first few days post stroke or TIA. However more recent trials have looked at antiplatelet combination therapy during the first 24–48 hours.

General considerations in secondary prevention

- The challenge of secondary prevention is to prevent a second stroke
- Approximately one in four strokes are recurrent events
- Ischaemic stroke may be considered part of a systemic vascular disease process. As such, patients with symptomatic vascular disease in other vascular beds such as the coronary arteries (angina or myocardial infarction (MI)) or leg arteries (claudication) should also be considered for secondary stroke prevention
- The lifestyle advice given to address risk factors for vascular disease and stroke in primary prevention (see ➔ Chapter 1) should always be reinforced. The difference in secondary prevention is that the risk of stroke recurrence is higher. There is no time to lose to address risk factor modification and this generally requires medical intervention and, in some cases, surgery. Lifestyle changes remain important but there is less time for them to take effect
- Secondary prevention is a lifelong commitment involving a close relationship between doctor, pharmacist, and patient. At the core is good patient education and medicine management to ensure compliance
- Compliance is key and all secondary prevention treatment regimens should be tailored to the patient
- Secondary prevention is about reducing the risk of recurrent stroke to its lowest value through relative risk (RR) reductions of individual

modifiable risk factors. The recurrent stroke risk will never be 0% but every patient should be given the opportunity of having the confidence that they are doing everything they reasonably can do to reduce their own risk of stroke. For the committed stroke physician, the scenario must not be: 'Should I lower this stroke patient's blood pressure?' or 'Should I put this stroke patient with atrial fibrillation (AF) on oral anticoagulation?' but rather 'How much can I lower this individual's blood pressure to maximize their risk reduction without making them ill?' and 'Why should I not be starting anticoagulation in a person with a stroke episode found to be in AF?'

- A clinical trial (PREVENTION, see ➔ Further reading) showed that active case management by a pharmacist produced a 12.5% absolute improvement in combined target BP and lipid control
- Stroke is a heterogenous condition and therefore it is no surprise that a 'one size' approach will not 'fit all'. It is important to try to identify what caused the stroke to best tailor appropriate secondary prevention. This will differ markedly according to the stroke subtype; for example, anticoagulation for stroke due to AF or endarterectomy for stroke due to carotid stenosis.

Non-compliance

- Remember, as the number of medications goes up, the compliance goes down
- If the drugs aren't working (e.g. the BP is still high on four medications), the patient may be treatment resistant, but it is more likely that they are not taking the medication
- You should bear non-compliance in mind but you should never be accusatory to your patient
- Ask about side effects. Poor compliance can be as much about fear of side effects as intolerance of common (often transient) unwanted symptoms associated with a drug.

Assessing and explaining benefit

Risk:benefit ratios

When considering any preventative measure, one should consider:

- How effective it is at preventing stroke?
- What are the risks of the treatment?

The best way to present data on treatment benefits is by using the number needed to treat (NNT). This is the number of patients needed to treat to prevent one additional bad outcome. It is calculated from the absolute risk reduction. It gives a good idea of the benefit of a treatment and is a simple and honest way to present the potential benefit of a treatment to a patient.

The potential benefit and NNT will depend on how high the risk of recurrent stroke is during the period of treatment.

- If the risk of stroke is 2% a year, and treatment prevents 50% of stroke (i.e. RR of 50%), treating 100 patients for 1 year will only prevent one stroke; i.e. NNT is 100
- If the risk of stroke is 20% over 1 year, and the treatment prevents 25% of strokes, treating 100 patients for 1 year will prevent five strokes; i.e. NNT is 20
- One can see that the less effective treatments prevent more strokes if applied to a high-risk group of patients
- This example shows how using RR to explain treatments to patients ('This treatment will half your risk of stroke') can be misleading.

Therefore, to assess benefit one needs to know the risk of stroke in the type of patient being treated.

Some rough estimates of stroke risk at different times post-stroke are given in Table 10.1.

Certain conditions present particularly high risk, e.g. symptomatic carotid stenosis and AF, and for these, specific data on risk are given in the relevant sections.

Table 10.1 Summary of the effectiveness of interventions for the primary and secondary prevention of stroke

Primary prevention strategies

Intervention	Risk ratio	Stroke risk per year (%)		Relative risk reduction (95% CI) (%)	Absolute risk reduction (%)
		Control	Intervention		
Nil		0.14			
Blood pressure–lowering (by 10-mmHg systolic)	1.54	0.22	0.13	41 (33–48)	0.09
LDL cholesterol–lowering (by 1.0 mmol/L)	1.27	0.18	0.14	21 (6–13)	0.04
Anticoagulation (for atrial fibrillation)	5.00	0.70	0.25	64 (49–74)	0.45
Cigarette `	1.45	0.20	0.14	31 (25–36)	0.06

Secondary prevention strategies

Intervention	Stroke risk per year (%)		Relative risk reduction (95% CI) (%)	Absolute risk reduction (%)
	Control	Intervention		
Blood pressure–lowering (by 5 mm Hg systolic)	3.3	2.9	13 (8–19)	0.4
LDL cholesterol–lowering (by 1 mmol/L LDL) with statin	2.4	2.1	12 (1–22)	0.3
Aspirin	2.5	2.1	19 (8–29)	0.4
Aspirin and ER dipyridamole (vs. aspirin)	4.3	3.5	18 (9–26)	0.8
Clopidogrel (vs. aspirin)	5.8	5.3	8.7 (0.3–16)	0.5
Aspirin and ER dipyridamole (vs. clopidogrel)	3.6	3.6	−1 (−11 to 8)	0.0
Anticoagulation for AF	12.0	4.7	66 (43 to 80)	7.3
PFO closure	2.0	0.3	87 (33 to 100)	0.17

(Continued)

Table 10.1 (*Contd.*)

Intervention	Stroke risk per year (%)			
	Control	Intervention	Relative risk reduction (95% CI) (%)	Absolute risk reduction (%)
Carotid revascularization for 70–99% symptomatic carotid stenosis	6.0	3.0	48 (38 to 60)	3.0

CI = confidence interval; LDL = low-density lipoprotein; ER = extended release; PFO = patent foramen ovale.

Reproduced from Diener HC, Hankey GJ. Primary and secondary prevention of ischemic stroke and cerebral hemorrhage: JACC focus seminar. *J Am Coll Cardiol.* 2020 Apr 21;75(15):1804–1818, with permission from Elsevier.

Lifestyle measures

A number of lifestyle measures are associated with increased stroke risk, and addressing them is an important part of secondary prevention. Their association with stroke is described in ➔ Chapter 1. However, there are fewer data on the extent to which modifying them reduces recurrent stroke risk, partly because randomized controlled trials (RCTs) in this area are difficult to perform.

Lifestyle measures to address include:
• healthy eating
• taking more exercise
• stopping smoking
• moderating alcohol consumption
• losing weight.

In addition to possible benefits for stroke risk, lifestyle modification is also worth pursuing because it provides a context in which the patient adjusts to the stroke and takes the secondary prevention medication. By giving the patient lifestyle measures to address, it also gives them some 'control' and responsibility over their condition.

Healthy eating

Outside of avoiding obesity, a healthy 'cardiovascular diet' is important. This should include:
• plenty of fruit and vegetables—at least five portions a day
• low levels of fat, particularly saturated fat
• low salt levels—avoid processed foods, many of which have large amounts of added salt. Also, look at the salt content of less obvious foods such as biscuits and bread—this can be surprisingly high
• low sugar diet (even for non-diabetics)
• high fibre intake—30 g/day (a lot more than you may think)
• oily fish may reduce cardiovascular risk.

A cardiovascular diet may reduce risk by multiple mechanisms, including lowering BP, reducing weight, lowering cholesterol, and improving glucose tolerance.

Data from an RCT in patients post-MI showed a Mediterranean diet was associated with a 50% reduction in recurrent MI, death, and other cardiovascular events. No such trials have been performed in stroke but there are likely to be similar benefits.

Details on many suitable diets and healthy eating advice for patients are widely available on the web. For example:
• British Heart Foundation 'Healthy eating' (🕮 https://www.bhf.org.uk/heart-health/preventing-heart-disease/healthy-eating)
• The DASH diet is a stringent diet aimed at reducing hypertension. It is rich in whole grain foods, fruit, vegetables, low-fat or non-dairy products, lean meat, fish, fowl, nuts, and some fats and sweets (🕮 http://www.dashdiet.orgz).

Physical activity

Physical activity improves many stroke risk factors. It may:
- lower BP
- lower weight
- improve glucose tolerance.

Overall, it reduces the risk of stroke by about a fifth.

Stroke risk is reduced more by vigorous exercise (within reason) than by moderate exercise.

We advise our post-stroke patient to undertake aerobic exercise (e.g. running, swimming, bicycling, fast walking) for 20–30 minutes at least three times a week.

Obesity

- Obesity is defined as a body mass index (BMI) of >30 kg/m^2
- It is an independent risk factor for stroke
- Obesity is related to several major risk factors, including hypertension, diabetes, hyperlipidaemia.

Losing weight:
- improves BP
- reduces fasting glucose
- reduces serum lipids
- improves physical fitness

Lifestyle measures are key to reducing obesity

However, in resistant cases interventional treatments include
- Bariatric surgery
- Glucagon-like-peptide-1 receptor analogues (GLP-1RAs)—➔ see under diabetes mellitus later in this chapter

Alcohol consumption

- Studies indicate that a reduction in alcohol intake is useful for primary prevention of stroke. There is no type of alcohol that is either more beneficial or harmful than another
- Chronic alcohol and heavy drinking are risk factors for all stroke subtypes
- Alcohol intake of >60 g per day causes an increased RR of all stroke of about 1.6, but over 2 for haemorrhagic stroke
- High alcohol intake may increase hypertension, hypercoagulability, and AF
- In the UK, the recommended limit for alcohol intake in international units is 14 units/week for men and women, with alcohol-free days in between and avoidance of 'binge' drinking of ≥8 units for men and 6 for women

Smoking

- The risk of ischaemic stroke in smokers is twice that of non-smokers
- The risk of haemorrhagic stroke in smokers is between two and four times higher than that of non-smokers
- After 2 years of stopping smoking, stroke reduces to about 50% and returns to near baseline by 5 years

- Patients are unable to smoke while in hospital; later, it is important to give them advice on how to stop and perhaps refer to a smoking cessation clinic. Some patients need nicotine replacement patches while in the stroke unit (see Tables 10.2 and 10.3)
- All stroke patients who smoke should be strongly advised to stop and offered appropriate counselling
- Comprehensive smoking ban legislation was associated with significantly lower rates of hospital admissions (or deaths) for coronary events, other heart disease, stroke (RR, 0.84) and respiratory disease.
- Use of eCigarettes is increasing. There are not enough studies available yet to take a view on their relevance to stroke.

Table 10.2 Nicotine products to help stop smoking

Product type	How it works
Nicotine gum	When you chew nicotine gum, the nicotine is absorbed through the lining of your mouth
Nicotine patches	Nicotine patches work well for most regular smokers and can be worn around the clock (24-hour patches) or just during the day (16-hour patches)
Nicotine microtabs	These are small tablets containing nicotine which dissolve quickly under your tongue
Nicotine lozenges	Lozenges are sucked slowly to release the nicotine and take about 20–30 minutes to dissolve
Nicotine inhalators	Inhalators look like a plastic cigarette. The inhalator releases nicotine vapour which gets absorbed through your mouth and throat. If you miss the 'hand-to-mouth' aspect of smoking, these may suit you
Nicotine nasal spray	The spray delivers a swift and effective dose of nicotine through the lining of your nose

Table 10.3 Other stop-smoking medicines that can help

Bupropion hydrochloride is a treatment which changes the way that your body responds to nicotine. You start taking bupropion 1–2 weeks before you quit and treatment usually lasts for a couple of months to help you through the withdrawal cravings. It is only available on prescription in the UK and is contraindicated in pregnancy

Varenicline works by reducing your craving for a cigarette and by reducing the effects you feel if you do have a cigarette. You set a date to stop smoking, and start taking tablets 1 or 2 weeks before this date. Treatment normally lasts for 12 weeks. It is only available on prescription in the UK and is contraindicated in pregnancy

Blood pressure

- Lowering BP is the single most important intervention in the secondary prevention of stroke
- BP is an independent risk factor for recurrent stroke and the higher the BP (systolic or diastolic) the higher the risk
- Antihypertensive treatment has been shown to reduce stroke risk in many trials and is associated with up to 40% stroke risk reduction
- Lifestyle modifications are part of the treatment of BP
- Initially, most data were from primary prevention trials. Some questioned whether reducing established hypertension in patients with stroke could worsen outcome, owing to reduced cerebral perfusion in patients with impaired cerebral autoregulation
- The Perindopril Protection Against Recurrent Stroke Study (PROGRESS) trial demonstrated that reducing BP was as beneficial in secondary prevention as in primary prevention (see Fig. 10.1):
  - In PROGRESS, 6105 patients with stroke or TIA within the previous 5 years were randomized to perindopril or perindopril plus indapamide
  - The risk of both haemorrhagic and ischaemic stroke was reduced from 14% to 10% (a RR reduction of 28%)
  - Combination therapy resulted in a greater BP reduction (mean 12/5 mmHg) and greater clinical benefit: 43% reduction in recurrent stroke
  - There was no benefit in giving perindopril alone but the BP drop was much less (5/3 mmHg)
  - A similar RR reduction was seen in patients with raised or *normal* BP
  - This has led to the suggestion that all patients with stroke should receive antihypertensive agents unless they have low BP
- Most guidelines recommend a target BP of 130/80 mmHg or below and we would aim for this in all stroke patients
- BP reduction is important for both ischaemic and haemorrhagic stroke
- The overall reduction in stroke and all vascular events is related to the degree of BP lowering achieved
- Variability or lability of BP is also related to stroke risk
- There is no definite evidence that one class of agent is better—it appears what is most important is the magnitude of the BP drop but some agents such as calcium channel blockers seem better at reducing BP variability
- We usually start a calcium channel blocker, angiotensin receptor blocker (ARB) or angiotensin-converting enzyme (ACE) inhibitor initially
- Outside of lowering BP to facilitate thrombolysis, it is still unclear as to when to start lowering BP in acute ischaemic stroke (see p. 247), but certainly after the first month all stroke patients should be considered to have their BP lowered. Recent data from INTERACT 4 study have demonstrated improved outcomes in acutely lowering systolic BP to 130–140 mmHg in ICH within 2 hours of onset and maintaining this.

For every 1 mmHg BP reduction, recurrent stroke risk is reduced approximately by 3%. Therefore, if BP is reduced by 10 mmHg, stroke risk is reduced by up to 30%.

Blood pressure reduction in special groups

- While there is often concern about lowering BP in patients with occlusive or stenotic extracranial disease for fear of reducing the perfusion above the stenosis, this is rarely an issue in clinical practice. In the minority of patients with carotid stenosis/occlusion and impaired haemodynamic reserve, haemodynamic symptoms may well be alleviated by reducing or stopping antihypertensive medication (this may be a useful temporary strategy while revascularization is considered).
- The SPS3 trial showed it was safe and possible to lower BP to <130 mmHg in stroke patients with small-vessel lacunar infarction.
- With the results of HYVET and other studies which confirmed the benefit of primary prevention of BP lowering in those over 80 years, it is reasonable to assume that all stroke patients, regardless of age, should be treated for persistent raised BP after stroke. Frail, older stroke patients are, however, likely to be more susceptible to side effects of antihypertensive drug treatments.

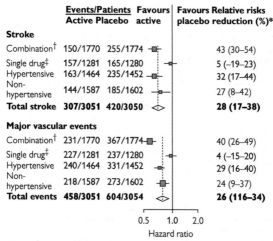

	Events/Patients Active Placebo		Favours active	Favours placebo	Relative risks reduction (%)*
Stroke					
Combination†	150/1770	255/1774			43 (30–54)
Single drug‡	157/1281	165/1280			5 (−19–23)
Hypertensive	163/1464	235/1452			32 (17–44)
Non-hypertensive	144/1587	185/1602			27 (8–42)
Total stroke	**307/3051**	**420/3050**			**28 (17–38)**
Major vascular events					
Combination†	231/1770	367/1774			40 (26–49)
Single drug‡	227/1281	237/1280			4 (−15–20)
Hypertensive	240/1464	331/1452			29 (16–40)
Non-hypertensive	218/1587	273/1602			24 (9–37)
Total events	**458/3051**	**604/3054**			**26 (116–34)**

0.5   1.0   2.0
Hazard ratio

*95% confidence interval in parentheses
†Perindopril plus indapamide
‡Perindopril alone

Fig. 10.1 Rate of stroke during follow-up in PROGRESS in the study group as a whole and in the different subgroups. Active treatment was either perindopril or perindopril and indaptamide. *95% CI in parentheses; †perindopril plus indapamide; ‡perindopril alone.

Reproduced from *Lancet*, 358, PROGRESS Collaborative Group, Randomised trial of a perindopril-based blood-pressure-lowering regimen among 6105 individuals with previous stroke or transient ischaemic attack, pp. 1033–1041, Copyright (2001), with permission from Elsevier.

Cholesterol

- Clinical trials have shown convincingly that reducing cholesterol with statins reduces ischaemic stroke risk (see Table 10.4). The benefits are most in those with an atherosclerotic stroke aetiology.
- Most trial data are from studies in patients with coronary heart disease or cardiovascular disease of all types rather than specifically in stroke. For example, the Heart Protection Study (HPS) randomized 20 000 individuals with a history of coronary heart disease, other occlusive arterial disease, or diabetes to either simvastatin 40 mg or placebo. Over a mean follow-up of 5 years, there were highly significant reductions in mortality (13%), major coronary events (27%), and stroke (25%). The reduction in stroke was in ischaemic stroke, with no reduction in cerebral haemorrhage
- The Stroke Prevention by Aggressive Reduction in Cholesterol Levels (SPARCL) study was the first trial of statin therapy (atorvastatin 80 mg) specifically in stroke patients. A total of 4731 patients with previous TIA or stroke were randomized.
- The statin group showed a significant reduction in recurrent stroke (absolute risk reduction of 2.2% over 5 years, hazard ratio (HR) risk reduction of 16%, NNT to save one recurrent stroke = 45).
- In SPARCL there was a slightly increased risk of recurrent haemorrhagic stroke in the treatment group, supporting the suggestion that high-dose statin therapy probably does not benefit such patients.
- The benefit seen in SPARCL is thought to be mediated through LDL reduction and, interestingly, subgroup analysis showed that those patients with large-vessel carotid disease stroke benefited most.
- The current UK stroke guidelines recommend starting lipid-lowering treatment in patients with ischaemic stroke and TIA to achieve a target (fasted) LDL of 1.8 mmol/L (70 mg/L) or less (unless a definite non-atherosclerotic cause has been diagnosed, such as dissection).
- Our current practice is to prescribe all ischaemic stroke patients atorvastatin 40–80 mg. If atorvastatin does not control cholesterol levels, we switch to an alternative agent such as rosuvastatin or add 10 mg ezetimibe (see Fig. 10.2).
- We would not routinely prescribe statins for haemorrhagic stroke unless patients had other established atherosclerotic disease, such as symptomatic coronary artery disease.
- For patients with both ischaemic and haemorrhagic cerebrovascular disease, we prescribe statins.
- Statins are thought to act primarily by cholesterol/LDL reduction, and the magnitude of benefit correlates with the degree of cholesterol reduction in clinical trials. It has also been suggested they may have other beneficial 'pleiotropic' effects, including:
  - plaque stabilization
  - improved endothelial function
- Unlike BP lowering, the evidence for aggressive lipid-lowering in older patients, especially over the age of 80 years, is sparse.

Other medications also used to treat hyperlipidaemia include:
- niacin
- fibrates
- cholesterol absorption inhibitors (e.g. ezetimibe).
- proprotein convertase subtilisin-kexin type 9 (PCSK9) inhibitors
  - PCSK9 plays a major regulatory role in cholesterol homeostasis.
  - PCSK9 binds to the epidermal growth factor-like repeat A (EGF-A) domain of the low-density lipoprotein receptor (LDLR), inducing LDLR degradation.
  - A number of monoclonal antibodies have been developed which bind to PCSK9 near the catalytic domain that interacts with the LDLR and hence inhibit the function of PCSK9. These include evolocumab, bococizumab, and alirocumab.
  - They have been shown in large RCTs (FOURIER and ODYSSEY) to reduce LDL levels further in those already taking statins, and reduce cardiovascular events including stroke.
  - PCSK 9 inhibitors are administered by injection and are expensive but should be considered in stroke patients with who are unable to otherwise achieve target values of LDL.
- Bempedoic acid (oral inhibitor of ATP citrate lyase) can be considered in statin-intolerant individuals. It is a pro-drug activated in the liver and not peripherally with less associated muscle cramps but in CLEAR— the major RCT of bempedoic acid including 13, 970 statin intolerant participants, bempedoic acid did not reduce stroke (fatal or non-fatal) despite reducing LDL and other coronary endpoints.

Table 10.4 Effect of cholesterol reduction of 1 mmol/L of LDL on all stroke, by risk factors and stroke type (any type of lipid-lowering medication)

Category	Trials	Events	Percent change in risk (95% CI)
All stroke	41	3319	−20 (−14 to −26)
All stroke in people with known vascular disease	32	2311	−22 (−28 to −16)
All stroke in people without known vascular disease	7	752	−6 (−22 to 14)
Thromboembolic stroke	8	1204	−28 (−35 to −20)
Haemorrhagic stroke	8	149	−3 (−35 to 47)
Fatal stroke	56	678	−2 (−17 to 16)
Non-fatal stroke	40	2519	−23 (−29 to −16)

Reproduced from *Lancet*, 370(9602), Prospective Studies Collaboration, Blood cholesterol and vascular mortality by age, sex and blood pressure: a meta-analysis of individual data from 61 prospective studies with 55 000 vascular deaths, pp. 1829–1839, Copyright (2007), with permission from Elsevier.

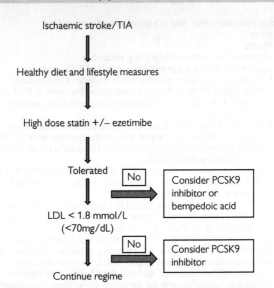

Fig. 10.2 Schematic approach to managing hyperlipidaemia in ischaemic stroke and TIA.

Diabetes

- Cerebrovascular disease is very common in diabetes and good diabetic control is essential to reduce the risk of further microvascular and macrovascular disease.

- In the order of 1 in 3 ischaemic stroke patients have diabetes but also 1 in 4 ICH patients. Diabetics have more severe strokes with increased risk of disability, death, recurrence, readmission, and dementia.

- Most of the available data on stroke prevention in patients with diabetes are on primary rather than secondary prevention of stroke. Intensive treatment addressing multiple risk factors, including control of hyperglycaemia, hypertension, and dyslipidaemia, have demonstrated reductions in the risk of cardiovascular events.

- Tighter glycaemic control has been shown to reduce the occurrence of microvascular complications (nephropathy, retinopathy, and peripheral neuropathy) in several clinical trials, and is recommended in multiple guidelines for both primary and secondary prevention of stroke and cardiovascular disease. Data on the efficacy of glycaemic control on macrovascular complications, including stroke, are more limited.

- Analysis of data from randomized trials suggest a continual reduction in vascular events with the progressive control of glucose to normal levels.

- Normal fasting glucose is defined as glucose <5.6 mmol/L (100 mg/ dL), impaired fasting glucose has been defined as levels between 5.6 and 6.9 mmol/L (100–126 mg/dL). Diabetes is defined by a fasting plasma glucose level >7.0 mmol/L (126 mg/dL) or a non-fasting plasma glucose >11.1 mmol/L (200 mg/dL).

- The glycosylated haemoglobin A_{1c} level is useful in monitoring diabetes control. A level >7% is considered as inadequate control of hyperglycaemia. Therefore, one should look for levels of haemoglobin A_{1c} of <7%.

- There is good evidence that vigorous control of BP in patients with diabetes mellitus reduces stroke risk. For example, in patients with diabetes randomized into the Hypertension Optimal Treatment (HOT) trial, there was a 51% reduction in major cardiovascular events in patients allocated to a target BP of 80 mmHg diastolic compared with those aiming for 90 mmHg.

- Although all major classes of antihypertensives are suitable for BP control in patients with diabetes, most patients will require more than one agent. ACE inhibitors and angiotensin receptor blockers are more effective in reducing the progression of renal disease and are recommended as first-choice medications for patients with diabetes mellitus.

- Trial evidence also supports reducing cholesterol in this patient group. The Heart Protection Study demonstrated the beneficial effect of simvastatin in diabetic patients. A total of 5963 people >40 years of age with diabetes were randomized to simvastatin 40 mg daily or placebo. Simvastatin was associated with a 28% (95% CI, 8–44) reduction in ischaemic stroke (3.4% vs. 4.7%; $P = 0.01$).

- More rigorous control of BP and lipids should be considered in all diabetic stroke patients.

- Glucagon-like-peptide-1 receptor analogues (GLP-1RAs) are a new class of diabetic treatment which may well have a direct action on the underlying mechanisms causing stroke. GLP-1 is an incretin hormone with a short half-life of 1- 2 minutes, secreted from the gut after eating in a glucose dependent manner to modulate insulin secretion. There are GLP-1 receptors throughout the gut but also in the brain.
- GLP-1RAs (e.g. liraglutide, semaglutiude, dulaglutide) cause weight loss, and improve glycaemic control (without the risk of hypoglacaemia as their action is glucose-dependent)
- They can also cross the blood–brain barrier (BBB) to act on GLP-1 receptors in the brain—reducing post-stroke inflammation and oxidative stress in animal models, and so may be neuroprotective.
- While there are little RCT data for use in acute stroke, long-term follow-up in a number of GLP-1RA RCTs (SUSTAIN-6, PIONEER-6, REWIND) has demonstrated a consistent class effect of reduction in stroke in diabetics on GLP-1 RA treatment.
- They can be considered in both difficult to control diabetes, and also obesity.

Homocysteine

- Hyperhomocysteinaemia is an independent risk factor for cardiovascular disease and stroke.
- Homocysteine levels can be reduced by vitamin B complex and folic acid treatment.
- However, whether reducing levels in stroke patients reduces risk of recurrent stroke is uncertain.
- The Vitamin Intervention for Stroke Prevention (VISP) study randomized patients with a stroke and mild to moderate hyperhomocysteinaemia (>9.5 μmol/L for men, 8.5 μmol/L for women) to receive either a high- or low-dose vitamin therapy (e.g. folate, vitamin B_6, or B_{12}) for 2 years. The mean reduction in homocysteine was greater in the high-dose group. However, there was no reduction in stroke rates in the patients given high-dose vitamins, with 2-year stroke rates of 9.2% in the high-dose and 8.8% in the low-dose arm. A possible confounding effect was that fortification of bread with folic acid was commenced during the study.
- The Vitamins to Prevent Stroke (VITATOPS) trial randomized 8164 patients within 7 months of stroke or TIA to placebo or vitamin B supplements—regardless of homocysteine levels. The composite endpoint after over 3 years of follow-up was cardiovascular death/MI or stroke. Taking vitamin B supplements was seen to be safe but had no significant effect on primary outcome. There was a borderline effect on reducing recurrent stroke in patients with lacunar stroke on a secondary analysis, and in an MRI substudy vitamin therapy was associated with reduced white matter hyperintensity progression.
- A large primary prevention trial in hypertensive individuals in China (CSPPT) showed a reduced stroke risk in those taking vitamin therapy to reduce homocysteine levels, but this was in patients without previous stroke and the Chinese diet may differ from other countries.
- Mendelian randomization studies suggest homocysteine is a risk factor for lacunar stroke and small-vessel disease but not for large-artery or cardioembolic stroke. Secondary analyses of the RCTs provide some additional evidence for this. Therefore, some authorities suggest treating elevated homocysteine in small-vessel stroke cases.
- Until more data become available, whether to treat elevated homocysteine is a matter of individual choice and has largely fallen out of guideline recommendations. In patients in whom we wish to lower it we give daily folic acid 5 mg and 250 mg vitamin B_6 (as part of strong vitamin B mixed tablet) supplements.
- The benefit of vitamins to reduce homocysteine is likely to be much greater in those countries with low folic intake, compared to countries where there is folate fortification in foods such as bread.

Antiplatelet agents

- After an ischaemic stroke, all patients should be considered for antiplatelet therapy.
- Dual antiplatelet therapy (DAPT) is commonly used in acute stroke treatment (typically within 48 hours of diagnosis) and early secondary prevention in a time-limited regime described in ➔ Chapter 9 p. 240.
- However for the long-term prevention of stroke monotherapy is usually used.
- There are currently three options for **long-term** secondary prevention:
  - aspirin
  - aspirin and dipyridamole
  - clopidogrel.
- All three drugs inhibit platelet activation and aggregation but by different mechanisms:
  - aspirin by inhibiting cyclo-oxygenase and thromboxane A2
  - dipyridamole by increasing plasma adenosine and inhibiting platelet phosphodiesterase
  - clopidogrel by blocking adenosine diphosphate (ADP) receptors.
  - Dipyridamole—used in its modified-release formula is now difficult to obtain and has largely been replaced by clopidogrel treatment.
  - There are other antiplatelets routinely used in coronary disease that have either been trialled or are in the process of being investigated in stroke disease listed as follows:

Aspirin

- In an Antithrombotic Trialists' Collaboration, meta-analysis of results of 21 randomized trials comparing antiplatelet therapy with placebo in 18 270 patients with prior stroke or TIA, antiplatelet therapy was associated with a 28% relative odds reduction in non-fatal strokes and a 16% reduction in fatal strokes.
- Aspirin in doses ranging from 50 to 1300 mg/day appears to prevent recurrent ischaemic stroke.
- Higher (1200 mg/day) or lower (75–300 mg/day) doses have similar effects on stroke prevention.
- However, higher doses produce more side effects.
- Therefore, a dose in the range 75–300 mg daily is recommended.

Clopidogrel

- Clopidogrel monotherapy (75 mg once daily) appears to be as good, or slightly more effective, than aspirin.
- If required, to rapidly achieve plasma levels a 300 mg loading dose once daily is used.
- Clopidogrel resistance is a potential issue to its efficacy. Resistance is thought to be partly bioavailability and genetic polymorphisms. The presence of a gene polymorphism resulting in loss of function of the drug-metabolizing enzyme CYP2C19 was found to be an important factor.

CAPRIE
- The efficacy of clopidogrel monotherapy was compared with that of aspirin in the Clopidogrel versus Aspirin in Patients at Risk of Ischemic Events (CAPRIE) trial.
- More than 19 000 patients with stroke, MI, or peripheral vascular disease were randomized to aspirin 325 mg/day or clopidogrel 75 mg/day.
- The primary end point, a composite outcome of ischaemic stroke, MI, or vascular death, occurred in 8.7% fewer patients treated with clopidogrel compared with aspirin ($P=0.043$).
- However, in a subgroup analysis of those patients with prior stroke, the risk reduction with clopidogrel was slightly smaller and was not significant.

MATCH
- The Management of Atherothrombosis With Clopidogrel in High-Risk Patients With TIA or Stroke (MATCH) trial showed the combination of clopidogrel and aspirin had no benefit over clopidogrel alone.
- Patients with prior stroke or TIA plus additional risk factors ($n = 7599$) were allocated to clopidogrel 75 mg or clopidogrel plus aspirin 75 mg once daily.
- The primary outcome was the composite of ischaemic stroke, MI, vascular death, or rehospitalization secondary to ischaemic events.
- There was no significant benefit of combination therapy compared with clopidogrel on the primary outcome or any of the secondary outcomes.
- The risk of major haemorrhage was increased in the combination group compared with clopidogrel alone, with a 1.3% absolute increase in life-threatening bleeding. Although clopidogrel plus aspirin is recommended over aspirin for acute coronary syndromes, the results of MATCH do not suggest a similar risk:benefit ratio for long-term secondary prevention in stroke and TIA survivors.

Dipyridamole
- Limited data suggest that dipyridamole monotherapy is probably about as effective as aspirin. Considerable evidence suggests that the combination of aspirin and dipyridamole is better than aspirin alone.
- The European Stroke Prevention Study 2 (ESPS-2) randomized 6602 patients with prior stroke or TIA in a factorial design using a different dipyridamole formulation and aspirin dose compared with ESPS-1. The treatment groups were:
  - aspirin 50 mg/day plus extended-release dipyridamole 400 mg/day
  - aspirin alone
  - extended-release dipyridamole alone
  - placebo.
- The risk of stroke was significantly reduced, by 18% on aspirin alone, 16% with dipyridamole alone, and 37% with a combination of aspirin plus dipyridamole.

The ESPIRIT study confirmed this:
- Patients within 6 months of a TIA or minor stroke of presumed arterial origin were randomized to aspirin (30–325 mg daily) with (n = 1363) or without (n = 1376) dipyridamole (200 mg twice daily).
- Treatment was open, but auditing of outcome events was blinded.
- Mean follow-up was 3.5 years (standard deviation (SD) 2.0).
- Primary outcome events (the composite of death from all vascular causes, non-fatal stroke, non-fatal MI, or major bleeding complication, whichever happened first) occurred in 13% of patients on aspirin and dipyridamole and in 16% on aspirin alone (HR 0.80, 95% CI 0.66–0.98; absolute risk reduction 1.0% per year, 95% CI 0.1–1.8).
- Patients on aspirin and dipyridamole discontinued medication more often than those on aspirin alone (470 versus 184), mainly because of headache:
  - If dipyridamole is used, the modified-release preparation (200 mg twice daily) should be given as this was the formulation shown to be beneficial in trials.
  - If the patient is being fed nasogastrically, or in those countries where the slow-release preparation is not available, the standard preparation (100 mg three times daily) can be given. It is available as a liquid.
  - Headache is the most common side effect of dipyridamole. If it occurs, reduce the dose to 200 mg once daily and it may pass after a few days, when the dose can be increased. In 10–20% of cases, headache prevents continued use.

Clopidogrel versus aspirin + dipyridamole
- The PRoFESS results randomized stroke patients between 25 mg of aspirin plus 200 mg extended-release dipyridamole twice daily or clopidogrel 75 mg once daily.
- A total of 20 332 patients were followed for a mean of 2.5 years.
- Recurrent stroke occurred in 916 (9.0%) receiving aspirin + dipyridamole and in 898 (8.8%) receiving clopidogrel (HR, 1.01; 95% CI 0.92–1.11).
- There were more major haemorrhagic events in the aspirin + dipyridamole group (4.1 versus 3.6%, HR, 1.15; 95% CI, 1.00–1.32), including intracranial haemorrhage (HR, 1.42; 95% CI, 1.11–1.83).
- The net risk of recurrent stroke or major haemorrhagic event was similar in the two groups (aspirin + dipyridamole 11.7% versus 11.4% with clopidogrel, HR, 1.03; 95% CI, 0.95–1.11).

Which regimen should you use?
- Globally, low-dose aspirin is still commonly most commonly prescribed for long-term secondary stroke prevention.
- Our current practice is to use clopidogrel as first-line therapy for all new stroke episodes.
- Some guidelines (e.g. UK NICE) recommend aspirin for the first two weeks and then switching to clopidogrel. This is based on the fact that the trials of antiplatelets in acute stroke used aspirin. However, starting clopidogrel on admission is likely to be as effective. If so we would load with a single dose of 300 mg and then continue with 75 mg od.

- During the acute phase, dual anti-platelet therapy with aspirin and clopidogrel is increasingly used in patients with TIA and minor stroke, following the POINT and CHANCE trial results (see next). This should normally be continued for 3–4 weeks, after which monotherapy with clopidogrel is given.
- In some patients with tight large-artery stenosis, in whom the risk of early recurrent stroke is particularly high, we give dual anti-platelet with aspirin and clopidogrel for a longer time, often 3 months.

Special situations

In certain situations, the combination of aspirin and clopidogrel is often used.

TIA and minor stroke during the first 24 hours.

The CHANCE and POINT trials both showed DAPT with aspirin and clopidogrel reduces the risk of recurrent stroke in patients with minor stroke and TIA when given within 24 hours of symptom onset (see ➔ Chapter 9 antiplatelet therapy, p. 240)

A meta-analysis suggested an optional period of DAPT, balancing the risk of recurrent stroke versus the risk of bleeding, was three weeks.

Carotid stenting

Most clinicians use clopidogrel and aspirin therapy perioperatively and usually for a period of 1–3 months post-stenting. This is based on trials in coronary stenting, although there are no trial data for carotid stenting.

Large-artery disease

Patients with large-artery disease (e.g. carotid stenosis, MCA stenosis) have a very high risk of early recurrent stroke. In this setting some clinicians use the combination of clopidogrel and aspirin. In the CARESS study in recently symptomatic carotid stenosis it was more effective than aspirin alone in reducing asymptomatic cerebral emboli detected on transcranial Doppler and there appeared to be a reduction in recurrent clinical events (although the study was not powered for this).

Similar results were obtained in the CLAIR trial looking at embolic signals in symptomatic intracranial stenosis. This is supported by data from Stenting and Aggressive Medical Management for Preventing Recurrent stroke in Intracranial Stenosis (SAMMPRIS), a study of stenting for intracranial stenosis, where the medical arm were given aspirin and clopidogrel and had a low recurrent stroke rate.

It is also supported by the CHANCE study. In the overall study comparing DAPT with aspirin 5170 patients with minor stroke or TIA within 24 hours of symptom onset, there was a significant reduction in recurrent stroke risk at 90 days with a HR of stroke-free survival of 0.68 (95% CI 0.57–0.81; P <0.001) compared to aspirin alone. In a subgroup analysis of those who had intracranial CTA the benefit was particularly marked in those with large-artery disease (primarily intracranial in this population) who had the highest recurrent stroke rate.

The combination of aspirin and clopidogrel may be used for:
- symptomatic high-grade carotid stenosis not amenable to intervention
- symptomatic intracranial stenosis
- while waiting for CEA.

Our policy is that in cases of recently symptomatic TIA or minor stroke due to large-artery stenosis (>50%) whether it is in the carotid, vertebral, or intracranial arteries intracranial stenosis we use the combination of aspirin 75 mg and clopidogrel 75 mg for 3–6 months only and then switch patients to clopidogrel monotherapy. We load patients with 300 mg clopidogrel.

Lacunar stroke/cerebral small-vessel disease

• There is concern over bleeding risk in this stroke subtype. Cerebral small-vessel disease pathology underlies lacunar stroke as well as many cases of subcortical intracranial haemorrhage. Furthermore, this is the stroke subtype most likely to have cerebral microbleeds on gradient echo MRI. Patients with radiological leucoaraiosis, a feature of cerebral SVD, are at increased risk of bleeding on warfarin.

• The SPS3 trial was a landmark double-blind, multicentre trial involving 3020 patients with recent symptomatic lacunar infarcts identified by MRI. It was the first large trial to evaluate treatment effects in lacunar stroke confirmed on MRI. Patients were randomly assigned to receive 75 mg of clopidogrel or placebo daily; patients in both groups received 325 mg of aspirin daily. The primary outcome was any recurrent stroke, including ischaemic stroke and intracranial haemorrhage. After a mean follow-up of 3.4 years, the risk of recurrent stroke was not significantly reduced with aspirin and clopidogrel (DAPT) but the risk of major haemorrhage was almost doubled with DAPT.

• Therefore, in lacunar stroke, monotherapy with aspirin or clopidogrel should be used, and we would not use the combination of aspirin and clopidogrel.

Testing for clopidogrel resistance

• Clopidogrel is a pro-drug. The *CYP2C19* gene encodes the CYP2C19 enzyme, which is needed to metabolize clopidogrel to its active form.

• The *CYP2C19* gene has many alternative versions (alleles) that produce variations of the CYP2C19 enzyme with different levels of activity. The function of each allele can be described as 'normal', 'completely absent', 'decreased' or 'increased', or the function may be uncertain.

• Clopidogrel is less effective in people with alleles that produce CYP2C19 enzymes with completely absent or decreased function.

• People with two loss-of-function alleles have no CYP2C19 enzyme activity. They cannot activate clopidogrel to its active form and are classed as 'poor metabolizers'. People with only 1 loss-of-function allele have reduced enzyme activity and are classed as 'intermediate metabolizers'.

• Loss-of-function alleles are more common in certain ethnic groups, such as people with an Asian ethnic background.

• There are a number of tests available to determine which CYP2C19 alleles a patient has; some of these are point of care.

• Carriers of *CYP2C19* loss-of-function alleles are at greater risk of stroke and composite vascular events than noncarriers among patients with ischaemic stroke or TIA treated with clopidogrel.

• One meta-analysis reported that among 15 studies of 4762 patients with stroke or TIA treated with clopidogrel, carriers of *CYP2C19* loss-of-function alleles were at increased risk of stroke in comparison with noncarriers (12.0% versus 5.8%; risk ratio, 1.92, 95% confidence interval, 1.57–2.35; P <0.001).

- In patient who have clopidogrel resistance an alternative antiplatelet agent can be given such as ticagrelor or aspirin.
- The Chinese CHANCE2 trial randomized 6412 subjects with minor ischaemic stroke or TIA within 24 hours of symptom onset, who carried *CYP2C19* loss-of-function alleles to ticagrelor (180 mg on day 1 followed by 90 mg twice daily on days 2 through 90) and placebo clopidogrel or to clopidogrel (300 mg on day 1 followed by 75 mg once daily on days 2 through 90) and placebo ticagrelor; both groups received aspirin for 21 days.
- Stroke occurred within 90 days in 191 patients (6.0%) in the ticagrelor group and 243 patients (7.6%) in the clopidogrel group (HR, 0.77; 95% confidence interval, 0.64 to 0.94; P = 0.008). The risk of severe or moderate bleeding did not differ between the two treatment groups, but ticagrelor was associated with more total bleeding events than clopidogrel.

In 2024 NICE in the UK recommended *CYP2C19* in patients in whom clopidogrel is being prescribed after TIA or stroke.
    ℞ https://www.nice.org.uk/guidance/dg59

Newer antiplatelet agents

Ticagrelor
- Ticagrelor is a related platelet aggregation inhibitor but is not a pro-drug and has a faster onset than clopidogrel but a shorter half-life—it has to be taken BD.
- The SOCRATES trial showed no superiority of ticagrelor over aspirin in the early management of TIA or minor ischaemic stroke but THALES demonstrated a benefit of combination ticagrelor and aspirin over aspirin but with an excess of bleeding complications in acute secondary prevention treatment (started under 24 hours). In THALES the aspirin dose was 300 mg—higher than in POINT or CHANCE.
- Ticagrelor can then be used in acute short-term secondary prevention in combination with aspirin as an alternative to clopidogrel and can be justified as long-term secondary prevention monotherapy in aspirin and clopidogrel intolerant individuals.

Prasugrel
- Prasugrel is a third-generation thienopyridine with a more consistent and efficient metabolism than clopidogrel:
  - It becomes active within 30 minutes.
  - It binds irreversibly to the platelet P2Y12 receptor.
  - In the Japanese PRASTRO-I RCT of low-dose prasugrel (3.75 mg compared to the usual 10 mg used in coronary disease) against clopidogrel (75 mg) in 3747 stroke patients aged over 75 yrs, non-inferiority was unproven and there was no safety benefit in terms of bleeding of the low-dose prasugrel.
  - Prasugrel is not routinely used in stroke secondary prevention currently.

Cilostazol
- Cilostazol is a phosphodiesterase 3 inhibitor (dipyridamole is a PDE5 inhibitor) metabolized by cytP450 in the liver and independent of the P2Y12 receptor and cyclooxygenase pathways used by clopidogrel (ticagrelor, prasugrel) and aspirin.
- PDE3 is found throughout the body and cilostazol has mechanisms of action outside of platelet and endothelial cells, including reduction in systemic inflammation, reduction in triglycerides, and increase in HDL.
- Cilostazol is licenced in Europe and the U.S. to treat claudication in peripheral arterial disease and has been commonly used in Asian Pacific countries for non-cardioembolic stroke secondary prevention.
- In the Cilostazol Stroke Prevention Study CSPS, subsequent CSPS 2, cilostazol reduced stroke compared with placebo and then aspirin. Patients in CSPS 2 were Asian and the majority had lacunar infracts.
- Headache, dizziness, and GI upset are frequent side effects—more so than dipyrimadole, but bleeding complications are less than with dipyrimadole.
- Long-term (over 3.5-year follow-up) secondary prevention with cilostazol in combination with aspirin or clopidogrel was found to be superior compared to monotherapy, with no increase in bleeding complications in one Japanese study of high-risk patients.
- It has been suggested that cilostazol may be particularly effective in small-vessel disease, acting via vasoactive rather than anti-platelet effects. A recent small factorial designed RCT of cilostazol and isosorbide mononitrate for secondary prevention in lacunar stroke (LACI-2) within a UK population has shown a possible effect and cilostazol is now being tested in the larger LSCI-3.

Anticoagulation

Anticoagulation used to be widely used in stroke secondary prevention. However, trials have shown that antiplatelet agents are the better choice except for certain specific situations:

- AF
- Mechanical prosthetic heart valves
- Certain other high-risk cardioembolic sources of embolism
- Some hypercoagulable states.

Anticoagulation in the prevention of all ischaemic stroke

- A number of trials have shown that anticoagulation has less or similar efficacy to antiplatelet agents, but that it has a higher risk. Therefore antiplatelet agents are the treatment of choice except in specific circumstances.
- The Stroke Prevention in Reversible Ischemia Trial (SPIRIT) was stopped early because of increased bleeding among those treated with high-intensity oral anticoagulation (INR 3.0–4.5) compared with aspirin (30 mg/day) in 1316 patients. Intracerebral bleeding was particularly increased in patients with leucoaraiosis on brain imaging.
- This demonstrated that high levels of anticoagulation were not beneficial, but trials with lower INRs were then performed.
- The Warfarin Aspirin Recurrent Stroke Study (WARSS) compared the efficacy of warfarin (INR 1.4–2.8) with aspirin (325 mg) for the prevention of recurrent ischaemic stroke among 2206 patients with a non-cardioembolic stroke. This randomized, double-blind, multicentre trial found no significant difference between the treatments for the prevention of recurrent stroke or death (warfarin, 17.8%; aspirin, 16.0%).
- Rates of major bleeding were not significantly different between the warfarin and aspirin groups (2.2% and 1.5% per year, respectively).
- The European–Australian Stroke Prevention in Reversible Ischemia Trial (ESPRIT) randomly assigned patients within 6 months of TIA or minor stroke of presumed arterial origin to anticoagulants (target INR range 2.0–3.0; $n = 536$) or aspirin (30–325 mg daily; $n = 532$). The mean follow-up was 4.6 years (SD 2.2).
- The primary outcome was the composite of death from all vascular causes, non-fatal stroke, non-fatal MI, or major bleeding complication, whichever occurred first.
- The mean achieved INR was 2.57 (SD 0.86).
- A primary outcome event occurred in 19% patients on anticoagulants and in 18% of patients on aspirin (HR 1.02, 95% CI 0.77–1.35).
- The HR for ischaemic events was 0.73 (0.52–1.01), and for major bleeding complications, 2.56 (1.48–4.43).

Specific diseases and warfarin

Cardioembolic stroke and AF are dealt with on ➲ p. 289.

Intracranial stenosis
- The Warfarin–Aspirin Symptomatic Intracranial Disease (WASID) trial was designed to test the efficacy of warfarin with a target INR of 2–3 (mean 2.5) versus aspirin for those with angiographically documented intracranial stenosis of >50%.
- It was stopped prematurely for safety concerns among those treated with warfarin.
- At the time of termination, warfarin was associated with significantly higher rates of adverse events and was no better than aspirin.
- During a mean follow-up of 1.8 years, adverse events in the two groups were death (aspirin, 4.3%; warfarin, 9.7%; HR, 0.46; 95% CI 0.23–0.90; $P = 0.02$), major haemorrhage (aspirin, 3.2%; warfarin, 8.3%; HR, 0.39; 95% CI 0.18–0.84; $P = 0.01$).
- The primary endpoint (ischaemic stroke, brain haemorrhage, and non-stroke vascular death) occurred in 22% of patients in both treatment arms (HR, 1.04; 95% CI 0.73–1.48; $P = 0.83$).
- Therefore, antiplatelets are preferred in intracranial stenosis.

Carotid and vertebral dissection
- Two phase two trials (CADISS 250 recruits) and TREAT-CAD (194 recruits) compared aspirin to warfarin in secondary prevention after symptomatic carotid and vertebral dissection. They showed no difference between the two treatments. An individual patient pooled analysis of data from both trials showed no difference.
- In the STOP-CAD large observational study in 3636 patients (11.1% received exclusively anticoagulation and 67.5% received exclusively antiplatelets), there was no significant difference in recurrent stroke rate by 30 days in the two groups, although there was a non-significant trend to lower stroke rates with anticoagulation.
- Therefore either antiplatelets or anticoagulants can be used (see ➡ Chapter 11 for more on the treatment of cervical dissection).

Atrial fibrillation

- Anticoagulation should be considered in all patients with AF. It is such an effective treatment that one should only not prescribe it if there is a good reason not to do so.
- The mainstay of treatment has traditionally been warfarin, although this is now being replaced by direct-acting oral anticoagulants (DOACs).
- Multiple clinical trials have demonstrated the superior therapeutic effect of warfarin compared with placebo in the primary prevention of thromboembolic events among patients with non-valvular AF.
- These trials did not include patients with cardiac valve disease and AF because it was thought that withholding warfarin was unethical.
- An analysis of pooled data from five primary prevention trials of warfarin versus control showed consistent benefits across studies, with an overall RR reduction of 68% (95% CI 50–79) and an absolute reduction in annual stroke rate from 4.5% to 1.4%.
- This absolute risk reduction indicates that 31 ischaemic strokes will be prevented each year for every 1000 patients treated.
- Overall, warfarin use was relatively safe, with an annual rate of major bleeding of 1.3% for patients on warfarin compared to 1% for patients on placebo or aspirin.
- The European Atrial Fibrillation Trial confirmed that there was a similar benefit in the secondary prevention of stroke, i.e. in using warfarin in patients who have already had a stroke.
- The optimal intensity of oral anticoagulation for stroke prevention in patients with AF appears to be 2.0–3.0.
- The efficacy of oral anticoagulation declines significantly below an INR of 2.0.
- Both persistent AF and paroxysmal AF are potent risk factors for first and recurrent stroke and both should be treated similarly.
- Evidence supporting the efficacy of aspirin is substantially weaker than that for warfarin.
- A pooled analysis of data from three trials resulted in an estimated RR reduction of 21% compared with placebo (95% CI 0–38).
- The ACTIVE W trial showed that warfarin was more effective than the combination of aspirin and clopidogrel.
- There is no evidence that combining anticoagulation with an antiplatelet agent is of benefit compared to anticoagulant therapy alone in AF.
- Direct oral anticoagulants (DOACs) have been shown to be at least as efficacious as warfarin in preventing stroke in patients with non-valvular AF and safer.
- The DOACs are oral medications with rapid-onset anticoagulation and require no routine monitoring of therapeutic dose (one of the major advantages over warfarin, which has a narrow therapeutic range and requires regular INR monitoring to ensure efficacy). Recent large-scale RCTs have shown them to be as effective as warfarin in the prevention of stroke in individuals with AF.
- The first DOAC to be licenced was the direct thrombin inhibitor dabigatran in the RELY trial. This was followed by two similar large-scale RCTs of the factor Xa inhibitors rivaroxaban (ROCKET AF) and apixaban

(ARISTOTLE). In all three trials, the comparator was warfarin and in each trial the DOACs proved 'non-inferior' to warfarin. In fact, the DOACs were in general safer and as, or more, efficacious than warfarin.

- The direct thrombin inhibitor DOAC dabigatran has a reversal agent (the monoclonal FAB fragment idarucizumab) and Xa inhibitor anticoagulant effect for all the drugs in that class of DOAC, which can be reversed with Andexanet-alpha. The anticoagulant effect of Warfarin can be reversed with 4 Factor PCC and vitamin K— although this is often done poorly in practice.

Therefore, unless a clear contraindication exists, AF patients with a recent stroke or TIA should receive long-term anticoagulation rather than antiplatelet therapy.

Predictors of risk in AF

- Data from the AF clinical trials show that age, recent congestive heart failure, hypertension, diabetes, and prior thromboembolism identify high-risk groups for arterial thromboembolism among patients with AF.
- This can be estimated in any individual using the CHA_2DS_2-VASc score (see Tables 10.5 and 10.6).
- While the CHA_2DS_2-VASc score helps predict the annualized stroke risk, the HAS-BLED score can be used to estimate the risk of bleeding complications (see Table 10.7). This is important when individualizing choice of anticoagulation in patients and counselling in general with regard to the risk/benefit of anticoagulation in each patient assessed. Remember that in CHA_2DS_2-VASc, any history of hypertension scores 1, while in HAS-BLED 1 is scored only in the context of poorly controlled BP (systolic BP >160 mmHg). Therefore, HAS-BLED is a good routine checklist for the key modifiable risk factors for haemorrhagic complications with anticoagulation.

Table 10.5 CHA_2DS_2-VASc score

Risk factor	Score
Congestive heart failure/ LV dysfunction	1
Hypertension	1
Age ≥75 y	2
Diabetes mellitus	1
Stroke/TIA/TE	2
Vascular disease (prior myocardial infarction, peripheral artery disease, or aortic plaque)	1
Age 65–74 y	1
Sex **c**ategory (i.e. female)	1

LV= left ventricular; TE= thromboembolism; TIA= transient ischaemic attack

Reproduced from Lip GY, Nieuwlaat R, Pisters R, Lane DA, Crijns HJ. Refining clinical risk stratification for predicting stroke and thromboembolism in atrial fibrillation using a novel risk factor-based approach: the euro heart survey on atrial fibrillation. *Chest.* 2010; 137: 263–272, Copyright © 2010 The American College of Chest Physicians, with permission from Elsevier.

Table 10.6 Stroke or other thromboembolism events per patient year based on the CHA$_2$DS$_2$VASc scoring system

CHA$_2$DS$_2$ VASc score	N	No. of TE events/PY	TE rate during 1 year (95% CI)	TE rate during 1 year, adjusted for warfarin use*
1	422	3/653	0.46 (0.10, 1.34)	1.3
2	1230	15/1913	0.78 (0.44, 1.29)	2.2
3	1730	31/2673	1.16 (0.79, 1.64)	3.2
4	1718	38/2665	1.43 (1.01, 1.95)	4.0
5	1159	42/1732	2.42 (1.75, 3.26)	6.7
6	679	36/1016	3.54 (2.49, 4.87)	9.8
7	294	15/436	3.44 (1.94, 5.62)	9.6
8	82	3/125	2.41 (0.53, 6.88)	6.7
9	14	1/18	5.47 (0.91, 27.0)	15.2
Total	7329	184/11 233	P value for trend	P<0.0001

*Theoretical TE rates without therapy: assuming that warfarin provides a 64% reduction in TE risk, based on Hart et al.**. CI indicates confidence interval.

** Hart RG, Pearce LA, Aguilar MI. Meta-analysis: antithrombotic therapy to prevent stroke in patients who have nonvalvular atrial fibrillation. Ann Intern Med. 2007;146:857–867.

Reproduced from Lip GYH, Frison L, Halperin JL, Lane DA. Identifying patients at high risk for stroke despite anticoagulation. Stroke. 2010 Dec;41(12):2731–2738. doi:10.1161/strokeaha.110.590257. Copyright © 2010 American Heart Association, with permission from Wolters Kluwer Health, Inc.

- The other key issue with regard to risk and anticoagulation with warfarin relates to time in the therapeutic window (TTR). As INR drifts above 3, so does the risk of haemorrhagic complication, while at the same time sub-therapeutic INR below 2 offers inadequate protection against cardiac embolism in AF. A TTR of 70% or more is the target for optimum anticoagulation with warfarin. A TTR of below 50% has been shown to be no more efficacious than a placebo control.
- In this context, DOACs are simpler to use for both the patient and the physician as the dose does not have to be individually tailored using INR measurement.

Difficult management situations

- There has been uncertainty around when to initiate oral anticoagulation in a patient with AF after a stroke or TIA. However, we now have data from a number of RCTs, including OPTIMAS, ELAN, and TIMING. An individual patient data analysis of these trials has been performed by the CATALYST investigators. This demonstrates that transformation starting DOACs early in the first few days is safe, at least as good as waiting for 2 weeks and is probably better. This is also applied even

Table 10.7 HAS-BLED score for estimating bleeding risk in patients anticoagulated for atrial fibrillation

Risk factor	Score	HAS-BLED score	Bleeding rate (%/year)
Hypertension	1	0	1.13
Abnormal renal/hepatic function	1 (each)	1	1.02
Stroke	1	2	1.88
Bleeding	1	3	3.74
Labile INRs	1	4	8.70
Elderly (≥65 years)	1	≥5	Insufficient data
Drugs or alcohol use	1 (each)		

to patients with minor haemorrhagic transformation. and is probably beneficial Therefore, our practice is to start DOACs soon after stroke, rather than waiting for 2 weeks.

- For patients with AF who suffer an ischaemic stroke or TIA despite therapeutic anticoagulation, there are no data to indicate that either increasing the intensity of anticoagulation or adding an antiplatelet agent provides additional protection against future ischaemic events. In addition, both strategies are associated with an increase in bleeding risk. Switching anticoagulant agent is pragmatic e.g. from Xa inhibitor to a direct thrombin inhibitor or to warfarin but unproven in RCTs compared to continued current therapy. In such a scenario, it is important to assess compliance, correct dose, and for any drug interactions that may undermine the therapeutic effect of an OAC.
- Patients with confluent leucoaraiosis on brain imaging have a markedly increased risk of bleeding on warfarin. In many of these cases, microbleeds can be seen on gradient echo (GRE) MRI but whether this allows one to identify those who are at high risk of warfarin-related bleeding is uncertain.
- About one-third of patients who present with AF and an ischaemic stroke will be found to have other potential causes for the stroke such as carotid stenosis. For these patients, treatment decisions should focus on the presumed most likely stroke origin. In some cases, it will be appropriate to initiate anticoagulation, because of the AF, and additional therapy (such as CEA).

Warfarin or DOACs in older people

- Anticoagulation is often underused in older people owing to fears of bleeding complications.
- The risk of these is of the order of 2% per annum.
- Many physicians have then been deterred from prescribing warfarin in the frail elderly with stroke because of the view that this trial figure, where INRs are closely monitored, is likely to be an underestimate.

However, the reality seems to be that anticoagulation is generally well tolerated in older people—exactly the group with the highest incidence of AF and the greatest risk of recurrent stroke. This was well shown in the Birmingham AF treatment in the aged (BAFTA) study, which randomized almost 1000 patents with an average age of 81 years between warfarin and aspirin. The aspirin group suffered more strokes and the same small number of bleeding complications as the anticoagulation group.

- It has been estimated that an elderly patient taking warfarin would have to fall approximately 300 times per year for the risk of bleeding complications from falling to outweigh the benefits for prevention of embolic stroke.
- The key issue is then, not so much a crystal ball estimate of a perceived falls risk in older patients, but more the practicality of a patient having appropriate compliance; in this setting use of a DOAC rather than warfarin is much simpler.

Secondary stroke prevention in AF patients unable to be anticoagulated

- In practice, such a scenario is rare as the risk of recurrent cardioembolic stroke usually outweighs the risk of bleeding, but there will always be individual cases where this arises.
- For such patients, left atrial appendage occlusion (LAAO) may be an option as the left atrial appendage is the most common (but not the only) source of embolism in AF.
- In the LAAOS III RCT of surgical LAAO in 4770 AF patients otherwise undergoing cardiopulmonary bypass surgery, cardioembolic stroke was significantly reduced over 5 years of follow-up (4.6% occlusion group compared to 6.9% no occlusion HR 0.67, CI 0.52–0.84), although most subjects in both groups were still taking antithrombotic treatment.
- Less invasive percutaneous or endovascular LAAO may be technically possible depending on the 'shape' of the LAA. The commonest shape is the 'chicken wing' followed by the 'cactus', 'windsock', and 'cauliflower'. The latter is most associated with embolic stroke.
- A number of devices—Amplatzer Plug and Amulet, Watchman, and Watchmen FLX—have been trialled, mostly in unrandomized open-label studies, but the results of the heterogeneous PROTECT AF and PREVAIL RCTS and the Watchman device registry, saw the FDA approve LAAO in AF patients with a high risk of bleeding on OAC in 2015.
- All patients undergoing LAAO will need to take a single antiplatelet as a minimum for 6 months until the device is well endothelialized.
- Access to LAAO is highly variable across countries and demographics but remains an option for stroke secondary prevention for highly selected patients.

Anticoagulation for other cardioembolic sources

Valvular heart disease

- Recurrent embolism occurs in 30–65% of patients with *rheumatic mitral valve* disease who have a history of a previous embolic event—therefore anticoagulation is frequently given, ideally before the onset of AF, which is a frequent complication of late-stage disease.

- The risk of stroke is high in untreated patients with *mechanical heart valve prostheses* and lifelong warfarin anticoagulation is standard therapy. DOACs are not licenced for this indication, and long-term warfarin is the preferred option because in the RE-ALIGN study, 252 patients underwent randomization: 168 were assigned to receive dabigatran and 84 were assigned to warfarin. The trial was terminated prematurely because of an excess of thromboembolic and bleeding events in the dabigatran group. Stroke occurred in 5% of the dabigatran group and none of the warfarin group; major bleeding occurred in 4% and 2%, respectively.

- The risk of stroke is lower with *bioprosthetic cardiac valves* and antiplatelet agents alone are often prescribed in the long term. Some clinicians use anticoagulants for the first few months post-valve insertion, although there are no trial data for this approach.

- *Mitral valve prolapse* is the most common form of valve disease in adults but its embolic risk is low and it does not usually merit anticoagulation.

- Systemic embolism in isolated *aortic valve disease* is increasingly recognized because of thrombi or calcium emboli, but antiplatelet therapy is usually used.

Acute MI and left ventricular thrombus

- Stroke or systemic embolism is less common among uncomplicated MI patients but can occur in up to 12% of patients with acute MI complicated by an LV thrombus.

- The incidence of embolism is highest in the first 1–3 months after MI.

- Thrombus may persist for 2 years in a quarter of cases but is rarely associated with late embolic events.

- For patients with an ischaemic stroke or TIA caused by an acute MI in whom LV mural thrombus is identified by echocardiography, oral anticoagulation is reasonable.

- It is also reasonable to anticoagulate patients with akinetic left ventricular segments on echocardiography although again there are no good trial data on which to base this.

Cardiomyopathy

- The incidence of stroke seems to be inversely proportional to ejection fraction.

- Figures from the Survival and Ventricular Enlargement (SAVE) study showed:
  - for an ejection fraction of about 32%, a stroke rate of 0.8% per year
  - for an ejection fraction of about 23%, a stroke rate of 1.7% per year.

- Warfarin, or a DOAC, is sometimes prescribed to prevent cardioembolic events in patients with cardiomyopathy. However, there are no RCT data to substantiate this.

Anticoagulation for embolic stroke of undetermined source (ESUS)

- ESUS was historically thought to be largely driven by undiagnosed paroxysmal AF or other cardioembolic sources.
- Two large, well-conducted RCTs of DOACs investigating both dabigatran (RE-SPECT- ESUS) and rivaroxaban (NAVIGATE-ESUS) showed no significant benefit over conventional antiplatelet therapy in preventing recurrent stroke.
- The subsequent apixaban to prevent recurrence after cryptogenic stroke in patients with atrial cardiopathy (ARCADIA) trial of 1015 participants also failed to show the benefit of DOAC over aspirin, in a potentially enriched cardio-embolic population of ESUS patients.
- Therefore there is no evidence for using anticoagulation in ESUS, and antiplatelet therapy is the first-line therapy.

Is there a role for combined antiplatelet therapy and anticoagulation in stroke secondary prevention?

- It is rare for a patient to have a clear indication for long-term antiplatelet and anticoagulation due to the risk of bleeding in cerebrovascular disease. Uncomplicated MI and AF can be managed with a DOAC but if a patient with AF undergoes acute coronary stenting, they will need antiplatelet therapy for a fixed time.
- For patients with advanced but stable atherosclerotic disease—coronary and peripheral (including >50% carotid), evidence from the COMPASS RCT of 27,395 participants, saw an overall mortality benefit in patients taking **low-dose** DOAC (rivaroxaban 2.5 mg BD) and 100 mg aspirin OD compared to aspirin alone. It is important to note that none of the participants of COMPASS had recent stroke at the time of inclusion.

New antithrombotic treatments in stroke secondary prevention—Factor XI inhibitors

- Factor XI inhibition within the contact (intrinsic) coagulation pathway prevents the amplification of thrombin production and pathological thrombi while the tissue factor (extrinsic) pathway can maintain thrombin formation for haemostasis. In this way, Factor XI inhibition is thought to provide anticoagulation but not cause bleeding.
- Two Factor XI inhibitors have been trialled to date in stroke secondary prevention—milvexian (AXIOMATIC-SSP) and asundexian (PACIFIC - AF, AMI, and -STROKE) as adjuncts to existing best medical treatment. Although there was not a significant reduction in ischaemic stroke in the treatment groups, there was no excess bleeding.
- Asundexian is currently being further tested as stroke secondary prevention against best medical treatment in atherosclerotic causes of ischaemic stroke in the OCEANIC-STROKE study.

Treatment of patent foramen ovale and stroke

For many years, while PFO was clearly a risk factor for stroke, no trials had shown that PFO closure actually reduced the risk of further stroke.

Ultimately, this was shown to be because when other risk factors were present, these were much more important than the PFO itself. Only when patients with no other risk factor apart from a PFO were treated were positive results obtained.

- Initial RCTs did not verify the superiority of PFO closure over conservative management (PC and RESPECT trials).
- Subsequent Trials with an 'enriched' study population, showed a marked reduction in stroke risk following PFO closure (CLOSE and REDUCE trials).
- In the CLOSE trial, no patient in the intention-to-treat PFO closure group had a stroke, while stroke occurred in 14 patients in the antiplatelet-only arm (HR 0.03; 95% CI 0 to 0.26; P <0.001). The composite secondary outcome of stroke/TIA or systemic embolism occurred in significantly fewer patients in the PFO closure group compared with the antiplatelet-only group (3.4% vs. 8.9%; HR 0.39; 95% CI 0.16 to 0.82; $P = 0.01$).
- In the REDUCE trial, recurrent ischaemic stroke occurred in six patients (1.4%) in the PFO closure group compared with 12 (5.4%) in the antiplatelet-only group (HR 0.23; 95% CI 0.09 to 0.62; $P = 0.002$)
- Meta-analysis of trials with an average follow-up of 3.8 years reported the NNT with PFO closure to prevent one stroke overall was 37 (95% CI 26 to 68) and 21 in patients with high-risk PFO features (95% CI 16 to 61).
- A recent trial, DEFENSE-PFO (Device Closure vs. Medical therapy for Cryptogenic Stroke Patients With High-Risk PFO), studied a similar cohort as CLOSE and REDUCE and reported a 2-year ischaemic stroke rate of 10.3% in the medical group (5 out of 60 subjects) compared with zero (out of 60) in the closure group ($P = 0.013$).
- Our current practice is to make the decision to perform PFO closure in cryptogenic stroke with a multidisciplinary team, comprising a neurologist or stroke physician and a cardiologist.

The typical patient we would refer is:

Younger (<60 years old)

Has no other risk factors for stroke (uncontrolled hypertension, diabetes, cholesterol, major other cardiac disease, or AF, thrombophilia, continued heavy smoking or drug use).

Has no indication of anticoagulation

Carotid endarterectomy

Symptomatic carotid artery stenosis is associated with a high risk of early recurrent stroke. Two large trials, the North American Symptomatic Carotid
Endarterectomy Trial (NASCET) and the European Carotid Surgery Trial
(ECST), have shown that CEA is highly effective at preventing recurrent
stroke in patients with severe recently symptomatic carotid stenosis.

Management depends on the degree of stenosis, as indicated in the following sections. The degree of stenosis varies according to the method
used to measure it (Fig. 10.3), and the following advice is given for measurements made using the NASCET method.

≥70% symptomatic stenosis

- Removing the stenosis by endarterectomy almost abolishes the risk of
  recurrent ipsilateral stenosis.
- This has to be balanced against the risk of surgery—about 5% stroke
  risk in good units—but the benefits greatly outweigh the risk.
- The 2-year (3-year in ECST) risk of all stroke and perioperative death
  was reduced by CEA from 32.3% to 15.8% in NASCET, and from 21.9%
  to 12.3% in ECST.
- The risk of stroke, if untreated, and therefore the benefit, decline
  markedly in the first weeks after stroke. Therefore, to maximize the
  benefit, the operation needs to be done urgently.

50–69% stenosis

- There is less benefit to operating in this group; the trial showed a small
  benefit for this group if CEA was carried out soon after symptoms
  (within 2 weeks), but not if treatment was delayed.
- It is reasonable to treat a patient with this degree of stenosis if they
  have other indicators of high risk, and particularly if they can be
  operated on within the first 2 weeks of symptoms.

<50% stenosis

For patients with carotid stenosis, the trials showed no benefit and operation should not be routinely performed. If a patient has clear evidence
of embolic infarction and no other embolic source and a highly ulcerated
unstable plaque CEA may be still be reasonable to discuss—acknowledging
this sits outside of evidence base from RCTs.

Indicators of high risk

- Age >75 years
- Male gender
- Recent symptoms
- Ulcerated plaque on angiography
- Hemispheric symptoms rather than transient monocular blindness
- Stroke (rather than TIA).

Indicators of lower risk

- Opposite of high-risk indicators listed earlier
- Distal collapse of the ICA.

Timing of CEA

- The chances of recurrent stroke are greatest in the first few weeks after the initial event, and much of the benefit of CEA is lost if surgery is delayed.
- A pooled analysis of data from both NASCET and ECST data has made this very clear.
- Therefore, for all patients with TIA, operation should be performed urgently.
- For patients with stroke, particularly those with larger stroke, some surgeons like to wait 2–4 weeks before operating as the operative risk is higher and there is a risk of reperfusion injury and haemorrhage into the acute infarct after reopening the stenosed carotid artery. There is no good evidence to guide what to do here. We tend to operate urgently when the stroke is small on brain imaging (<1–2 cm maximum dimension) but delay 2 weeks if it is larger.

Table 10.8 shows the absolute risk reduction with CEA for symptomatic carotid stenosis from the pooled analysis of RCTs. It shows that the benefit of operation declines as the time since last symptoms increases, is greater in males, and is greater in older people.

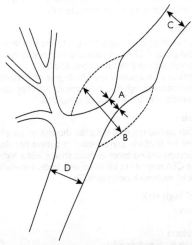

Fig. 10.3 Measurement of carotid stenosis. The degree of stenosis will vary according to the methods used. The advice given here is for measurement using the NASCET method. The ECST method has become less popular because one has to 'guess' where the arterial lumen prior to the stenosis was. The common carotid method (CCM) is simple.

NASCET method: C − A/C × 100

ECST method: B − A/B × 100

CCM: D − A/D.

NASCET stenosis can be approximately converted to ECST by using the simple form.

Table 10.8 The absolute risk reduction with surgery in 5-year actual risk of ipsilateral carotid ischaemic stroke and any stroke or death within 30 days after surgery from the pooled analysis of the RCTs

Factor	All patients
Time since last event (weeks):	Surgical vs. medical (ARR; 95% CI)
<2	85/627 vs. 122/558 (9.2; 4.7 to 13.7)
2–4 weeks	63/602 vs. 72/452 (6.4; 2.1 to 10.7)
4–12 weeks	147/1257 vs. 148/1055 (2.9; 0.0 to 5.8)
Gender:	
Male	253/2307 vs. 301/1868 (6.0; 3.8 to 8.2)
Female	134/929 vs. 107/789 (−0.4; −3.8 to 3.0)
Age in years:	
<65	186/1645 vs. 163/1255 (2.2; −0.3 to 4.7)
65–74	169/1303 vs. 180/1105 (4.1; 1.2 to 7.1)
≥75	32/288 vs. 65/297 (11.9; 5.7 to 18.1)

Adapted from *Lancet*, 361(9352), Rothwell PM, Eliasziw M, Gutnikov SA, et al. Analysis of pooled data from the randomised controlled trials of endarterectomy for symptomatic carotid stenosis, pp. 107–116, Copyright (2003), with permission from Elsevier.

Choosing a patient for CEA

When deciding whether to operate on a patient with symptomatic stenosis, a number of considerations are important:

- Does the patient have a severe stenosis (>70%)?
- If not, does the patient have a 50–69% stenosis and are they at particularly high risk as indicated by the earlier-mentioned markers?
- What is the estimated life expectancy of the patient? This needs to be at least 2 years to obtain reasonable benefit from CEA for symptomatic disease (see ➲ Interim life tables, Table 1.5, p. 26)?
- Can the patient be operated on soon? If there is a delay then any benefit of surgery may be negated.
- Does the surgeon have an acceptable operative risk (not more than 5–7%) and do they do enough CEAs to maintain experience? It is important that outcome figures from units are audited, ideally by an independent physician. Outcome is better for patients looked after in larger specialist units.
- In patients with larger strokes, one needs to balance the expected life expectancy and whether there is much function left to lose in that ICA territory if further strokes occur. For this reason, we would not operate in very large MCA strokes, but limit intervention to patients with TIA or small to moderate-sized stroke and moderate disability.

Complications of carotid endarterectomy

Despite having definite benefit, CEA has risks although these are much reduced in specialized units. Causes of stroke include:

- dislodgement of embolic material during carotid manipulation and dissection
- haemodynamic ischaemia during clamping of the carotid artery
- embolism from the site of CEA, which is denuded of endothelium and thrombogenic
- cerebral haemorrhage and seizures owing to reperfusion injury.

Other complications include cranial nerve injuries, particularly hypoglossal nerve injury.

Carotid stenting (CAS)

- This offers an alternative to CEA
- Potential advantages are its less invasive nature, with the lack of an incision and potential for cranial nerve palsies
- Initial studies used angioplasty alone, but restenosis rates were very high, and the standard is now to use stenting
- It allows treatment of more distal stenosis inaccessible to surgery.

A number of trials have compared angioplasty and stenting with CEA but as yet no clear benefit for stenting has been shown.

Carotid and vertebral artery transluminal angioplasty study (CAVATAS)

- This randomized trial compared angioplasty with surgical therapy among 504 symptomatic carotid patients, in whom only 26% received stents.
- Major outcome events within 30 days did not differ between endovascular treatment and surgery groups, with a 30-day risk of stroke or death of 10.0% and 9.9%, respectively.
- Restenosis was significantly more common in the angioplasty arm.

Stent-protected angioplasty versus carotid endarterectomy in symptomatic patients (SPACE)

- A total of 1200 patients with symptomatic carotid artery stenosis were randomly assigned within 180 days of TIA or moderate stroke to carotid artery stenting ($n = 605$) or CEA ($n = 595$)
- The primary end point, the rate of death, or ipsilateral ischaemic stroke from randomization to 30 days after the procedure, was 6.84% with carotid artery stenting and 6.34% with CEA (absolute difference 0.51%, 90% CI −1.89–2.91%, $P = 0.09$)
- This trial showed no significant difference but a small trend towards better outcome with CEA.

EVA-3S

- A randomized trial comparing stenting with endarterectomy in patients with a symptomatic carotid stenosis ≥60%.
- The trial was stopped prematurely after the inclusion of 527 patients for reasons of both safety and futility.
- The 30-day incidence of any stroke or death was 3.9% after endarterectomy (95% CI 2.0–7.2) and 9.6% after stenting (95% CI 6.4–14.0); RR of stenting compared with endarterectomy of 2.5 (95% CI 1.2–5.1).
- Why this trial showed such a poor outcome for stenting while SPACE showed no significant difference is uncertain.

International Carotid Stenting Study (ICSS)

- This trial randomized 1700 patients with symptomatic carotid stenosis between CEA and carotid stenting
- The primary end point was any stroke, death, or peri-procedural MI

- The 120-day primary end point was more common in the stenting group compared with the CEA group: 8.5% vs. 5.1%, odds ratio 1.73 (1.18–2.52)
- The final results showed that after a median follow-up for both procedures of 4.2 years there was no significant difference primary outcome of fatal or disabling stroke HR of 1.08 (95% CI 0.73–1.60; $P = 0.69$)
- CEA was significantly more efficacious than carotid artery stenting in preventing any form of stroke more than 30 days after completion of treatment, (excluding the perioperative period). At 1 year, the rate of any stroke was 1.8% vs. 2.9%, respectively, and at 5 years, the rate was 5.8% vs. 9.2%, respectively.

Carotid Revascularization Endarterectomy Versus Stenting Trial (CREST)

- 2502 patients with symptomatic or asymptomatic carotid stenosis were randomized to carotid artery stenting or CEA
- The primary end point was stroke, MI, or death from any cause during the periprocedural period, or any ipsilateral stroke within 4 years after randomization
- Over a median follow-up period of 2.5 years, there was no significant difference in the estimated 4-year rates of the primary end point between the stenting group and the endarterectomy group (7.2% and 6.8%, respectively $P = 0.51$)
- The 4-year rate of stroke or death was 6.4% with stenting and 4.7% with endarterectomy ($P = 0.03$); the rates among symptomatic patients were 8.0% and 6.4% ($P = 0.14$); the rates among asymptomatic patients were 4.5% and 2.7% ($P = 0.07$), respectively
- Periprocedural rates for stroke were (4.1% vs. 2.3%, $P = 0.01$), and for MI (1.1% vs. 2.3%, $P = 0.03$)
- After this period, the incidences of ipsilateral stroke with stenting and with endarterectomy were similarly low (2.0% and 2.4%, respectively; $P = 0.85$).

Current recommendations

- Taken together, the trials show that the risk of periprocedural stroke is slightly higher after stenting than CEA, although many of these strokes are non-disabling.
- Our interpretation is that carotid stenting should only be performed in patients who are unsuitable for CEA
- It may be used in selected patients in whom stenosis is difficult to access surgically, when medical conditions that greatly increase the risk for surgery are present, or other specific circumstances exist such as radiation-induced stenosis or restenosis after CEA
- Initially it was thought that it might be particularly suitable for more elderly patients, but data from SPACE and the run-in phase to the CREST trial have suggested the risk of stenting is in fact higher in older people.

Asymptomatic carotid stenosis

- Treatment of asymptomatic carotid stenosis is primary not secondary prevention but is covered here as it is an important area
- The situation differs greatly from symptomatic carotid stenosis because the risk of stroke if it is treated medically is much lower— 1–2% per annum compared with 20–30% in the first year for symptomatic stenosis
- Although trials have shown that CEA results in a large RR reduction, the benefit to an individual patient, or absolute risk reduction, is much lower. This is because the risk of stroke in these patients is much less than that in symptomatic stenosis
- The benefit may be even less than that found in trials because, with the widespread use of more effective secondary prevention drugs such as statins, the annual risk of stroke in medically treated patients may now be nearer 1% compared with the approximately 2% found in the RCTs.

Two large randomized trials, summarized in Table 10.9, have compared the best medical therapy with the operation for asymptomatic carotid stenosis.

Asymptomatic Carotid Atherosclerosis Study (ACAS)

- Between 1987 and 1993, 1662 patients with asymptomatic carotid artery stenosis with ≥60% stenosis were randomized to CEA or medical therapy
- After a median follow-up of 2.7 years, with 4657 patient-years of observation, the aggregate risk estimated over 5 years for ipsilateral stroke and any perioperative stroke or death was 5.1% for surgical patients and 11.0% for patients treated medically (aggregate risk reduction of 53% (95% CI 22–72%))
- The perioperative risk for CEA was very low (1.5%, excluding risk of angiography), and this made some question how generalizable these results were. However, a similar benefit was found in the larger ACST study.

Asymptomatic Carotid Surgery Trial (ACST)

- Between 1993 and 2003, 3120 asymptomatic patients were randomized between immediate CEA (half underwent CEA by 1 month, 88% by 1 year) and indefinite deferral of any CEA (only 4% per year underwent CEA), and were followed for a mean of 3.4 years
- Including perioperative strokes, the 5-year risk of stroke was 6.4% for CEA versus 11.8% for medical treatment, and 3.5% for CEA versus 6.1% for medical treatment for fatal or disabling strokes
- The absolute risk reduction was similar in ACAS (2.7%) and ACST (2.5%)
- As can be seen, although the RR reduction is large, the absolute risk reduction is very small, i.e. a lot of operations need to be done to prevent one stroke

A meta-analysis of the two trials suggested that the group who particularly benefit are younger men (see Fig. 10.4).

Table 10.9 The main outcomes from the Asymptomatic Carotid Surgery Trial

			Outcomes from ACAS and ACST					
Trial	n	Operative risk (%)	Risk of stroke with BMT (%)	Risk of stroke with CEA* (%)	ARR with CEA (%)	RRR with CEA (%)	NNT with CEA	Strokes prevented per 1000 CEAs
5-year outcomes								
ACAS	1662	2.3	11.0	5.1	5.9	54	17	59
ACST	3120	2.8	11.8	6.4	5.4	46	19	53
10-year outcomes								
ACST	3120	2.8	17.9	13.4	4.6	26	22	46

*The 5-year and 10-year CEA data include the 30-day risk of death or stroke. ACAS, Asymptomatic Carotid Atherosclerosis Study; ACST, Asymptomatic Carotid Surgery Trial; ARR, absolute risk reduction in stroke; BMT, best medical therapy; CEA, carotid endarterectomy; NNT, number needed to treat to prevent one stroke; CEA, carotid endarterectomy; NNT, number needed to treat to prevent one stroke; RRR, relative risk reduction in stroke.

Reproduced from *Nat Rev Cardiol*, 9(2), Naylor AR, Time to rethink management strategies in asymptomatic carotid artery disease, pp. 116–124, Copyright (2011), with permission from Macmillan Publishers Ltd.

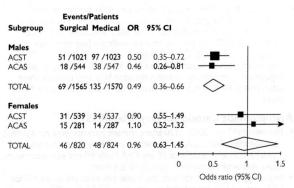

Fig. 10.4 The effect of endarterectomy for asymptomatic carotid stenosis on the risk of any stroke and operative death by sex in ACST and ACAS.

Reproduced from *Stroke*, 35, Rothwell PM, Goldstein LB, Carotid endarterectomy for asymptomatic carotid stenosis: Asymptomatic Carotid Surgery Trial, pp. 2425–2427, Copyright (2004), with permission from Wolters Kluwer Health, Inc.

Second asymptomatic carotid surgery trial (ACST2)

- This RCT compared CEA and CAS for asymptomatic carotid stenosis.
- It did not include a best medical therapy arm so cannot tell us whether CAS is beneficial compared with not operating.
- Between 15 January 2008 and 31 December 2020, 3625 patients in 130 centres were randomly allocated, 1811 to CAS and 1814 to CEA, with a mean 5 years of follow-up.
- Overall, 1% had a disabling stroke or death procedurally (15 allocated to CAS and 18 to CEA) and 2% had a non-disabling procedural stroke (48 allocated to CAS and 29 to CEA).
- Kaplan–Meier estimates of 5-year non-procedural stroke were 2.5% in each group for fatal or disabling stroke, and 5.3% with CAS versus 4.5% with CEA for any stroke (rate ratio [RR] 1.16, 95% CI 0.86–1.57; $P = 0.33$).
- There was no significant difference between CAS and CEA.
- The stroke risk rate with either, putting the operative and long-term risk together, was about 5% over 5 years, or 1% per annum. This is similar to the recent estimate of stroke risk in medically treated asymptomatic stenosis.

Evidence that stroke risk in asymptomatic carotid stenosis is falling

- There is increasing evidence that, with current best medical therapy, the risk of stroke in asymptomatic carotid stenosis is falling.
- In the ACST it was approximately 2% per annum.
- Analysis of more recent prospective studies shows it may now be 1% (see Fig. 10.5).
- In fact, this parallels findings from ACST and ACAS in which the risk of stroke in the medically treated arm fell over time. In 1995, the 5-year risk of any stroke in ACAS was 3.5% per annum in the medical therapy arm. When the data from ACST were reported in 2004, the first 5-year risk of any stroke in medically treated patients had fallen to 2.4% per annum. In 2010, the 10-year data from ACST showed that the second 5-year risk of any stroke in medically treated patients had fallen further to 1.4% per annum.
- If the risk is 1% there is little benefit from operating for unselected patients with asymptomatic carotid stenosis.

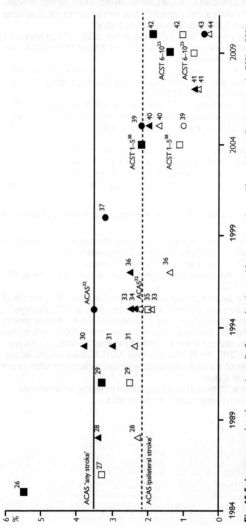

Fig. 10.5 Average annual stroke rates in medically treated patients with asymptomatic carotid stenosis. ν indicates any stroke 70% to 99% stenosis; λ, any stroke 60% to 99% stenosis; π, any stroke 50% to 99% stenosis; Υ, ipsilateral stroke 70% to 99% stenosis; □, ipsilateral stroke 60% to 99% stenosis; ρ, ipsilateral stroke 50% to 99% stenosis.

Who should one operate on for asymptomatic stenosis?

- Different clinicians have different views
- It is essential to give patients true information about the potential benefit using data based on the absolute risk reduction or NNT
- We explain to patients that for every 100 patients operated on, over the next 5 years five disabling strokes or deaths will be avoided. This means that 95% will have no benefit over that time period. Many patients feel that this is too small a benefit to warrant intervention
- There is great interest in identifying predictors of stroke risk, which would allow a high-risk group to be selected.
  - In the multicentre Asymptomatic Carotid Emboli Study (ACES) study it has been shown that embolic signals on TCD predict stroke risk.
  - Plaque morphology on ultrasound particularly hypolucency was shown to predict stroke risk in the asymptomatic carotid stenosis and risk of stroke (ACSRS) study
  - Plaque morphology on MRI, including intraplaque haemorrhage has been shown to predict risk in observational studies
- However these risk markers have not yet been incorporated into large RCTs of asymptomatic carotid stenosis versus best medical therapy and are not widely used in the clinical setting
- There is no evidence to support routine CEA in patients with asymptomatic ICA stenosis undergoing coronary artery bypass grafting (CABG) surgery.

Carotid occlusion

- The risk of stroke in carotid occlusion is less than that with tight carotid stenosis but is nevertheless increased
- The risk is highest soon after the occlusion. Presumably with time, collaterals occur and/or those high-risk patients with poor collaterals have strokes, leaving a lower-risk group
- CEA is not possible in this patient group
- It is possible to bypass the occlusion by an extracranial–intracranial (EC–IC) bypass. In this operation, an anastomosis is made between the superficial temporal branch of the external carotid artery and an intracranial branch of the internal carotid artery through a burr hole in the skull
- However, the EC–IC bypass study showed no benefit for this operation in patients with carotid occlusion, stenosis, or occlusion of the MCA. The perioperative risk of stroke was high
- Therefore EC–IC bypass is not routinely performed
- Studies have shown that only a small proportion of patients with carotid occlusion have impaired cerebral haemodynamics and, in prospective follow-up, it is this group that is at high risk of recurrent stroke
- This has led to the suggestion that EC–IC bypass may benefit this subgroup. No estimate of haemodynamic status was performed in the EC–IC bypass
- Cerebral haemodynamics can be measured using PET, or with estimation of cerebral blood flow (with xenon, CT perfusion, or TCD before and after a vasodilatory stimulus such as increased inspired carbon dioxide or IV acetazolamide)
- This approach with a selection of patients with impaired haemodynamics for EC–IC bypass was tested in the Carotid Occlusion Surgery Study (COSS). Of 195 patients with arteriographically confirmed carotid occlusion causing hemispheric symptoms within 120 days and haemodynamic cerebral ischaemia identified by ipsilateral increased oxygen extraction fraction measured by PET, 97 were randomized to receive surgery and 98 to no surgery. The trial was terminated early for futility
- Two-year rates for ipsilateral ischaemic stroke were 21.0% (95% CI 12.8–29.2%; 20 events) for the surgical group and 22.7% (95% CI 13.9–31.6%; 20 events), i.e. no significant difference between the two groups.
- Moya-Moya (➔ see unusual causes, Chapter 11) is characterized by intracranial ICA occlusion—often bilateral, with associated fragile new vessel formation. Management of this condition is covered in ➔ Chapter 11.

Vertebral stenosis

- One in four strokes occur in the posterior circulation and, after stenosis of the internal carotid artery, stenosis of the vertebral artery is the second commonest site of focal atherosclerotic disease in the cerebral circulation
- The vertebral artery is conventionally divided into four segments. The first (V1) is from the origin of the vertebral artery to where it enters the foramen in the transverse process of the fifth or sixth cervical vertebra. The second segment (V2) is the part that courses cranially through the transverse foramina, until the artery emerges beside the lateral mass of the atlas. The last extracranial segment (V3) then forms a loop that allows free movement of the head. The intracranial segment (V4) begins where the artery pierces the atlanto-occipital membrane, the dura mater, and the arachnoid mater, and ends when the two vertebral arteries fuse to form the basilar artery ventral to the medullopontine junction.
- Within the vertebral artery, the most frequent site for stenosis is the origin of the vessel but it can also involve the distal (intracranial) vertebral artery
- It has been shown in prospective studies that symptomatic vertebral stenosis is associated with a high risk of recurrent stroke—comparable to that of high-grade symptomatic internal carotid artery stenosis
- As for carotid stenosis, the recurrent stroke risk is highest in the first few weeks
- The risk is much higher for intracranial compared with extracranial stenosis. In a prospective study of patients with posterior circulation TIA or stroke, all of whom had angiographic imaging with CTA or MRA of their posterior circulation, 24.6% of patients with vertebral or basilar stenosis had recurrent stroke within 90 days versus 7.2% in those without (odds ratio, 4.2; 95% CI 2.1–8.6; P <0.0001). Ninety-day stroke risk was higher (33%) with intracranial than extracranial stenosis (16.2%).

Stenting for vertebral stenosis

- Unlike the extracranial internal carotid artery, the vertebral artery is surgically inaccessible and endarterectomy is fraught with complications (to access the vessel the surgeon has to remove part of the clavicle, and pneumothorax and interruption of the sympathetic chain are common complications). The vessel is, however, easily accessible endovascularly in the majority of cases
- Similarly, the vertebral artery is far more technically challenging to image with duplex ultrasound compared to the internal carotid artery, leading to problems with (under)diagnosis of such lesions. Improvements with non-invasive imaging by CEMRA and CTA show promise for routine screening of all posterior circulation ischaemic stroke patients
- Large case series have shown that endovascular angioplasty of the extracranial vertebral artery is a technical success and reasonably safe with perioperative stroke risk of about 1–2% for extracranial stenosis and 5–10% for intracranial stenosis

- Published experience to date has seen up to a 30% 2-year re-stenosis rate for extracranial vertebral stenosis treated with angioplasty alone and, following both carotid and coronary endovascular experience, expandable vertebral artery-specific wall stents have now been developed
- Two RCTs have examined stenting in both extracranial and intracranial stenosis
  - VAST showed no difference between patients with vertebral stenosis treated with stenting or medical therapy but this was only in 115 patients.
  - VIST recruited 182 patients (85% extracranial, 17% intracranial). Patients with recently symptomatic vertebral stenosis were randomized between best medical treatment plus angioplasty/ stenting or best medical treatment alone. Although underpowered there seemed to be a reduced stroke risk with stenting. The HR for the primary endpoint (stenting vs. no stenting) was 0.4 (95% CI 0.14– 1.13; $P = 0.08$), with an absolute risk reduction of 25 strokes per 1000 person-years. After adjustment for days between last symptoms and randomization the HR was 0.34 (95% CI 0.12–0.98; $P = 0.046$).
- Two RCTS (SAMMPRIS and VISSIT) examined stenting in intracranial vertebral stenosis only as part of larger trials including intracranial stenosis in multiple vessels. Both showed no benefit for intracranial stenosis as a whole with outcomes better with best medical therapy. Only SAMMPRIS allowed the presentation of results separately for vertebral stenosis. For both basilar and intracranial vertebral stenosis outcome was worse with stenting than medical therapy.
- An individual patient analysis of the VIST, VAST, and SAMMPRIS data found that in the stenting group, the frequency of periprocedural stroke or death was higher for intracranial stenosis than for extracranial stenosis (ten (16%) of 64 patients vs. one (1%) of 121 patients; P <0.0001).
- During 1036 person-years of follow-up, the HR for any stroke in the stenting group compared with the medical treatment group was 0.81% CI 0.45–1.44; $P = 0.47$).
- For extracranial stenosis alone the HR was 0.63 (95% CI 0.27–1.46) and for intracranial stenosis alone it was 1.06 (0.46–2.42)
- The conclusions were:
  - There is no benefit for stenting of intracranial stenosis due to the high intraoperative stroke risk for stenting in this location.
  - Stenting for extracranial stenosis might be beneficial, but further larger trials are required to determine the treatment effect in this subgroup. The ongoing Chinese VISTA trial is examining stenting in extracranial vertebral stenosis, using a drug eluting stent to reduce risk of restenosis.

Intracranial stenosis

- Data from prospective studies show that patients with symptomatic intracranial atherosclerosis have a high risk of recurrent stroke.
- The Warfarin Aspirin Symptomatic Intracranial Disease (WASID) study showed warfarin was no better than aspirin in secondary stroke prevention.
- It is possible to stent intracranial stenoses but this has a significant risk.
- The SAMMPRIS trial found that intracranial stenting, with the Wingspan stent, was associated with a worse outcome compared with best medical therapy.
- Early results showed that, by 30 days, 33 (14.7%) of 224 patients in the stenting group and 13 (5.8%) of 227 patients in the medical group had died or had a stroke.
- This difference persisted in longer-term follow-up with similar longer-term stroke rates in the two groups. During a median follow-up of 32.4 months, 34 (15%) of 227 patients in the medical group and 52 (23%) of 224 patients in the stenting group had a primary end point event. Beyond 30 days, 21 (10%) of 210 patients in the medical group and 19 (10%) of 191 patients in the stenting group had a primary end point.
- Best medical therapy was intensive with aspirin (325 mg per day) for the duration of follow-up, clopidogrel (75 mg per day) for 90 days after enrolment, management of the primary risk factors (targeting systolic BP lower than 140 mm Hg (<130 mm Hg if diabetic) and LDL-cholesterol lower than 1.81 mmol/L, and management of secondary risk factors (diabetes, non-HDL cholesterol, smoking, weight, exercise) with the help of a lifestyle modification programme.
- The results of SAMMPRIS were reproduced in the 112 patients in the VISSIT study, which used a different balloon mounting stenting system (a potential criticism of SAMMPRIS was the type of stenting—Wingspan® system used) and confirmed the benefit of intensive medical treatment over endovascular intervention.
- Intraoperative stroke risk was particularly high when those arteries with perforator arteries coming off them were stented; the basilar and middle cerebral arteries.
- Stenting should only now be an option considered for those individual patients with recurrent events despite optimal medical management as described in SAMMPRIS and VISSIT.
- We recommended that such patients receive intensive medical management, following the protocol adopted in SAMMPRIS.

Further reading

Introducing stroke prevention

McAlister FA, Majumdar SR, Padwal RS, *et al.* (2014). Case management for blood pressure and lipid level control after minor stroke: PREVENTION randomized controlled trial. *CMAJ* **186**, 698.

Lifestyle measures

de Lorgeril M, Salen P, Martin J-L, *et al.* (1999). Mediterranean diet, traditional risk factors, and the rate of cardiovascular complications after myocardial infarction. Final Report of the Lyon Diet Heart Study. *Circulation* **99**, 779–785.

Edjoc RK, Reid RD, Sharma M (2012). The effectiveness of smoking cessation interventions in smokers with cerebrovascular disease: a systematic review. *BMJ Open* **2**, e002022.

Tan CE, Glantz SA (2012). Association between smokefree legislation and hospitalizations for cardiac, cerebrovascular and respiratory diseases: a meta-analysis. *Circulation* **126**, 2177–2183.

Blood pressure

Beckett NS, Peters R, Fletcher AE, et al. (2008). Treatment of hypertension in patients 80 years of age or older. *N Engl J Med* **358**, 1887–1898.

Boan AD, Lackland DT, Ovbiagele B (2014). Lowering of blood pressure for recurrent stroke prevention. *Stroke* **45**, 2506–2513.

Lawes CM, Bennett DA, Feigin VL, Rodgers A (2004). Blood pressure and stroke: an overview of published reviews. *Stroke* **35**, 1024.

Powers WJ (2014). Lower stroke risk with lower blood pressure in hemodynamic cerebral ischemia. *Neurology* **82**, 1027–1032.

PROGRESS Collaborative Group (2001). Randomised trial of a perindopril-based blood-pressure-lowering regimen among 6105 individuals with previous stroke or transient ischaemic attack. *Lancet* **358**, 1033–1041.

The SPS3 Study Group (2013). Blood-pressure targets in patients with recent lacunar stroke: the SPS3 randomised trial. *Lancet* **382**, 507–515.

Cholesterol

Blom DJ, Hala T, Bolognese M, et al. (2014). DESCARTES Investigators. A 52-week placebo-controlled trial of evolocumab in hyperlipidemia. *N Engl J Med* **370**, 1809–1819.

Ridker PM (2014). LDL cholesterol: controversies and future therapeutic directions. *Lancet* **384**, 607–617.

Robinson JG, Farnier M, Krempf M, et al. (2015). Efficacy and safety of alirocumab in reducing lipids and cardiovascular events. *N Engl J Med* **372**, 1489–1499.

The Stroke Prevention by Aggressive Reduction in Cholesterol Levels (SPARCL) investigators (2006). High-dose atorvastatin after stroke or transient ischaemic attack. *N Engl J Med* **355**, 549–559.

Homocysteine

Hankey GJ, Eikelboom JW, Yi Q, et al. (2012). Antiplatelet therapy and the effects of B vitamins in patients with previous stroke or transient ischaemic attack: a post-hoc subanalysis of VITATOPS, a randomised, placebo-controlled trial. *Lancet Neurol* **11**, 11512–11520.

Huo Y, Li J, Qin X, et al. (2105). Efficacy of folic acid therapy in primary prevention of stroke among adults with hypertension in China: the CSPPT randomized clinical trial. *JAMA* **313**, 1325–1335.

Toole JF, Malinow MR, Chambless LE, et al. (2004). Lowering homocysteine in patients with ischemic stroke to prevent recurrent stroke, myocardial infarction, and death: the Vitamin Intervention for Stroke Prevention (VISP) randomized controlled trial. *JAMA* **291**, 565–575.

Spence JD, Hankey GJ (2022). Problem in the recent American Heart Association guideline on secondary stroke prevention: B vitamins to lower homocysteine do prevent stroke. *Stroke* **53**, 2702–2708.

Antiplatelet agents

Aspirin

Antithrombotic Trialists' Collaboration (2002). Collaborative meta-analysis of randomised trials of antiplatelet therapy for prevention of death, myocardial infarction, and stroke in high risk patients. *BMJ* **324**, 71–86.

CAPRIE Steering Committee (1996). A randomised, blinded, trial of clopidogrel versus aspirin in patients at risk of ischaemic events (CAPRIE). *Lancet* **348**, 1329–1339.

Clopidogrel versus aspirin + dipyridamole

Sacco RL, Diener HC, Yusuf S, et al. (2008). Aspirin and extended-release dipyridamole versus clopidogrel for recurrent stroke. *N Engl J Med* **359**, 1238–1251.

The ESPRIT Study Group, Algra A (2007). Medium intensity oral anticoagulants versus aspirin after cerebral ischaemia of arterial origin (ESPRIT): a randomised controlled trial. *Lancet Neurol* **6**, 115–124.

Aspirin and clopidogrel dual antiplatelet treatment in minor stroke/high-risk TIA

Gao Y, Chen W, Pan Y, et al. INSPIRES Investigators (2023). Dual antiplatelet treatment up to 72 hours after ischemic stroke. *N Engl J Med* **389**(26), 2413–2424.

Pan Y, Chen W, Xu Y, et al. (2017). Genetic polymorphisms and clopidogrel efficacy for acute ischemic stroke or transient ischemic attack: a systematic review and meta-analysis. *Circulation* **135**(1), 21–33.

Pan Y, Elm JJ, Li H, Easton JD, et al. (2019). Outcomes associated with clopidogrel-aspirin use in minor stroke or transient ischemic attack: a pooled analysis of clopidogrel in high-risk patients with acute non-disabling cerebrovascular events (CHANCE) and platelet-oriented inhibition in new TIA and minor ischemic stroke (POINT) trials. *JAMA Neurol* **76**, 1466–1473.

SPS3 Investigators, Benavente OR, Hart RG, et al. (2012). Effects of clopidogrel added to aspirin in patients with recent lacunar stroke. *N Engl J Med* **367**, 817–825.

Wang Y, Zhao X, Liu L, et al. (2013). Clopidogrel with aspirin in acute minor stroke or transient ischemic attack. *N Engl J Med* **369**, 11–19.

Ticagrelor versus clopidogrel in addition to aspirin

Lun R, Dhaliwal S, Zitikyte G, Roy DC, Hutton B, Dowlatshahi D (2022). Comparison of ticagrelor vs clopidogrel in addition to aspirin in patients with minor ischemic stroke and transient ischemic attack: a network meta-analysis. *JAMA Neurol* **79**(2), 141–148.

Wang Y, Meng X, Wang A, et al. CHANCE-2 Investigators (2021). Ticagrelor versus clopidogrel in CYP2C19 loss-of-function carriers with stroke or TIA. *N Engl J Med* **385**(27), 2520–2530.

Anticoagulation

Chimowitz MI, Lynn MJ, Howlett-Smith H, et al. (2005) Comparison of warfarin and aspirin for symptomatic intracranial arterial stenosis. *N Engl J Med* **352**, 1305–1316.

ESPRIT Study Group, Halkes PH, van Gijn J, et al. (2007). Medium intensity oral anticoagulants versus aspirin after cerebral ischaemia of arterial origin (ESPRIT): a randomised controlled trial. *Lancet Neurol* **6**, 115–124.

Gorter JW (1999). Major bleeding during anticoagulation after cerebral ischemia: patterns and risk factors. Stroke Prevention In Reversible Ischemia Trial (SPIRIT). European Atrial Fibrillation Trial (EAFT) study groups. *Neurology* **53**, 1319–1327.

Hariharan NN, Patel K, Sikder O, et al. (2022) Oral anticoagulation versus antiplatelet therapy for secondary stroke prevention in patients with embolic stroke of undetermined source: A systematic review and meta-analysis. *Eur Stroke J* **7**(2), 92–98.

SPIRIT (1997). Randomized trial of anticoagulants versus aspirin after cerebral ischemia of presumed arterial origin. The Stroke Prevention in Reversible Ischemia Trial (SPIRIT) Study Group. *Ann Neurol* **42**, 857–865.

Atrial fibrillation

Atrial Fibrillation Investigators (1994). Risk factors for stroke and efficacy of antithrombotic therapy in atrial fibrillation: analysis of pooled data from five randomized controlled trials. *Arch Intern Med* **154**, 1449–1457.

ACTIVE Writing Group (2006). Clopidogrel plus aspirin versus oral anticoagulation for atrial fibrillation in the Atrial fibrillation Clopidogrel Trial with Irbesartan for prevention of Vascular Events (ACTIVE W): a randomised controlled trial. *Lancet* **367**, 1903–1912.

Eikelboom JW, Connolly SJ, Brueckmann M, et al. (2013). Dabigatran versus warfarin in patients with mechanical heart valves. *N Engl J Med* **369**, 1206–1214.

Ntaios G, Papavasileiou V, Diener HC, Makaritsis K, Michel P (2012). Nonvitamin-K-antagonist oral anticoagulants in patients with atrial fibrillation and previous stroke or transient ischemic attack: a systematic review and meta-analysis of randomized controlled trials. *Stroke* **43**, 3298–3304.

Pollack C, Reilly P, Eikelboom J, et al. (2015). Idarucizumab for dabigatran reversal. *N Engl J Med* **373**, 511–520.

Sellers MB, Newby LK (2011). Atrial fibrillation, anticoagulation, fall risk, and outcomes in elderly patients. *Am Heart J* **161**, 241–246.

Seiffge DJ, Cancelloni V, Räber L, et al. (2024) Secondary stroke prevention in people with atrial fibrillation: treatments and trials. *Lancet Neurol* **23**(4), 404–417.

Carotid stenting

AbuRahma, Ali F, et al. (2022). Society for Vascular Surgery clinical practice guidelines for management of extracranial cerebrovascular disease. *J Vasc Surg* **75**(1), 4S–22S.

Bonati LH, Dobson J, Featherstone R, et al. (2015). Long-term outcomes after stenting versus endarterectomy for treatment of symptomatic carotid stenosis: the International Carotid Stenting Study (ICSS) randomised trial. *Lancet* **385**, 529–538.

Brott TG, Hobson RW, Howard G, et al. (2010). Stenting versus endarterectomy for treatment of carotid-artery stenosis. *N Engl J Med* **363**, 11–23.

Coelho A, Peixoto J, Mansilha A, et al. (2022). Timing of carotid intervention in symptomatic carotid artery stenosis: a systematic review and meta-analysis. *Eur J Vasc Endovasc Surg* **63**(1), 3–23.

Liu ZJ, Fu WG, Guo ZY, et al. (2012). Updated systematic review and meta-analysis of randomized clinical trials comparing carotid artery stenting and carotid endarterectomy in the treatment of carotid stenosis. *Ann Vasc Surg* **26**, 576–590.

Mas JL, Chatellier G, Beyssen B, et al. EVA-3S Investigators (2006). Endarterectomy versus stenting in patients with symptomatic severe carotid stenosis. *N Engl J Med* **355**, 1660–1671.

SPACE Collaborative Group (2006). 30 day results from the SPACE trial of stent-protected angioplasty versus carotid endarterectomy in symptomatic patients: a randomised non-inferiority trial. *Lancet* **368**, 1239–1247.

Asymptomatic carotid stenosis

AbuRahma A (2024). An analysis of the recommendations of the 2022 Society for Vascular Surgery clinical practice guidelines for patients with asymptomatic carotid stenosis. *J Vasc Surg* **79**(5), 1235–1239.

Executive Committee for the Asymptomatic Carotid Atherosclerosis (ACAS) Study (1995). Endarterectomy for asymptomatic carotid artery stenosis. *JAMA* **273**, 1421–1428.

Halliday A, Harrison M, Hayter E, et al. (2010). Asymptomatic Carotid Surgery Trial (ACST) Collaborative Group. 10-year stroke prevention after successful carotid endarterectomy for asymptomatic stenosis (ACST-1): a multicentre randomised trial. *Lancet* **376**, 1074–1084.

Halliday A, Bulbulia R, Bonati LH, et al. ACST-2 Collaborative Group (2021). Second asymptomatic carotid surgery trial (ACST-2): a randomised comparison of carotid artery stenting versus carotid endarterectomy. *Lancet* **398**, 1065–1073.

Naylor AR (2011). Time to rethink management strategies in asymptomatic carotid artery disease. *Nat Rev Cardiol* **9**, 116–124.

Nicolaides AN, Kakkos SK, Kyriacou E, et al. Asymptomatic Carotid Stenosis and Risk of Stroke (ACSRS) Study Group (2010). Asymptomatic internal carotid artery stenosis and cerebrovascular risk stratification. *J Vasc Surg* **52**(6), 1486–1496.

Carotid occlusion

EC/IC Study group (1985). Failure of extracranial-intracranial bypass to reduce the risk of ischaemic stroke. Results of an international randomized trial. *N Engl J Med* **313**, 1191–1200.

Nguyen VN, Motiwala M, Elarjani T, et al. (2022). Direct, indirect, and combined extracranial-to-intracranial bypass for adult moyamoya disease: an updated systematic review and meta-analysis. *Stroke* **53**(12), 3572–3582.

Reinhard M, Schwarzer G, Briel M, et al. (2014). Cerebrovascular reactivity predicts stroke in high-grade carotid artery disease. *Neurology* **83**, 1424–1431.

Powers WJ, Clarke WR, Grubb RL, et al. (2011). Extracranial-intracranial bypass surgery for stroke prevention in hemodynamic cerebral ischemia: The Carotid Occlusion Surgery Study: a randomized trial. *JAMA* **306**, 1983–1992.

Vertebral stenosis

Gulli G, Marquardt L, Rothwell PM, Markus HS (2013). Stroke risk after posterior circulation stroke/transient ischemic attack and its relationship to site of vertebrobasilar stenosis: pooled data analysis from prospective studies. *Stroke* **44**(3), 598–604.

Markus HS, van der Worp HB, Rothwell PM (2013). Posterior circulation ischaemic stroke and transient ischaemic attack: diagnosis, investigation, and secondary prevention. *Lancet Neurol* **12**, 989–998.

Markus HS, Harshfield EL, Compter A, et al. Vertebral Stenosis Trialists' Collaboration. (2019). Stenting for symptomatic vertebral artery stenosis: a preplanned pooled individual patient data analysis. *Lancet Neurol* **18**(7), 666–673.

Intracranial stenosis

Derdeyn CP, Chimowitz MI, Lynn MJ, et al. (2014). Stenting and aggressive medical management for preventing recurrent stroke in intracranial stenosis trial investigators. Aggressive medical treatment with or without stenting in high-risk patients with intracranial artery stenosis (SAMMPRIS): the final results of a randomised trial. *Lancet* **383**, 333–341.

Luo J, Wang T, Yang K, et al. (2023). Endovascular therapy versus medical treatment for symptomatic intracranial artery stenosis. *Cochrane Database Syst Rev* **2**(2), CD013267.

Zaidat OO, Fitzsimmons BF, Woodward BK (2015). VISSIT Trial Investigators. Effect of a balloon-expandable intracranial stent vs. medical therapy on risk of stroke in patients with symptomatic intracranial stenosis: the VISSIT randomized clinical trial. *JAMA* **313**, 1240–1248.

Unusual causes of stroke and their treatment

Introduction

Rare causes of stroke make up a small proportion of stroke cases but it is important that they are recognized because they may require very specific treatment.

Most are more important in younger individuals (in whom conventional risk factors and atherosclerosis are less common). A few (e.g. temporal arteritis) are commoner in older people.

In many cases, specific investigations and a high index of suspicion are required to make the diagnosis.

Rare causes of stroke may be:
- isolated stroke syndromes
- part of a more widespread neurological disease: other neurological features, e.g. migraine, encephalopathy, seizures, or dementia, may occur
- part of a systemic disease, e.g. systemic vasculitis.

Carotid and vertebral artery dissection

Carotid and vertebral artery dissection are important causes of stroke, particularly in the young.

Epidemiology

- Accounts for up to 10% of young adult stroke (<45 years) and 20–25% (<30 years)
- It has been estimated that one-third of cases of dissection will present with stroke or TIA.

Pathogenesis

- Most carotid and vertebral dissections are extracranial. Intracranial dissections have unique features (see later in topic)
- The initial event is usually an intimal tear, allowing blood to track along planes in the arterial wall
- Carotid dissection often tracks upwards as far as the skull base, resulting in a characteristic tapering and angiographic appearance
- Consequences of the dissection include the following:
  - Thrombus formation at the site of the intimal tear, which may result in thromboembolism and stroke
  - Reduction in luminal diameter secondary to extrinsic compression from intramural haemorrhage. This may result in vessel occlusion and haemodynamic compromise
  - Pseudoaneurysm formation—this is common but pseudoaneurysms are usually asymptomatic although occasionally may cause local pressure symptoms. They do not rupture.
- Most stroke due to dissection is believed to be embolic. This is supported by radiographic patterns suggesting multiple emboli and the detection of asymptomatic emboli using transcranial Doppler ultrasound
- Intracranial dissections are most common in the supraclinoid carotid artery, MCA, fourth segment of the vertebral artery, and the basilar trunk. Intracranial vertebral artery dissection may result in subarachnoid haemorrhage caused by leakage of blood into the CSF.

Causes

- Vertebral and carotid dissection may occur following major penetrating and non-penetrating trauma
- A history of minor trauma is common but whether it relates to the dissection or not is sometimes unclear
- In approximately half of dissections no history of trauma is present
- A number of diseases affecting the arterial wall increase the risk of dissection, including fibromuscular dysplasia and Ehlers–Danlos syndrome type IV
- Minor connective tissue abnormalities on electron microscopy of skin biopsies have been reported in a high proportion of patients with spontaneous dissection in some but not all studies
- Genetic variants increasing the risk of apparently sporadic dissection have been recently identified.

Classification of causes of cervical artery dissection

Major trauma
- Penetrating trauma
- Blunt trauma.

Major trauma causing carotid dissection
- Basal skull fracture
- Stretching across the lateral processes of C2–C3
- Strangulation
- Peritonsillar trauma
- Mandibular fracture.

Major trauma causing vertebral dissection
- Atlanto-axial subluxation
- Cervical spine fracture
- Cervical spine hyper-rotation and hyperextension.

Minor trauma
- Chiropractic manipulation
- Neck turning (e.g. during a parade)
- Violent coughing
- Fairground rides
- Sporting activities
- Hyperextension during hairdressing (vertebral dissection).

Iatrogenic trauma
- Endovascular procedures (e.g. angiography, interventional procedures)
- Neckline insertion.

Underlying arterial disease
- Fibromuscular dysplasia
- Ehlers–Danlos syndrome type IV (vascular variant)
- Cystic medial degeneration
- Marfan syndrome
- Pseudoxanthoma elasticum.
- Loeys–Dietz syndrome

Idiopathic.

Clinical features of cervical artery dissection

Extracranial carotid dissection
- Headache—usually ipsilateral and localized to the side of dissection in the neck, face, orbit, and cheek
- Horner's syndrome—partial ptosis and pupillary constriction resulting from compression and interruption of sympathetic fibres running along the internal carotid artery
- TIA and stroke—TIA and stroke in the carotid territory and/or amaurosis fugax or retinal artery infarction. Presenting feature in approximately one-third of carotid dissections. Almost all strokes/TIAs occur within 1 month of dissection onset and most within 1 week
- Cranial nerve palsies—most commonly hypoglossal palsy owing to compression of the hypoglossal nerve immediately below its exit

through the anterior condylar canal. Glossopharyngeal and vagal nerve palsies occur less commonly.

Extracranial vertebral dissection
- Pain in posterior neck, occipital region, and around the ears
- TIA and stroke in vertebrobasilar territory.

Intracranial dissection
- TIA and stroke in the relevant arterial territory
- Subarachnoid haemorrhage, particularly in vertebrobasilar dissection
- A difficult diagnosis and often only made at postmortem.

Diagnosis
- A high index of suspicion in young stroke patients, even in the absence of a history of trauma, is essential
- Duplex carotid ultrasound may show stenosis, occasionally a flap, appearances consistent with occlusion, or high resistance damped Doppler flow signals consistent with distal stenosis. However, ultrasound has a low sensitivity (perhaps only 50%), and MRI-based techniques are better
- MRA may show tapering occlusion or pseudo-occlusion (Figs. 11.1 and 11.2)
- Structural MRI with cross-sectional fat-suppressed inversion recovery views through the extracranial carotid or vertebral artery, in combination with MRA, is now the investigation of choice. The axial (cross-sectional) images must go down through the neck. Those available in a normal brain MRI do not go low enough. A hyperintense signal, usually semilunar-shaped, in the wall of the artery in both T1- and T2-weighted imaging is seen in the first week, indicating the presence of mural haematoma
- CTA shows similar appearances to MRA; newer scanners have high sensitivity to detect diagnostic angiographic features
- Digital subtraction angiography is rarely necessary but may show intimal flaps, and appearances of vessel compression and tapering
- Vertebral dissection is more difficult to diagnose than carotid dissection on MRI owing to the smaller vessel lumen. The intramural hyperintense signal is often less clear.

Treatment
- Anticoagulation—many authorities have recommended anticoagulation with heparin and then warfarin to reduce the risk of thromboembolism, usually continued for 3–6 months.
- Other authorities suggest antiplatelet agents are adequate.
- Meta-analysis (of data from observational studies) found no evidence of a difference between anticoagulation and antiplatelet agents
- Two phase two trials, CADISS (250 recruits) and TREAT-CAD (194 recruits), compared aspirin to warfarin in secondary prevention after symptomatic carotid and vertebral dissection. They showed no difference between the two treatments. An individual patient pooled analysis of data from both trials showed no difference.

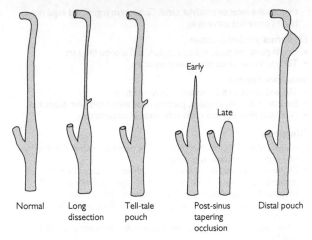

Fig. 11.1 Schematic diagram of different angiographic appearances seen in carotid dissection.

Adapted from Brown MM, Markus H, Oppenheimer S, *Stroke Medicine*, Copyright (2006), with permission from CRC Press.

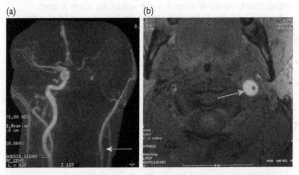

Fig. 11.2 Carotid artery dissection on MRI and MRA. An MRI sequence from a patient with acute left proximal internal carotid artery dissection. (a) MRA demonstrating apparent left internal carotid artery occlusion. This is in fact a pseudo-occlusion caused by compression from thrombus in the false lumen. (b) Axial view through the internal carotid artery in the neck demonstrating a high signal within the arterial wall (recent thrombus) surrounding a small residual lumen (low signal). © Hugh Markus.

- In the STOP-CAD large observational study in 3636 patients (11.1% received exclusively anticoagulation and 67.5% received exclusively antiplatelets), there was no significant difference in recurrent stroke rate by 30 days in the two groups, although there was a non-significant trend to lower stroke rates with anticoagulation.
- Therefore either antiplatelets or anticoagulants can be used (➲ see Chapter 11 for more on treatment of cervical dissection).
- Surgical treatments (tying the carotid artery to prevent embolization) and interventional treatment (stenting) have been used but there is no evidence for these. Arteries usually recanalize spontaneously. Very rarely, surgical treatment or stenting is required for very large expanding pseudoaneurysms.

Prognosis

- Some natural history data suggest the risk of recurrent stroke is highest in the first week and very low after 1 month, but CADISS data suggest the risk by the time patients present is low at only 2%
- Spontaneous recanalization frequently occurs over the first few weeks or months
- The risk of recurrent dissection is very low (<1%) unless there is an underlying disorder (e.g. Ehlers–Danlos)
- Pseudoaneurysms are common and usually persist but require no specific treatment and have a very low risk of complications.

Fibromuscular dysplasia

- A non-atherosclerotic disease of medium-sized arteries that can present with arterial stenosis, beading, dissection, and aneurysm (see Fig. 11.3)
- Fibromuscular dysplasia (FMD) can affect arteries throughout the body. It does not affect the venous system
- Renal arteries are most commonly affected and this can cause renal artery stenosis and hypertension. The hypertension is often early onset and/or difficult to control. In the US FMD Registry almost 80% of individuals had renal FMD
- Cerebrovascular FMD is more common than previously appreciated; in the US FMD Registry almost three-quarters had carotid FMD, and 37% vertebral FMD
- Other reported sites include mesenteric arteries, iliac arteries, intracranial arteries, and brachial arteries
- Multivessel involvement is common; in the US Registry 65% of individuals with renal FMD who underwent cerebrovascular imaging had evidence of carotid or vertebral involvement
- Most common in young and middle-aged women; in the US Registry 92% of cases were in women
- Often asymptomatic: mild degrees in asymptomatic individuals have been reported in as many as 1% of angiograms
- Symptoms and signs depend on the arteries involved and the severity of the arterial lesions
- Distal cervical extracranial internal carotid artery is the most common cerebral site
- Can present with carotid dissection, which may be recurrent
- Dissection may present with stroke or TIA; occasionally, stenosis can cause TIA or stroke, without dissection
- Pulsatile tinnitus is a more common symptom than previously appreciated being reported as a presenting symptom of 32% of patients in the US Registry
- Other features can include headache, neck pain, and a neck bruit
- Can be diagnosed on contrast MRA and CTA but sometimes requires formal intra-arterial angiography.

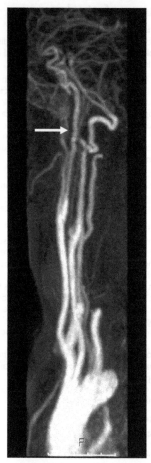

Fig. 11.3 Fibromuscular dysplasia appearance on contrast-enhanced MRA. There is a narrowing of the right ICA shortly after its origin. Distal to this can be seen the characteristic beading of the artery (arrowed). © Hugh Markus.

Genetic causes of stroke

Genetic predisposition to stroke may be:
- monogenic (an abnormality in a single gene results in disease)
- polygenic (multiple genes contribute to stroke risk and frequently interact with environmental factors).

Monogenic causes of stroke are rare, but important on an individual patient basis. Polygenic/multifactorial contribution to stroke risk is much more important on a population basis but less important for the individual patient.

Diagnosing monogenic causes of stroke can be important because:
- the clinical syndromes can represent difficult diagnostic problems
- some monogenic causes of stroke have specific treatments
- there are implications for other family members, including the possibility of pre-natal testing.

Monogenic diseases causing stroke can:
- cause stroke alone (e.g. CADASIL), sometimes with other neurological features (e.g. migraine)
- cause stroke as part of a systemic disease (e.g. sickle cell disease).

Diagnosing monogenic causes of stroke

- Always take a family history of stroke and other diseases
- We recommend specifically asking individual first-degree relatives—parents and siblings—about a history of stroke, cardiovascular disease, dementia, and other neurological disease
- Remember when interpreting family history, diagnoses in other family members may be incorrect (e.g. multiple sclerosis misdiagnosed as CADASIL or vascular dementia diagnosed as Alzheimer's disease)
- Remember, a negative family history does not exclude monogenic stroke. Parents may have died young or disease may not be fully penetrant
- Diagnose the stroke subtype and then identify which monogenic diseases cause that subtype. Most monogenic causes of stroke result in one stroke subtype.
- Look for specific clues (e.g. migraine with aura or MRI evidence of anterior temporal pole involvement for CADASIL).

Monogenic causes of stroke

- Small-vessel disease:
  - CADASIL
  - CARASIL autosomal recessive *HTRA1*
  - CADASIL2 autosomal dominant *HTRA1*
  - COL4A1 and -2 small-vessel arteriopathy
  - Other much rarer causes.
- Large-artery atherosclerosis and other arteriopathies:
  - Familial hyperlipidaemias
  - Moyamoya disease
  - Pseudoxanthoma elasticum
  - Neurofibromatosis type I.
- Large-artery disease—dissection:
  - Ehlers–Danlos syndrome type IV

- • Marfan syndrome
- • Fibromuscular dysplasia.
- Disorders affecting both small and large arteries:
  - • Fabry disease
  - • Homocysteinuria
  - • Sickle cell disease.
- Cardioembolism:
  - • Familial cardiomyopathies
  - • Familial arrhythmias
  - • Hereditary haemorrhagic telangiectasia.
- Prothrombotic disorders
- Mitochondrial disorders:
  - • MELAS.
- Familial hemiplegic migraine.

CADASIL (cerebral autosomal dominant arteriopathy with subcortical infarcts and leukoencephalopathy)

CADASIL is an autosomal dominant condition causing cerebral small-vessel disease. It is the most common monogenic condition causing stroke without systemic features.

Pathogenesis

- A systemic arteriopathy with changes in vessels throughout the body (including skin and muscle) but clinical features are only seen in the brain
- Results in lacunar infarction and diffuse regions of ischaemia corresponding to radiological confluent white matter hyperintensities (neuronal loss, gliosis, ischaemic demyelination)
- Affects perforating arteries and arterioles within the brain and similarly sized vessels elsewhere in the body
- Results from mutations in the *NOTCH3* gene, which encodes a transmembrane protein involved in cell–cell signalling during development
- Arterial smooth muscle cell degeneration occurs, with deposition of granular osmiophilic material (GOM) seen only on electron microscopy. The aberrant extracellular portion of the NOTCH3 protein is deposited adjacent to GOM
- Mechanisms linking genetic defect to disease are not fully understood but most evidence suggests mutations do not cause disease by an alteration in enzyme function
- Recent experimental studies have led to the NOTCH3 cascade hypothesis. This suggests that aggregation/accumulation of the extracellular portion of the NOTCH3 protein in the brain vessels is a central event, promoting the abnormal recruitment of functionally important extracellular matrix proteins that may ultimately cause multifactorial toxicity
- Impaired cerebral autoregulation has been demonstrated in animal models and humans.

Clinical features

- Recurrent lacunar strokes: onset usually 40–70 years but may be later
- Migraine with aura (in about 60%): onset usually 20–30 years. Ninety per cent of migraine is with aura (in contrast, migraine in the population is 90% without aura). Auras include visual, sensory, and dysphasic. Confusional episodes may occur as part of the migraine attack
- Depression: may precede the onset of stroke
- Dementia: usually onset is at 60–70 years but is variable
- Encephalopathy: reversible reduction in conscious level usually following migraine with aura attack, fully reversible with conservative treatment. May occur in up to 10%
- Epilepsy may occur in 5-10%. Variable types
- Premature death: age variable, usually 60–75 years.

The clinical phenotype is highly variable even within families. Factors accounting for this variation are not fully understood but include:

- Position of mutation; mutations located more proximally and encoding epidermal growth factor repeats (EGFR) 1-6 are associated with more severe disease
- cardiovascular risk factors, including hypertension and smoking
- genetic modifiers.

Diagnosis

- Clinical phenotype with family history
- A family history of young-onset stroke, dementia, or migraine with aura is often present but is not present in a significant proportion of cases. Remember that a family history of Alzheimer's may in fact be CADASIL vascular dementia, and a family history of multiple sclerosis may be CADASIL
- MRI demonstrates confluent white matter hyperintensities (WMH) with multiple lacunar infarcts. Specific features of CADASIL include anterior temporal pole WMH involvement (sensitivity 90%, specificity 90%) and confluent external capsule involvement (sensitivity 90%, specificity 50%). Involvement of the corpus callosum may often occur (remember uncommon in sporadic small-vessel disease but common in multiple sclerosis) (see Fig. 11.4)
- Anterior temporal pole changes may often be seen on CT if marked. On MRI, these changes are frequent from age 30 onwards and may occur earlier
- Punch skin biopsy can be performed as an outpatient procedure. It must be examined under electron microscopy. Characteristic GOM is seen in 60–80% of cases. Sensitivity 100% (see Fig. 11.5). However, this is now less used due to the wider availability of genetic testing
- Genetic testing—there are large numbers of mutations which can occur in any of 22 exons encoding extracellular portions of the NOTCH3 protein. Almost all are point mutations (few deletions) and all alter a cysteine residue, disrupting cysteine–cysteine bonds in epidermal growth factor-like repeats in the extracellular portion of proteins. Mutations cluster in certain exons: over half are found in exon 4. The distribution of mutations varies in populations. For example, screening exons 3, 4, 5, 6, 8, 11, and 22 in a UK population identifies 90% of CADASIL cases. Some laboratories used to start by screening only the most commonly affected exons and screen the other exons only if this is negative and the clinical suspicion is high. However next generation sequencing panels it is usually more efficient to screen the whole gene, and other gene that can cause monogenic SVD (e.g. *HTRA1*) at the same time.

Treatment

- There is no specific treatment for the underlying genetic disorder. Symptomatic treatments are effective for many complications
- There is strong evidence that cardiovascular risk factors (particularly smoking and hypertension) are associated with earlier onset of stroke and more rapid progression of MRI disease. Therefore, tight cardiovascular risk factor prevention is recommended
- Aspirin or clopidogrel is usually given to patients who have suffered stroke

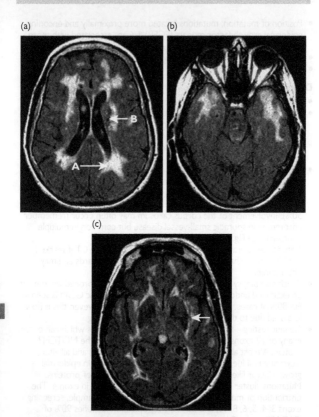

Fig. 11.4 FLAIR MRI appearances of CADASIL: (a) showing both confluent white matter hyperintensities (arrowed A) and focal lacunar infarction (arrowed B); (b) typical involvement of the anterior temporal pole can be seen in a CADASIL patient; (c) this scan shows involvement of the external capsule (arrowed). © Hugh Markus.

- Anticoagulation with warfarin or dual antiplatelet therapy with aspirin and clopidogrel is best avoided owing to the risk of haemorrhage (microbleeds are frequently seen on gradient echo MRI)
- Migraine—attacks are usually infrequent and therefore prophylaxis is usually not necessary. However, usual prophylaxis approaches (e.g. propranolol, pizotifen, etc.) are effective if necessary. Triptans may help attacks. Although there has been some concern over their use

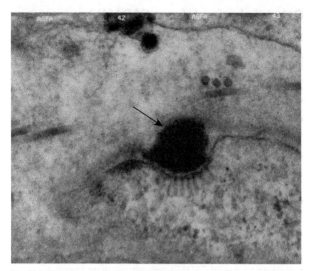

Fig. 11.5 Skin biopsy appearances in CADASIL. A definitive diagnosis of CADASIL is made by demonstrating mutations in the *NOTCH3* gene. However, skin biopsy may also be useful in diagnosis and in over half of individuals shows characteristic granular osmiophilic material (GOM) as arrowed. This appearance can only be seen on electron microscopy; light microscopy appearances are not diagnostic. © Hugh Markus.

in patients with underlying cerebrovascular disease a recent analysis reported they were well-tolerated in CADASIL and effective in about 50% of cases.
- Depression—responds to standard treatment with antidepressants in the same way as non-CADASIL depression
- Epilepsy—responds to normal antiepileptic medication.

Genetic testing
- Standardized protocols with genetic counselling should be used, particularly when testing asymptomatic family members or individuals with migraine alone. In such cases, it is recommended that counselling is followed by a period of at least 1 month for reflection and decision-making. Remember, an MRI may be considered as a genetic test if it detects specific signs such as anterior temporal pole involvement.
- Pre-natal testing with pre-implantation genetic diagnosis (this uses IVF techniques, and an embryo unaffected by the mutation is selected and reimplanted) can be offered to affected individuals planning a child
- Patient information leaflets are useful to provide information on the disease. One can be obtained from the following web address: http://www.cadasil.co.uk.

Other inherited (non-CADASIL) small-vessel arteriopathies

A number of other single-gene disorders causing monogenic small-vessel arteriopathies have been identified. All are much rarer than CADASIL. The commonest are:

- CARASIL and CADASIL—due to HTRA1 mutations
- COL4A1 and -2 small-vessel arteriopathy

CADASIL 2 – autosomal dominant HTRA1 disease

- Due to mutations in the *HTRA1* gene. HTRA1 protein is a serine protease that represses signalling by TGF-beta family members
- This is the same gene causing CARASIL—see below
- One mutation causes a milder autosomal dominant disease (CADASIL2), while two mutations cause more severe recessive disease (CARASIL)
- Second most common cause of monogenic SVD after CADASIL
- Similar clinical picture to CADASIL with migraine with aura, lacunar stroke, encephalopathy, and early onset dementia
- Imaging appearances similar to CADASIL including involvement of the anterior temporal pole
- Cannot be differentiated from CADASIL without genetic testing
- Management is as for CADASIL with tight risk factor control.

COL4A1 and COL4A2 small-vessel arteriopathy

- Mutations in the gene encoding type IV collagen α1 (*COL4A1 or A2*), a basement membrane protein
- Clinical features include:
  - Intracerebral haemorrhage
  - Lacunar stroke.
- Can cause neonatal porencephaly perhaps due to inter-uterine cerebral haemorrhage but can present with stroke in mid-life symptoms in the absence of any childhood problems
- MRI: confluent WMH, ICH. lacunes, and prominent cerebral microbleeds.

Cerebral autosomal recessive arteriopathy with subcortical infarcts and leukoencephalopathy (CARASIL)

- Mostly described in Japan; very rare
- Autosomal recessive *HTRA1* mutation—same gene as CADASIL2
- Cerebral small-vessel arteriopathy in combination with alopecia and orthopaedic problems (degenerative disc disease)
- Central nervous system (CNS) onset is usually 20–40 years with stroke (50%) and/or progressive subcortical dementia
- MRI lacunar stroke and confluent WMH.

Sickle cell disease

Stroke is a frequent complication of homozygous sickle cell disease (HbSS), particularly in children.

Pathogenesis

- Monogenic disease resulting in substitution of valine for glutamic acid at position 6 of the globin β chain
- Secondary to this, polymerization of the abnormal HbS haemoglobin occurs in regions of low oxygen saturation
- Polymerized haemoglobin deforms red cells, reducing their resilience and impairing their ability to pass through capillaries without becoming impacted
- Patients with full disease are homozygous. Heterozygous HbS individuals have 'sickle cell trait' and are not usually at increased risk of stroke
- Stroke may also complicate haemoglobin C sickle cell disease (HbSC)
- Sickle crises occur
- Haematological crises (sudden exacerbation of anaemia)
- Infectious crises (defective immunity owing to dysfunctional spleen)
- Vaso-occlusive crises (organ ischaemia owing to vessel occlusion).

Cerebrovascular complications in sickle cell disease

- Asymptomatic small-vessel disease
- Stenoses of large extracranial or intracranial vessels, particularly the MCA, secondary to fibrous proliferation of the intima
- Formation of aneurysms
- Moyamoya-like syndrome is secondary to basal intracerebral vessel occlusion.

Clinical features

Cerebrovascular
- Ischaemic stroke
- Intracerebral haemorrhage and subarachnoid secondary to new vessel formation (in patients with moyamoya-like syndrome)
- Cognitive impairment.

Non-cerebrovascular
- Haematological crises (sudden exacerbation of anaemia)
- Infectious crises (defective immunity owing to dysfunctional spleen)
- Vaso-occlusive crises (organ ischaemia owing to vessel occlusion).

Diagnosis

- Brain imaging (CT and MRI) may show territorial infarcts and/or small-vessel disease
- Extracranial and intracranial stenoses may be detected by transcranial Doppler ultrasound, MRA, CTA, or angiography
- Full blood count—anaemia with a high reticulocyte count. On a peripheral blood film, one can observe features of hyposplenism, i.e. target cells and Howell–Jolly bodies
- Haemoglobin electrophoresis shows HbS.

Treatment

- Exchange transfusion together with hydration and oxygen therapy for acute episodes
- Prophylactic exchange transfusion has been shown to reduce recurrent stroke risk in patients with MCA stenosis due to sickle cell disease detected using TCD
- Hydroxyurea is used to increase foetal haemoglobin (HbF) which reduces HbS polymerization
- Bone marrow transplant: This procedure can cure some people with sickle cell disease. It involves replacing the patient's bone marrow with healthy stem cells from a donor. It has significant risks (e.g. mortality in under 16 of 5% and in over 16s of about 9%). It works much better if the donor is well-matched. It is used in severe cases only
- Gene therapy: The patient's own bone marrow stem cells are genetically modified; for example, to cause foetal haemoglobin to remain switched on meaning the patient does not produce the globin β chain which sickles. Similar to a bone marrow transplant, "conditioning" chemotherapy or radiation is required prior to reinfusion of the genetically modified cells. to make space in the bone marrow. Initial results in small numbers have been dramatic, with a huge reduction in sickle crises. It was licensed by the FDA in the US in 2023 and the NHS in the UK in 2024. It is very expensive.

Fabry disease

- Fabry disease is a rare, sex-linked, recessive lysosomal storage disease caused by deficiency of α-galactosidase A
- It results in accumulation of glycosphingolipids in vascular endothelial smooth muscle cells and other cell types, including renal glomerular epithelial cells, dorsal root and autonomic neurons, and myocardial cells.

Clinical features

Non-cerebrovascular

- Burning neuropathic limb pain (acroparaesthesia) caused by lipid accumulation in sensory nerves
- Skin angiokeratosis
- Joint pain
- Corneal dystrophy (visible as cloudy streaks in the cornea)
- Renal failure
- Myocardial involvement.

Cerebrovascular involvement

- Small-vessel disease—lacunar infarction and WMH on MRI
- Large-artery disease preferentially affecting vertebrobasilar system with ectatic changes, dilatation, and stenoses
- Stroke can occur in patients with known Fabry disease
- A study in young cryptogenic stroke (18–55 years) found Fabry in 4.9% of men and 2.4% of women
- However, further studies have failed to find such a high frequency and suggest that Fabry disease is very rare in patients with young-onset stroke.

Diagnosis

- In men: α-galactosidase enzyme levels and genetic testing if abnormal
- In women: levels may be unhelpful (because sex-linked) and genetic testing is necessary.

Treatment

- IV enzyme replacement therapy is now available
- Very expensive
- Reduces painful symptoms
- No evidence yet that it reduces recurrent stroke risk.

Mitochondrial disorders and MELAS

Mitochondrial DNA mutations result in a variety of systemic syndromes that may include involvement of the neurological system. Some of these cause stroke-like episodes. The archetypical stroke phenotype is mitochondrial encephalopathy with lactic acidosis and stroke-like episodes (MELAS).

Clinical features

- Recurrent stroke-like episodes usually occur in childhood or young adulthood
- Episodes are often accompanied by epilepsy with partial and/or secondary generalized seizures
- Good recovery is often made from initial episodes with marked radiological recovery
- Recurrent episodes are associated with progressive disability and dementia
- Other clinical features include:
  - sensorineural deafness
  - migraine
  - episodic vomiting
  - other features of mitochondrial disorders, including proximal muscle weakness, cardiomyopathy, external ophthalmoplegia, retinopathy, ataxia.
- Overlap may occur with other mitochondrial disorders.

Imaging appearances

- Infarction involves the occipital cortex (most commonly) and posterior parietal and posterior temporal regions
- Distribution does not always correspond to cerebral arterial territories
- 'Infarcts' may dramatically improve or disappear over weeks to months (see Fig. 11.6)
- Increased diffusion (in contrast to restricted diffusion in ischaemic stroke) is often seen in DWI
- Magnetic resonance spectroscopy (MRS) may demonstrate lactate both within the normal and abnormal-appearing brain (remember this occurs in any acute ischaemic stroke within a lesion)
- White matter hyperintensities and subcortical changes may also occur.

Other diagnostic tests

- Raised CSF lactate on CSF examination
- Mitochondrial DNA analysis may show mutation: this is most common (in 80% of cases, it is the A>G3243 mutation) in the transfer RNA *leu* gene
- Genetic analysis on blood may not detect diagnosis caused by unusual mutations or heteroplasmy (genetic abnormality is only present in some cells)
- Muscle biopsy: may show ragged red fibres. DNA analysis on muscle may be positive when negative on blood owing to heteroplasmy.

Treatment

- No proven treatments
- Supportive therapy and treatment of epilepsy during acute episodes.

(a) (b)

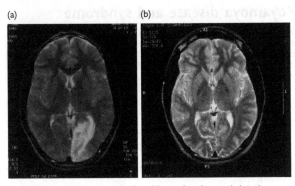

Fig. 11.6 One pattern seen in MELAS is of 'large infarcts', particularly in the occipitoparietal regions and posterior temporal regions. These may not obey arterial boundaries. A typical example is shown in this boy presenting with right homonymous hemianopia in whom a left occipital high signal lesion is seen on T2-weighted MRI (a). A characteristic feature of these MELAS 'infarcts' is that remarkable resolution of the MRI abnormalities may occur, as on this repeat scan some months later (b). © Hugh Markus.

Moyamoya disease and syndrome

Stenosis and occlusion of the basal intracerebral arteries (terminal ICA, proximal ACA, and MCA) occurs, usually in childhood. These occlusions result in ischaemia and secondary new vessel formation with many small collateral lenticulostriate arteries forming to bypass the occlusion (see Fig. 11.7). This pattern looks like a puff of smoke on angiogram: hence its name moyamoya, meaning 'puff of smoke' in Japanese.

Moyamoya disease is an idiopathic condition, most frequent in Japan and East Asia, but rare in the western hemisphere (although it can occur). Intimal thickening in walls occurs. There is a familial pattern in some cases. It has an autosomal dominant inheritance and incomplete penetrance has been suggested, but the underlying genes(s) are unknown.

Moyamoya syndrome can result from any condition that occludes basal intracerebral arteries in childhood or early adulthood with secondary new vessel formation.

Clinical features

- In childhood with stroke secondary to vessel occlusion
- Cognitive problems owing to additional silent infarction may occur
- In adulthood, subarachnoid or intracerebral haemorrhage is caused by bleeding from collateral vessels (the most common presentation)
- In idiopathic moyamoya, involvement of the posterior circulation is rare
- The incidence is approximately 1 per million in Japan
- Diseases causing secondary moyamoya syndrome include sickle cell disease, basal meningeal infection, and vasculitis.

Treatment

- Extracranial-to-intracranial (EC-IC) bypass has been suggested on the assumption that it improves collateral supply and reduces secondary new vessel formation.
- EC-IC bypass is widely practised, particularly in East Asia, although there is not strong RCT data to support this.
- A number of case series support this use, but there has been only one RCT, the Japan MMD trial.
- This enrolled 80 adult patients who experienced haemorrhage within 1 year, and allocated patients to bilateral direct STA-MCA revascularization ($n=42$) with or without additional indirect revascularization *versus* conservative therapy alone ($n=38$). The mean duration of observation was 4.32 years. No postoperative vascular (infarction or haemorrhage) or mortality complications occurred. Surgical patients experienced substantially fewer recurrent haemorrhages (11.9% vs. 31.6%, $P=0.052$), but numerically more infarctions (2.4% *versus* 0%, $P=$ ns) than the medically treated group. Outcome adjudication was not masked, and low enrolment prevented achieving the initial target goal of 160 patients, limiting statistical power.
- A criticism of this study was in regard to the 0% complication rate among 84 operated hemispheres, which is very different from EC-IC bypass in non-MMD trials: 15% in the Carotid Occlusion Stroke Study (COSS) and 12% in the External Carotid Internal Carotid (EC-IC) Bypass Study and raised concerns about the reliability of the report.

- A recent overview concluded more trial data was needed, but based on what is currently available, concluded revascularization seems superior to conservative therapy in adult patients presenting with haemorrhage, and in preventing future haemorrhages. Conversely, evidence that surgery is superior to medical therapy is not convincing in adult patients presenting with cerebral ischaemia, or for the prevention of future ischaemic events.
- Prior to new vessel formation, antithrombotic agents are frequently given. Following new vessel formation, their use is uncertain and could potentially increase haemorrhage risk.
- Control of blood pressure to reduce haemorrhage risk is necessary at all stages of the disease.

(a)   (b)

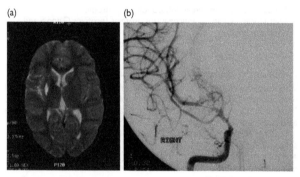

Fig. 11.7 A case of Moyamoya presenting with a left hemiparesis. (a) A right-sided subcortical infarct can be seen on T2-weighted MRI. (b) On the intra-arterial angiogram, a tight middle artery stenosis can be seen with new vessel formation bypassing it. © Hugh Markus.

Prothrombotic disorders in stroke

'Prothrombotic state' and 'thrombophilia' are both terms used to describe an increased tendency to clinical thrombosis associated with laboratory evidence of coagulation pathway abnormalities.

Frequently tested for in young stroke, the evidence linking them to sporadic arterial stroke is weak.

They appear to be more important in childhood stroke.

Whether it is worth testing for them in stroke in young adults is controversial. In our experience, testing for anticardiolipin antibody/lupus coagulant is worthwhile in young adults with ischaemic stroke but testing for protein C and S, APC resistance, and antithrombin III rarely alters management.

Causes of thrombophilia

- Lupus anticoagulant and antiphospholipid syndrome.
- Deficiencies of natural anticoagulant proteins (proteins C and S and antithrombin III)
- Activated protein C (APC) resistance which is usually associated with the factor V Leiden polymorphism

Lupus anticoagulant and anticardiolipin antibodies

These are closely related antibodies which react with proteins associated with phospholipids, including the phospholipid moieties of DNA or RNA. Most common in patients with SLE but may also occur without SLE and be associated with both arterial and venous thrombosis.

Features of the antiphospholipid antibody syndrome occurring in the absence of SLE include:

- stroke and other arterial thrombosis
- venous thrombosis, including cerebral venous thrombosis
- pulmonary embolism
- livedo reticularis skin appearance
- cardiac valve vegetations
- thrombocytopenia
- amaurosis fugax in absence of carotid stenosis
- ischaemic anterior optic neuropathy, probably caused by *in situ* thrombosis of the posterior ciliary artery
- other CNS involvement.
- recurrent miscarriage.

Diagnosis

- Lupus anticoagulant is detected in blood by prolongation of clotting time, probably as a result of interference with procoagulant effects of membrane phospholipids interacting with platelets and clotting
- Prolongation of kaolin cephalin time (KCT) and Russell viper venom test. Adding normal plasma to blood fails to correct this
- Anticardiolipin antibody detected by ELISA
- Remember, anticardiolipin antibodies can occur secondary to other conditions, e.g. malignancy, HIV infection, and are sometimes transiently associated with stroke. If elevated antibodies are found, repeat the level in the convalescent phase.

Treatment
- Anticoagulation with heparin and warfarin is usually recommended. Warfarin rather than a DOAC is usually recommended
- Where association is less certain, antiplatelet agents are often used
- Subcutaneous heparin during pregnancy may prevent recurrent miscarriage.

Protein C and S deficiency

- Protein C and S are synthesized by the liver before being released into the general circulation; involved in degradation of factors V and VIII, which play roles in the thrombotic cascade
- Deficiency may be inherited or acquired
- Inherited protein C and S deficiency occurs in approximately 0.4% of the population
- Large studies in sporadic stroke have found no association with ischaemic stroke. Smaller studies in young stroke (<40 years) have suggested a possible association
- Overdiagnosis often occurs because:
  - levels may fall post-stroke and during systemic illness—therefore, repeat 3 months after acute episode to confirm
  - ethnic differences in levels—for example, the normal levels are lower in Black, compared with white, individuals
  - levels fall on warfarin therapy.
- If association with stroke is suspected, treatment is anticoagulation with warfarin. Warfarin should *not* be started without additional heparin cover for the first week because it reduces protein C and S concentrations before other vitamin K-dependent coagulation factors
- Warfarin-induced skin necrosis appears to be more common in individuals with protein C deficiency.

Activated protein C resistance

- This is the most common inherited prothrombotic state
- There is functional resistance to the anticoagulation effects of activated protein C, resulting from a point mutation in factor V at the site (Arg 506) where APC cleaves and inactivates the Va procoagulant. The genetic polymorphism is called the Leiden factor V mutation
- Small studies have suggested an association with sporadic stroke but larger studies have not confirmed this
- Possibly stronger associations have been reported in younger patients (<40 years) and specific families
- Heterozygote form (associated with APC resistance) is present in 5% of the normal population; therefore, in clinical practice association may occur by chance
- It is the most common inherited predisposing factor to venous thrombosis (including cerebral venous thrombosis)
- If found in stroke, look for possible paradoxical embolism from venous thrombosis (via PFO)
- Treatment is anticoagulation.

Cerebral vasculitis

Stroke can occur as part of many vasculitic connective tissue disorders, including polyarteritis nodosa (PAN), SLE, rheumatoid arthritis, and Behçet's disease. In these diseases, stroke usually occurs in patients with already diagnosed systemic disease, although occasionally they can present with stroke. In contrast, stroke is often the presenting feature in giant cell arteritis (temporal arteritis) and Takayasu arteritis.

Cerebral vasculitis is both over-suspected clinically and under-diagnosed—it may require microscopic examination (biopsy of vessel or brain) to confirm. Biopsy—including stereotactic-guided brain biopsy under local anaesthetic—can be required to differentiate between vasculitis and other rare but treatable conditions such as intravascular lymphoma.

Cerebral vasculitis can be classified by the size of the vessel involved and/or mode of clinical presentation (see Tables 11.1 and 11.2).

Giant cell arteritis (temporal arteritis)

Pathophysiology
- Affects any medium-sized or large artery but by far most commonly involves the ophthalmic artery and branches of the external carotid artery
- On biopsy, characteristic giant cells are seen (hence its name) accompanied by other changes of vasculitis

Table 11.1 Classical presentations of cerebral vasculitis

Acute or subacute encephalopathy
Headache
Acute confusional state—may progress to drowsiness and coma
Intracranial mass lesion
Headache
Drowsiness
Focal signs
Sometimes raised intracranial pressure
Superficially resembling atypical multiple sclerosis
Relapsing–remitting course
Features such as optic neuropathy, brainstem episodes, seizures, headaches, and stroke episodes
Stroke
May be recurrent
May be (but not always) associated with systemic disease and raised inflammatory markers

Adapted from *Quarterly Journal of Medicine*, 90(1), Scolding NJ, Jayne DR, Zajicek JP et al., Cerebral vasculitis—recognition, diagnosis and management, pp. 61–73, Copyright (1997), with permission from Oxford University Press.

Table 11.2 Classification of cerebral vasculitis by size of vessel involved

Large-vessel vasculitis

Takayasu arteritis

Giant cell (temporal) arteritis

Medium-vessel vasculitis

Polyarteritis nodosa

Granulomatosis with polyangiitis (formerly Wegener's granulomatosis)

Isolated CNS vasculitis

Small-vessel vasculitis

Churg–Strauss arteritis

Essential cryoglobulinaemic vasculitis

Vasculitis secondary to connective tissue disorders: SLE, rheumatoid arthritis, relapsing polychondritis, Behçet's disease, and other connective tissue disorders

Vasculitis secondary to viral infection—usually due to hepatitis B and C, HIV, cytomegalovirus, Epstein–Barr virus, and parvo B19 virus

- Posterior circulation may be involved
- Pathological studies show vasculitis only involves extracranial vessels up to the level of the dura, suggesting intracranial vascular symptoms result from embolism.

Clinical features
- A disease of older people, usually aged over 60 years
- Most commonly presents with headache—throbbing or boring and affecting predominantly a temporal location
- May present with uniocular visual loss. This is usually permanent (in contrast to amaurosis fugax secondary to carotid atherosclerosis), but initially may be transient
- Facial pain and scalp tenderness from external carotid artery involvement
- Occasionally there is jaw claudication (pain on exercising the jaw, i.e. eating)
- On examination, there is tenderness and nodularity or absent pulses on palpation of temporal arteries
- Overlap with polymyalgia rheumatica which presents with malaise and myalgia, particularly affecting the shoulder and hip girdles
- Stroke may occur and the posterior circulation is more involved.

Diagnosis
- ESR usually markedly raised
- All elderly patients presenting with temporal headache or visual loss should have urgent ESR
- Liver function tests, particularly alkaline phosphatase, may be elevated
- Chronic normocytic anaemia may occur
- Definitive diagnosis is on temporal artery biopsy. Lesions may be skip lesions—therefore at least a 2-cm length of artery must be biopsied.

There is vasculitis with mononuclear cell infiltrate or granulomatous inflammation, usually with multinucleated giant cells.

Treatment
- To prevent permanent blindness, urgent confirmation of diagnosis and treatment is required
- Start high-dose steroids (prednisolone 40–80 mg/day) as soon as diagnosis is suspected, and before biopsy (which can be delayed by a couple of days and still give diagnostic information). Remember to give osteoporosis protection with steroids
- Symptoms of headache, facial pain, and polymyalgia rapidly resolve
- Slowly reduce prednisolone over the next few months, but low-dose treatment is often needed for 1–2 years
- The British Society for Rheumatology suggests the following tapering regimen:
  - 40–60 mg prednisolone continued for 4 weeks (until resolution of symptoms and laboratory abnormalities)
  - then the dose is reduced by 10 mg every 2 weeks to 20 mg
  - then by 2.5 mg every 2–4 weeks to 10 mg
  - then by 1 mg every 1–2 months, provided there is no relapse
- Self-limiting disease, which usually lasts 1–2 years, although it has a variable duration
- In some cases, additional immunosuppressive agents (e.g. azathioprine) are required
- Serial ESRs can be used to monitor asymptomatic relapse during steroid withdrawal, although occasionally symptomatic relapses have been reported with a normal ESR.

Other cerebral vasculitides

Isolated CNS angiitis
- By definition this is a vasculitis or angiitis affecting only the CNS
- Histology may show granuloma in the arteriolar walls—this led to the older name for the disease, granulomatous angiitis
- Small intracranial vessels are involved
- It presents with progressive dementia, multiple strokes affecting small arteries, and encephalopathy
- By definition, systemic involvement does not occur, although there is an overlap with systemic vasculitis
- ESR may be increased or normal
- CT or MRI scanning shows multiple areas of infarction, particularly in the white matter
- CSF may show an increase in protein concentration and a slight increase in lymphocyte count
- Angiography is often normal because small vessels are involved beyond the resolution of the technique
- Diagnosis is often only made at brain biopsy or postmortem
- There are no treatment trials or good data on optimal treatment approaches
- Case reports suggest immunosuppressive agents, particularly cyclophosphamide, may be beneficial.

Behçet's disease

- Systemic disorder which may involve the brain
- Most common in individuals from Turkey and Mediterranean regions
- Systemic features include arthritis, urogenital ulceration, uveitis, and recurrent phlebitis
- Neurological involvement includes:
  - stroke due to vasculopathy affecting medium-sized and small vessels, particularly in the brainstem
  - chronic aseptic meningitis
  - cerebral venous thrombosis.
- MRI appearances show preferential brainstem involvement
- Treatment with steroids and immunosuppressive agents
- Frequency of HLA-B51 increased.

Takayasu arteritis

- Large-vessel arteritis predominantly affecting the aorta and its branches at their origin
- Results in regions of vessel irregularity, focal stenosis, and occlusion in these vessels
- Most commonly affects young women, especially from the Far East
- Common features include systemic illness with fever, weight loss, arthralgias, night sweats, malaise, and raised ESR
- Stenoses in vessels arising from the aortic arch may result in brain ischaemia, arm ischaemia (claudication), and occasionally ischaemia in the kidneys and lower limbs
- Aortic regurgitation and coronary artery ischaemia may occur
- Clues on examination include reduced or absent radial pulses or reduced blood pressure, which may be asymmetrical
- The type of stroke will depend upon the vessels involved, but both carotid and vertebral territories can be affected
- Diagnosis is usually made on the pattern of involvement of aortic arch vessels seen on CTA, MRA, or intra-arterial angiography
- Treatment is with corticosteroids. This is usually required for a few years
- Prognosis is good with treatment: 5-year survival is 80%.

Diagnostic criteria

At least three out of six criteria are reported to yield sensitivity and specificity of 90.5% and 97.8%:

- Onset <40 years
- Claudication of extremities
- Decreased pulsation of one or both brachial arteries
- At least 10 mmHg systolic difference in both arms
- Bruit over one or both carotid arteries or abdominal aorta
- Arteriographic narrowing of the aorta, its primary branches, or large arteries in the upper or lower extremities.

Polyarteritis nodosa (PAN)

- Systemic necrotizing vasculitides includes three related disorders: PAN, granulomatosis with polyangiitis (formerly Wegener's granulomatosis), and Churg–Strauss syndrome. PAN is a systemic necrotizing vasculitis

and aneurysm formation affecting both medium and small arteries. If only small vessels are affected, it is called microscopic polyangiitis, although it is more associated with granulomatosis with polyangiitis than classic PAN
- Vasculitis affects medium-sized vessels. Involvement of cerebral circulation can occur and cause stroke, TIA, or vascular dementia
- Occasionally disease presents with stroke
- Other features include mononeuropathy or polyneuropathy (mononeuritis multiplex), livedo reticularis, renal involvement, myalgias, weakness, weight loss
- Eosinophilia is often present
- Arteriographic abnormalities and arterial biopsy (if performed) shows polymorphonuclear cells
- Antineutrophil cytoplasmic antibody (pANCA) is often elevated
- Treatment is with steroid and immunosuppressive therapy.

Granulomatosis with polyangiitis
- Systemic vasculitis of medium and small arteries, including venules and arterioles. It produces granulomatous inflammation of the respiratory tracts and necrotizing, pauci-immune glomerulonephritis
- There is nasal or oral inflammation (oral ulcers or purulent/bloody nasal discharge) which may be painful. There may be saddle nose deformity (nose flattened because of destruction of nasal septum by granulomatous inflammation)
- Abnormal CXR showing nodules, infiltrates, cavities
- Microscopic haematuria or RBC casts
- Vessel biopsy shows granulomatous inflammation
- Almost all patients with granulomatosis with polyangiitis have c-ANCA, but not vice versa
- The current treatment of choice is cyclophosphamide.

Systemic lupus erythematosus
- A systemic disorder which can involve both central and peripheral nervous systems
- Stroke may occur because of:
  - vasculitis/vasculopathy involving the small vessels
  - associated lupus anticoagulant syndrome causing thrombosis in large and medium-sized vessels
  - aseptic endocarditis (Liebman–Sacks) causing cerebral embolization
  - hypertension due to renal disease
  - cerebral venous thrombosis.
- Other involvement of the CNS includes headache, psychiatric presentations, seizures, and encephalopathy
- Systemic involvement includes rashes (photosensitive butterfly facial and discoid), arthralgia and arthritis, renal disease, pleuritis and pericarditis, Raynaud's, and leukopenia
- ESR is raised, complement may be reduced
- Diagnosis is on antibody testing: dsDNA (antibodies to genetic material in cells) and anti-Sm antibody (Sm is a protein found in the cell nucleus)
- Anticardiolipin antibody and lupus anticoagulant may be present.

Illicit drug use

- An important cause of stroke, particularly in younger individuals
- The strongest association appears to be with cocaine but there are also reports with amphetamines and sympathomimetic agents and occasionally other illicit drugs
- In some communities, as many as 10% of young strokes may be associated with drug abuse. How much of this is causal and how much is merely innocent association is unclear
- Drug screening should be performed in young stroke patients in whom illicit drug abuse is suspected.

Cocaine

- Associated with both ischaemic and haemorrhagic stroke
- Proposed mechanisms causing stroke include hypertension, vasospasm, vasculitis, cardiac arrhythmias, MI, and increased platelet aggregation
- Stroke appears more common with crack cocaine.

Amphetamines

- Intracerebral and subarachnoid haemorrhage have been associated. Ischaemic stroke is less common but may occur
- Pathological animal studies show small haemorrhages, infarctions, microaneurysms, and perivascular cuffing in small to medium-sized vessels following repeated amphetamine injection
- Cerebral angiography may show segmental narrowing and dilatations ('beading') of medium-sized intracerebral arteries consistent with vasculitis.

Heroin

- Associated particularly with ischaemic stroke
- Possible mechanisms include infective endocarditis with septic embolism, HIV infection, emboli from contaminants introduced during intravenous injection, hypotension, and possibly a vasculitis.

Infection and stroke

Associations between infection and stroke include the following:
- Specific infections which can cause stroke
- Non-specific association between recent infection and stroke—many studies have found recent infection is associated with increased ischaemic stroke risk
- Chronic inflammation and infection (particularly with *Chlamydia pneumoniae*) with accelerated atherosclerosis. Trials of antibiotic therapy have failed to reduce cardiovascular event risk after MI
- Infection frequently complicates stroke and may worsen outcome.
- A list of specific infections is shown in Table 11.3
- Infective endocarditis is an important cause of stroke. Embolism can cause ischaemic stroke, while septic emboli can result in mycotic aneurysm and cerebral haemorrhage (see ➔ p. 415)
- Meningeal infection can cause secondary vasculitis and thrombosis in basal cerebral arteries as they pass through the meninges. Important causes include tuberculosis, syphilis, and fungi. Contrast-enhanced MRI may show basal meningeal enhancement, and CSF examination is often diagnostic. Acute bacterial meningitis less commonly causes stroke by similar mechanisms
- Some viruses are associated with cerebral vasculitis occurring following acute infection, particularly herpes zoster and, less frequently, chicken pox (especially in children)
- Rarely, inflammation of the internal carotid artery in the neck can cause secondary thrombosis and stroke. This can occur because of infections in the neck, including pharyngitis and tonsillitis, especially in children.

COVID-19 and stroke
- COVID-19 is associated with an increased risk of stroke at the time of, the infection.
- The increased risk is thought to be primarily due to the inflammatory and prothrombotic response.
- Typical strokes are large artery occlusions, often in multiple vascular territories, and are associated with higher NINDS score on admission and worse outcome.
- The risk of stroke is highest at the time of infection but a longer time follow-up in 150 000 individuals also reported an increased risk of stroke beyond the first 30 d after COVID-19 infection, hazard ratio (HR) = 1.52 (1.43, 1.62) resulting in about 4 extra strokes per 1000 persons at 12 months.
- The Astra Zeneca COVID vaccine was associated with an increased risk of stroke, particularly due to cerebral venous thrombosis. A 2024 analysis of Medicare data found the bivalent vaccines (Pfizer-BioNTech BNT162b2 and WT/OMI BA.4/BA) were not associated with any increased stroke risk.

Table 11.3 Infection and stroke

Infections directly causing stroke
Infective endocarditis
Meningitis
Chronic
Tuberculosis
Syphilis
Fungal (*Cryptococcus, Candida, Aspergillus*, mucormycosis)
Acute bacterial
Viral infections
Herpes zoster vasculitis
Chicken pox (varicella)
HIV
COVID-19
Carotid inflammation
Tonsillitis
Pharyngitis
Lymphadenitis
Other associations of infection with stroke
Chronic inflammation/infection associated with atherosclerosis
Recent acute infection associated with increased stroke risk

HIV and stroke

- Stroke incidence is increased in individuals with HIV
- The risk of ischaemic stroke appears to be particularly increased. Cerebral haemorrhage risk may also be increased to a lesser extent (see Table 11.4)
- Many different stroke mechanisms are responsible, making a full diagnostic work-up essential
- Cardioembolism, particularly cardiomyopathy, may account for as much as 20% of HIV ischaemic stroke
- Vasculitis is a more common cause than in non-HIV stroke. Potential mechanisms include basal cerebral artery involvement due to basal meningitis (e.g. tuberculosis), neurosyphilis, and herpes zoster
- The role of hypercoagulability is controversial. Protein S deficiency and lupus anticoagulant are both more common, but recent studies have suggested these abnormalities are as common in HIV patients without stroke. They may be non-specific markers of illness
- With increased survival, an increased incidence of atherosclerotic stroke is becoming evident. Possible mechanisms include direct HIV effects on endothelial cells, secondary lipid abnormalities, and anti-retroviral therapy. Treatment with combination anti-retroviral therapies (CART), particularly those containing protease inhibitors, has been associated with severe premature atherosclerosis, including MI and stroke
- Associated drug abuse is common and may contribute to stroke. Cocaine use is a particular risk
- Causes of cerebral haemorrhage in HIV include thrombocytopenia, hypertension, and mycotic aneurysm secondary to infective endocarditis
- Diagnostic work-up for HIV stroke should include a full young stroke work-up and often lumbar puncture for CSF examination. Prothrombotic disorders should be tested for but if abnormalities are found it should not be assumed that these have caused stroke, and other potential causes should also be sought.

Table 11.4 Mechanisms of stroke in HIV-positive patients

Ischaemic stroke	Cerebral haemorrhage
Cardioembolism	Vascular
Cardiomyopathy	Vasculitis
Endocarditis	Mycotic aneurysm secondary to endocarditis
Vascultis	Cocaine
Tuberculosis meningitis	Haematological
Neurosyphilis	Reduced platelets (thrombocytopenia)
Herpes zoster	Reduced coagulation factors due to liver disease
Fungal	Cocaine-induced brain haemorrhage
Accelerated atherosclerosis	
Proinflammatory effect on endothelial cells	
Indirect induction of lipid abnormalities	
Anti-retroviral therapy	
Hypercoagulability	
Protein S deficiency	
Lupus anticoagulant/antiphospholipid antibody (?causal)	
Associated substance abuse (leading to vasculitis)	
Cocaine	
Amphetamine	
Injection of particulate matter (used to dilute drugs)	

Cancer and stroke

- An increased risk of stroke has been associated with cancer. Both are common diseases and in many patients may be associated by chance. In some, the cancer itself causes the stroke often by inducing a prothrombotic state a causal relationship is likely.
- Possible mechanisms causing stroke in cancer patients are shown in Table 11.5. These include:
  - Hypercoagulability
  - associations with specific tumours
  - complications of therapy: drug, surgical, and radiotherapy.
- Population based studies have reported the risk of stroke is doubled in those with cancer.
- More common cancers associated with stroke include breast, colonic, prostate and lung (adenocarcinoma).

Table 11.5 Possible causes of stroke in cancer patients

Cerebral infarction
Hypercoagulable state
Non-bacterial endocarditis (marantic endocarditis)
Embolism of tumour (including atrial myxoma)
Treatment-related:
Radiation vasculopathy
Interventions, including surgery
Drug therapy
Direct compression of extracranial or intracranial arteries
Opportunistic infections
Cerebral haemorrhage
Haemorrhage into primary brain neoplasms
Haemorrhage into metastases:
Melanoma
Bronchial carcinoma
Choriocarcinoma
Hypernephroma
Thrombocytopenia and other coagulopathies
Tumour embolization with aneurysm formation and rupture
Cerebral venous thrombosis
Tumour infiltration of venous sinuses
Tumour compression of venous sinuses
Hypercoagulable state

- Clinical pointers to a diagnosis of cancer related stroke include : no other cause found for stroke, infracts in multiple cerebral arterial territories, thrombosis elsewhere in the body, systemic signs of illness.
- A markedly elevated D-dimer is a useful clue to an underlying cancer, although it is not specific.
- A good maxim is that if you cannot find a cause for someone's stroke despite full usual examinations, then think of cancer.
- In possible cases a CT scan of the thorax, abdomen, and pelvis can be a useful screening test.
- An echocardiogram may show vegetations consistent with marantic endocarditis.
- Radiation vasculopathy is a well-recognized complication of cancer therapy. Usually in the years after irradiation to the head or neck, vasculopathy may occur. It may involve extracranial cerebral arteries or intracranial vessels (including microvasculature). It presents with stroke (often recurrent) and dementia (particularly for intracranial small-vessel vasculopathy). Progress is often relentless (particularly for intracranial small-vessel vasculopathy) and there is no proven treatment.

Reversible cerebral vasoconstriction syndrome

- Also known as Call–Fleming syndrome, benign angiopathy of the CNS, and post-partum angiopathy
- Peaks at about 40 years
- More common in women than in men
- Reversible cerebral vasoconstriction syndrome (RCVS) tends to be an acute, self-limiting illness without new symptoms after 1 month
- Headache is the main symptom. Onset is acute often with a thunderclap headache
- Nausea, vomiting, photophobia, and phonophobia can occur
- Headache may be recurrent for a couple of weeks
- Can be triggered by sexual activity, straining during defecation, stressful or emotional situations
- Over half the cases are in post-partum women or those taking vasoactive drugs (e.g. selective serotonin reuptake inhibitors or nasal decongestants)
- Seizures can occur in up to 40% of cases
- Focal deficits occur in 10% of cases and are usually negative mimicking stroke. However, some can be positive, like migraine aura
- Blood tests including ESR are usually normal
- CSF examination is usually normal or shows a mildly raised protein and/or white cell count
- CT brain scans can be normal. However, using MRI and on repeated imaging up to 80% can be abnormal with convexity subarachnoid haemorrhage, cerebral infarcts, intracerebral haemorrhage, or reversible brain oedema visible
- To diagnose RCVS, intra-arterial angiography, CT, or MRA may show segmental narrowing and dilatation (string of beads) of one or more arteries. The abnormalities may take a week to develop so imaging may need to be repeated
- Biopsy is not useful and arterial histology has been normal with no active inflammation, vasculitis, or micro-thrombosis

  The following are the current diagnostic criteria for RCVS:
- Acute and severe headache (often thunderclap) with or without focal deficits or seizures (this is the key symptom to pick up in the history—particularly if the thunderclap headache has been recurrent)
- Uniphasic course without new symptoms more than 1 month after clinical onset
- Segmental vasoconstriction of cerebral arteries shown by indirect (e.g. magnetic resonance or CT) or direct catheter angiography—so-called string-of-sausages sign
- No evidence of aneurysmal subarachnoid haemorrhage
- Normal or near-normal CSF (protein concentrations <100 mg/dL, <15 white blood cells per μL)
- Complete or substantial normalization of arteries shown by follow-up indirect or direct angiography within 12 weeks of clinical onset
- Treatment is supportive, including nutrition, aggressive IV fluid hydration, correction of electrolyte imbalance, and analgesia

- There are no trials of the best medication. Nimodipine in the doses used to treat subarachnoid haemorrhage have helped reduce the headache but has not been shown to prevent complications or improve neurological outcome
- In most patients, headaches and angiographic abnormalities resolve within days or weeks, and most by 3 months
- Most strokes improve slowly
- Less than 5% have life-threatening strokes or brain oedema
- The combined case fatality is reported as less than 1%
- Recurrence of the syndrome is possible but the rate is unknown.

Further reading

Carotid and vertebral artery dissection

CADISS trial investigators (2015). Antiplatelet treatment compared with anticoagulation treatment for cervical artery dissection (CADISS): a randomised trial. *Lancet Neurol* **14**, 361–367.

Kaufmann JE, Harshfield EL, Gensicke H, *et al.* (2024). CADISS and TREAT-CAD Investigators. Antithrombotic treatment for cervical artery dissection: a systematic review and individual patient data meta-analysis. *JAMA Neurol* **81**, 630–637.

Yaghi S, Engelter S, Del Brutto VJ, *et al.* (2024). A scientific statement from the American Heart Association. *Stroke* **55**, e91–e106.

Fibromuscular dysplasia

Green IE, Southerland AM, Worrall BB (2020). Fibromuscular dysplasia and stroke. *Pract Neurol* January, 42–46.

CADASIL and other monogenic forms of small-vessel disease

Cho BPH, Jolly AA, Nannoni S, *et al.* (2022). Association of *NOTCH3* variant position with stroke onset and other clinical features among patients with CADASIL. *Neurology* **99**, e430–e439.

Mancuso M, Arnold M, Bersano A, *et al.* (2020). Monogenic cerebral small-vessel diseases: diagnosis and therapy. Consensus recommendations of the European Academy of Neurology. *Eur J Neurol* **27**, 909–927.

Tan RY, Markus HS (2016). CADASIL: migraine, encephalopathy, stroke and their inter-relationships. *PLoS One* **11**, e0157613.

Verdura E, Hervé D, Scharrer E, *et al.* (2015). Heterozygous HTRA1 mutations are associated with autosomal dominant cerebral small vessel disease. *Brain* **138**, 2347–2358.

Sickle cell disease

Light J, Boucher M, Baskin-Miller J, Winstead M (2023). Managing the cerebrovascular complications of sickle cell disease: current perspectives. *J Blood Med* **14**, 279–293.

Singh A, Irfan H, Fatima E, *et al.* (2024). Revolutionary breakthrough: FDA approves CASGEVY, the first CRISPR/Cas9 gene therapy for sickle cell disease. *Ann Med Surg (Lond)* **86**, 4555–4559.

Fabry disease

Fellgiebel A, Muller MJ, Ginsberg L (2006). CNS manifestations of Fabry's disease. *Lancet Neurol* **5**, 791–795.

Shi Q, Chen J, Pongmoragot J, *et al.* (2014). Prevalence of Fabry disease in stroke patients—a systematic review and meta-analysis. *J Stroke Cerebrovasc Dis* **23**, 985–992.

Moyamoya disease and syndrome

Guey S, Tournier-Lasserve E, Hervé D, Kossorotoff M (2015). Moyamoya disease and syndromes: from genetics to clinical management. *Appl Clin Genet* **8**, 49–68.

Miyamoto S, Yoshimoto T, Hashimoto N, *et al.* JAM Trial Investigators (2014). Effects of extracranial-intracranial bypass for patients with hemorrhagic moyamoya disease: results of the Japan Adult Moyamoya Trial. *Stroke* **45**, 1415–1421.

Moussouttas M, Rybinnik I (2020). A critical appraisal of bypass surgery in moyamoya disease. *Ther Adv Neurol Disord* **13**, 1756286420921092.

Prothrombotic disorders in stroke

Morris JG, Singh S, Fisher M (2010). Testing for inherited thrombophilias in arterial stroke: can it cause more harm than good? *Stroke* **41**, 2985–2990.

Rodziewicz M, D'Cruz DP (2020). An update on the management of antiphospholipid syndrome. *Ther Adv Musculoskelet Dis* **12**, 1759720X20910855.

COVID and stroke

Lu Y, Matuska K, Nadimpalli G, *et al*. (2024). Stroke risk after COVID-19 bivalent vaccination among US older adults. *JAMA* **331**, 938–950.

Nannoni S, de Groot R, Bell S, Markus HS (2021). Stroke in COVID-19: a systematic review and meta-analysis. *Int J Stroke* **16**, 137–149.

Xie Y, Xu E, Bowe B, *et al*. (2022). Long-term cardiovascular outcomes of COVID-19. *Nat Med* **28**, 583–590.

HIV and stroke

Benjamin LA, Bryer A, Emsley HC, *et al*. (2012). HIV infection and stroke: current perspectives and future directions. *Lancet Neurol* **11**, 878–890.

Du M, Wang Y, Qin C, *et al*. (2023). Prevalence and incidence of stroke among people with HIV. *AIDS* **37**, 1747–1756.

Cancer and stroke

Dardiotis E, Aloizou AM, Markoula S, *et al*. (2019). Cancer-associated stroke: pathophysiology, detection and management (Review). *Int J Oncol* **54**, 779–796.

Navi BB, Kasner SE, Elkind MSV, *et al*. (2021). Cancer and embolic stroke of undetermined source. *Stroke* **52**, 1121–1130.

Rioux B, Touma L, Nehme A, *et al*. (2021). Frequency and predictors of occult cancer in ischemic stroke: a systematic review and meta-analysis. *Int J Stroke* **16**, 12–19.

Reversible cerebral vasoconstriction syndrome

Singhal AB (2023). Reversible cerebral vasoconstriction syndrome: a review of pathogenesis, clinical presentation, and treatment. *Int J Stroke* **18**, 1151–1160.

Cerebral venous thrombosis

Introduction

- Cerebral venous thrombosis (CVT) can be a difficult diagnosis to make, but an important one, because anticoagulation is associated with improved outcomes and patients in a severe neurological state can still have a good outcome.
- Variable clinical presentations, including headache, papilloedema, seizures, focal deficits, intracerebral haemorrhage, and coma, make a high index of suspicion important.
- Underdiagnosed. 0.5–1.0% of stroke admissions. Three times commoner in women.
- MRI and MR venography (MRV), as well as CT venography (CTV), have greatly improved ease of diagnosis.
- Overall low acute mortality of around 2–4% in the largest cohort series published from the USA.

Anatomy

- Venous sinuses drain blood from the brain and bones of the skull.
- They are situated between the two layers of the dura mater.
- They are lined by endothelium, continuous with the veins.
- They contain no valves and the walls are devoid of muscular tissue.
- Connections exist between venous sinuses and veins of the face, scalp, spine, and neck. This provides a path by which pathological processes such as infection can spread into cerebral venous sinuses, as well as an alternate route for blood to leave the cranial cavity when obstruction occurs.
- A diagram of the anatomy of the cerebral venous sinuses is shown in Fig. 12.1.
- The frequency of occluded sinuses is:
  - Transverse sinus (44–73%)
  - Superior sagittal sinus (39–62%)
  - Sigmoid sinus (40–47%)
  - Deep venous system (10.9%)
  - Cortical veins (3.7–17.2%)
  - Cavernous sinus (1.3–1.7%).

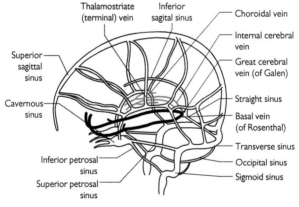

Fig. 12.1 The venous sinuses.

Aetiology

- Causes of CVT are shown in Table 12.1.
- Infection was, and in many parts of the world still is, a major cause of CVT. In developing countries, the proportion caused by infection has fallen from 40% in the 1960s to 10% or less currently.
- Infection is relatively more important for cavernous sinus thrombosis and lateral sinus thrombosis.
- Cavernous sinus thrombosis may originate via spread from the medial third of the face, nose, orbit, or paranasal sinuses, or by direct spread by ethmoid or sphenoid ear cells or through lateral sinuses from the ear. *Staphylococcus aureus* is the most common pathogen.
- Fungal infections may cause CVT, particularly in the cavernous sinus.
- Prothrombotic states and elevated blood homocysteine levels are risk factors. Leiden factor V (causing activated protein C resistance) is the most commonly associated risk factor.
- Increased risk is associated with pregnancy and particularly puerperium and contraceptive therapy is likely to be mediated via hypercoagulability.
- In closed head trauma there are a number of possible mechanisms of CVT:
  - Skull fractures or intracranial hematomas causing thrombosis by direct compression of the sinus
  - Compression of the sinuses from intracranial oedema
  - Endothelial injury within the sinus leading to the activation of the coagulation cascade
  - Intramural haemorrhages due to rupture of small sinusoids
  - Extension of the thrombus from injured emissary veins
- Frequently patients have more than one potential cause of CVT.

Table 12.1 Causes of cerebral venous thrombosis

Infective
Bacterial infections
Fungal infections
Non-infective
Inherited prothrombotic disorders:
APC resistance—factor V Leiden polymorphism
Antithrombin III deficiency
Protein C and S deficiency
Prothrombin gene mutation
Hyperhomocysteinaemia
Acquired prothrombotic state:
Pregnancy and puerperium
Lupus anticoagulant/anticardiolipin antibody
Vaccine-induced immune thrombotic thrombocytopenia (VITT)
Nephrotic syndrome
Dehydration
Inflammatory disorders and vasculitis:
Behçet's
Wegener's granulomatosis
SLE
Haematological conditions:
Polycythaemia
Anaemia, including paroxysmal nocturnal haemoglobinuria
Thrombocythaemia
Sickle cell anaemia
Thyrotoxicosis
Mechanical:
Head trauma
Neurosurgical or other interventional procedures
Neoplasia:
Usually haematogenous malignancies
Local compression, e.g. meningioma
Drugs: Oral contraceptives; COVID vaccination
Idiopathic

Clinical features

These may arise from:
- venous infarction which may be haemorrhagic;
- cerebral haemorrhage;
- impaired venous drainage leading to oedema and raised intracranial pressure.

Specific features include the following:
- Raised intracranial pressure with headache and papilloedema. This manifests particularly when the superior sagittal sinus is occluded owing to impaired absorption of cerebral spinal fluid (CSF) by the arachnoid villi.
- Headache owing to raised intracranial pressure or sometimes secondary to haemorrhage.
- Focal neurological deficits—these may fluctuate in severity. Hemiplegia is most frequent, and in superior sagittal sinus thrombosis the leg may be more affected than the face and arm.
- Seizures—these may occur in the absence of any other deficit although are more common in patients with focal neurological deficits.
- Cranial nerve palsy—particularly for cavernous sinus thrombosis.

Common patterns of presentation

Most presentations fall into a number of patterns with different rates of temporal progression (see Fig. 12.2):

- Abrupt onset of focal signs mimicking an arterial occlusion.
- Subacute onset of focal deficit with or without seizures or elevated intracranial pressure.
- Progressive rise in intracranial pressure. This occurs particularly with superior sagittal sinus thrombosis.
- Chronic presentations, which can be confused with a brain tumour.
- Progressive visual field impairment and headache—up to 10% of benign intracranial hypertension cases have underlying CVT.
- Sudden headache resembling subarachnoid haemorrhage.
- Asymptomatic, found on imaging in the context of head trauma and depressed skull fracture.

Whenever we see an unusual haemorrhage on brain imaging, we always think of CVT—especially in the context of associated seizures or insidious history of neurological deterioration

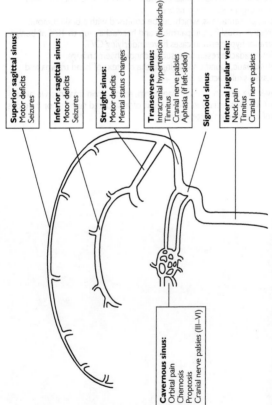

Superior sagittal sinus:
Motor deficits
Seizures

Inferior sagittal sinus:
Motor deficits
Seizures

Straight sinus:
Motor deficits
Mental status changes

Transverse sinus:
Intracranial hypertension (headache)
Tinnitus
Cranial nerve palsies
Aphasia (if left-sided)

Sigmoid sinus

Internal jugular vein:
Neck pain
Tinnitus
Cranial nerve palsies

Cavernous sinus:
Orbital pain
Chemosis
Proptosis
Cranial nerve palsies (III–VI)

Fig. 12.2 Major clinical syndromes according to location of cerebral venous thrombosis.
Reproduced from *Circulation* 125(13), Piazza G, Cerebral venous thrombosis, pp. 1704–9, Copyright (2012).

Cavernous sinus thrombosis

- This has a unique presentation owing to its anatomy (Fig. 12.3).
- It most commonly occurs secondary to infection in the middle third of the face, sphenoid, ethmoid or maxillary sinuses, and, less commonly, the oropharynx, teeth, neck, and ear.
- Presentation is related to venous obstruction, inflammation, and systematic infection.
- Headache is common.
- Proptosis and oedema of the eyelids and conjunctiva arise secondary to venous obstruction.
- Dilatation of facial veins may occur.
- Ophthalmoplegia with palsies of cranial nerves III, IV, and VI as they pass through the sinus may occur.
- Optic nerve involvement can result in impaired acuity and afferent pupillary defect.
- Papilloedema and retinal vein distension are often noted.
- The contralateral cavernous sinus may be affected because of midline communications through circular or intracavernous sinus.
- Facial numbness may be confined to the upper two-thirds of the face as the first two divisions of the trigeminal nerve are intracavernous. If the thrombosis or infection spreads into the inferior petrosal sinus, the third division of the trigeminal nerve may also be affected.
- The close proximity of cranial nerves III, IV, and VI and the first two divisions of the trigeminal nerve explains why palsies of these nerves are common in cavernous sinus thrombosis.

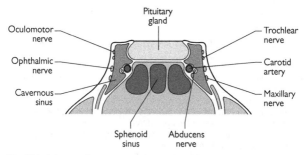

Fig. 12.3 A diagram of a cross-sectional view of a cavernous sinus showing close proximity to cranial nerves II, IV, VI, and Va and Vb.

Investigations

An elevated D-dimer supports the diagnosis of CVT, but a normal D-dimer level is not sufficient to exclude the diagnosis.

In any case where the suspicion of CVT is raised, e.g. an unusual intracerebral haemorrhage (ICH), maintain a low threshold for neuroimaging to exclude CVT.

Both MRI with MRV, and computed tomography angiography (CTA), can diagnose CVT.

CT and CTV

- CT may be abnormal in venous sinus thrombosis but the findings are often non-specific, particularly early in the disease course. Use of contrast enhancement can improve diagnostic yield.
- The posterior portion of the superior sagittal sinus can be directly visualized on CT.
- Specific features:
  - Delta sign—thrombosis of the superior sagittal sinus may appear as a dense triangle at the occiput on an unenhanced scan. Following contrast injection, the negative or empty delta sign may be seen (see Figs 12.4 and 12.5). This is a central lucency ascribed to sluggish or absent blood flow within the superior sagittal sinus surrounded by a margin of contrast enhancement.
  - Diffuse low density suggestive of oedema.
  - Generalized cerebral swelling.
  - Haemorrhagic infarcts—mixed hypodensity and increased density corresponding to ischaemia and haemorrhage.
  - Intracerebral haemorrhage.
- CTV can usually visualize the occluded sinus.

MRI and MRV

- Absence of normal 'flow void' in venous sinuses on T2-weighted imaging may be seen.
- Intravascular thrombus itself may be seen within the sinuses.
- MRI will also show similar consequences of venous thrombosis to those seen on CT, namely cerebral swelling, haemorrhagic infarction, and cerebral haemorrhage.
- The acute thrombus generally presents a hyposignal on gradient echo and susceptibility-weighted imaging (SWI) and a hypersignal on spin-echo T1, T2, diffusion-weighted imaging (DWI), and fluid-attenuated inversion recovery (FLAIR) sequences.
- MRV shows absent or reduced venous flow at the site of thrombosis.
- MRI and MRV or CTA can miss thrombosis in small sinuses or in the deep cerebral veins. This may require intra-arterial angiography to detect.

(a)   (b)

(c)   (d)

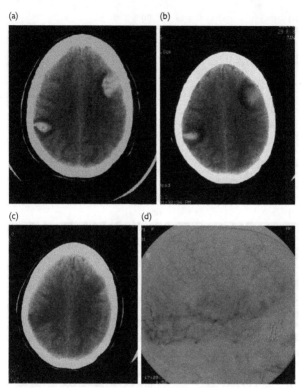

Fig. 12.4 Cerebral venous thrombosis may present with headache, focal neurological signs, and seizure, raised intracranial pressure, and impaired consciousness. This woman in her early thirties presented with reduced conscious level and seizures during the postpartum period. (a) CT scan showed haemorrhagic infarction in the left frontal region and right parietal region. (b) days after the first scan showed progressive resolution of the haemorrhages. She made a complete recovery. (c) Intra-arterial venography shows no filling in the superior sagittal sinus consistent with superior sagittal sinus thrombosis. She was treated with heparin, and serial CT scans 8 (d) and 19. © Hugh Markus.

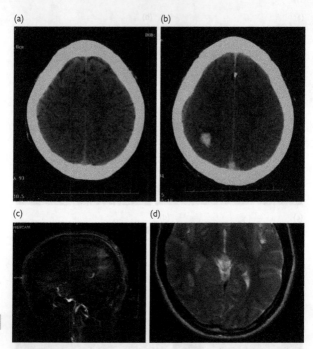

Fig. 12.5 This patient presented to the acute stroke unit with headache, nausea, and vomiting. (a) The initial CT showed no haemorrhage but a 'delta sign' was present, indicating thrombus in the posterior part of the superior sagittal sinus. (b) On CT scan at day 5, haemorrhage can now be seen in the right parietal lobe. (c) Magnetic resonance angiogram (MRA) confirmed the diagnosis, showing absence of flow in the superior sagittal sinus. (d) On MRI, a thrombus within the sagittal sinus can be seen. © Hugh Markus.

Treatment

- Any underlying provoking condition should be treated, e.g. infection.
- The standard recommended treatment is anticoagulation, although there are limited randomized data to support this—one small, very underpowered but positive trial. However, data from non-randomized studies suggest that even in patients with haemorrhagic infarction and intracerebral haemorrhage, dramatic improvements can occur with anticoagulation.
- Therefore, even in cases with ICH, anticoagulation should be started.
- Heparin, followed by warfarin for 3–6 months, is usually recommended. We use low molecular weight heparin acutely before switching to oral anticoagulation.
- DOACs are being increasingly used instead of warfarin. Small studies suggest they may be equivalent but there are no definitive large studies to show if they are better or worse.
- For unprovoked CVT, we would usually use anticoagulants for 6 months.
- If there are underlying abnormalities of coagulation on blood testing or other causes, longer-term anticoagulation may be necessary.
- Symptomatic treatment for epilepsy, raised intracranial pressure, etc. may be required including decompressive hemicraniectomy.
- Endovascular treatment (EVT), including thrombectomy and intrasinus thrombolysis, have been used to achieve recanalization. While recanalization rates of 90% have been reported, there is no clinical trial evidence that it improves outcomes. The TO-ACT trial showed no benefit over anticoagulation.
- Therefore, current guidelines recommend EVT is only used as a rescue treatment for patients who are experiencing clinical deterioration or failed or have contraindications to standard therapy.
- Hemicraniectomy may be considered a lifesaving procedure when there is a significant clinical risk that the intracranial pressure is so high the patient may cone.
- Bechet's disease is a special case. Here, first-line treatment is with high-dose steroids with anticoagulation, particularly if there is concomitant extra-CNS arterial or venous thrombosis.
- Most CVT in pregnancy occurs in the third trimester or puerperium. 80% occurs after delivery. Anticoagulation should be with low-molecular-weight heparin (LMWH).

Prognosis

- Early studies reported poor outcomes with high mortality and residual disability. More recent studies show improved outcomes.
- While most surviving patients do not have major physical disability, chronic symptoms such as headache, fatigue, neurocognitive deficits, and epileptic seizures can affect patients, and result in diminished quality of life.
- With aggressive treatment, the prognosis is often good. Dramatic improvement can be seen. The degree of improvement from focal deficits is more rapid and complete than that usually seen for ischaemic stroke.
- Prognosis is worse for thrombosis of the deep cerebral veins, older patients with underlying septicaemia and presenting with symptomatic brain haemorrhage or patients with underlying malignancy.
- In an inpatient cohort between 2001 and 2008 in the USA, 11 400 patients were hospitalized with CVT and 232 (2.0%) suffered in-hospital mortality.
- The high rate of recurrence (as much as 20%) emphasizes the importance of long-term anticoagulation where underlying prothrombotic states can be detected.
- Women with a history of CVT have an increased risk of CVT and other of thrombotic events (i.e. deep venous thrombosis, pulmonary embolism) in future pregnancies. Recent American Heart Association (AHA) guidelines suggest CVT is not a contraindication for future pregnancies, but that prophylaxis with LMWH during future pregnancies and the postpartum period is probably beneficial.

Vaccine-induced immune thrombotic thrombocytopenia

- CVT due to vaccine-induced immune thrombotic thrombocytopenia (VITT) after vaccination with adenoviral vector SARS-CoV-2 vaccine was a very rare complication of the COVID-19 vaccination programme.
- It was first described following administration of ChAdOx1 nCov-19 Astra Zeneca vaccine but has been described with other vaccines.
- No male/female bias.
- More common in young patients (generally, older patients did not receive this vaccine).
- Presentation is with venous or arterial thrombosis. Patients could be very sick with malaise, fever, headache, myalgia, nausea, vomiting, petechia or bleeding, and cerebral features of CVT.
- CVT symptoms could progress very rapidly.
- Diagnosis requires:
  - COVID vaccine recently
  - Any venous or arterial thrombosis (often cerebral or abdominal)
  - Thrombocytopenia (platelet count <150 × 10^9/L)
  - Positive platelet factor 4 'HIT' (heparin-induced thrombocytopenia) ELISA
  - Markedly elevated D-dimer (>4 times upper limit of normal)
- Treatment is with intravenous immunoglobulin or plasma exchange and a non-heparin anticoagulant (e.g. fondaparinux).

- Mortality rate is about 20%. The outcome depends on the severity of the presenting illness and subsequent complications.
- Once the acute episode has passed, the risk of further thrombosis is low (1–2%).

Further reading

General overview

Idiculla PS, Gurala D, Palanisamy M, *et al.* (2020). Cerebral venous thrombosis: a comprehensive review. *Eur Neurol* **83**, 369–379.

Diagnosis and management

Saposnik G, Bushnell C, Coutinho JM, *et al.* (2024). Diagnosis and management of cerebral venous thrombosis: a scientific statement from the American Heart Association. *Stroke* **55**, e77–e90.

Treatment

Yaghi S, Saldanha IJ, Misquith C, *et al.* (2022). Direct oral anticoagulants versus vitamin K antagonists in cerebral venous thrombosis: a systematic review and meta-analysis. *Stroke* **53**, 3014–3024.

Imaging

Sadik J-C, Jianu DC, Sadik R, *et al.* (2022). Imaging of cerebral venous thrombosis. *Life* **12**, 1215.

Cerebral haemorrhage

Introduction

Intracranial haemorrhage is classified according to the region into which the haemorrhage occurs:

- Extradural haemorrhage (EDH)
- Subdural haemorrhage (SDH)
- Subarachnoid haemorrhage (SAH)
- Intracerebral haemorrhage (ICH).

Cerebral haemorrhage only presents with clinical stroke if there is focal compression in an eloquent brain region, or secondary ischaemic change (e.g. vasospasm in the case of SAH). ICH usually presents with a clinical stroke.

Extradural haemorrhage (EDH)

- EDH is seldom a cause of a stroke syndrome
- It is caused by bleeding into the extradural space
- It usually occurs after head injury
- One of the extradural arteries (such as the middle meningeal artery) is ruptured and blood enters the extradural space (see Fig. 13.1)
- This compresses the brain from the outside, raising ICP acutely, and can be fatal if not recognized and treated promptly
- Ten per cent of EDHs are venous in origin
- It should be suspected in patients with head injury who have a reduced or reduced level of consciousness
- The diagnosis is easily confirmed on brain imaging with CT or MRI
- EDH is a neurosurgical emergency
- EDH patients need urgent scanning and urgent neurosurgical treatment by evacuation of the haematoma, either through burr holes or a craniotomy.

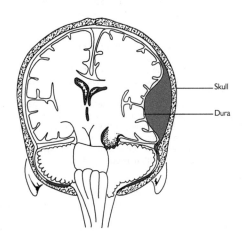

Fig. 13.1 Location of an extradural haemorrhage.

Subdural haematoma (SDH)

- Bleeding occurs in the subdural space (see Fig. 13.2).
- In acute SDH, fragile veins that bridge the subdural space may tear and blood flows at low pressure into the subdural space.
- It is more common in the presence of brain atrophy, particularly in older people and also in chronic alcoholics.
- It is normally thought to be caused by trauma, although the actual incident may not be recalled by the patient at the time that the SDH is diagnosed.
- In chronic SDH, even minor trauma may trigger leakage of blood from the dural border cell layer, which then causes an inflammatory response. Inflammatory mediators stimulate angiogenesis. New fragile vessels can then bleed into regions of the subdural space, forming chronic loculated areas of SDH.

Clinical presentation

- A variety of presentations can occur depending on how acute the subdural haemorrhage is, its size, and its location
- Clinical presentation is often insidious
- It can present as:
  - a stroke with focal symptoms—most commonly hemiparesis, but other cortical signs can occur
  - reduction in consciousness level owing to raised ICP
  - worsening neurological/confusional state, often insidious, particularly in older people
- A high index of suspicion should be present in an elderly patient who is having progressive problems such as a deteriorating gait
- Diagnosis is made on brain imaging with CT or MRI (see Fig. 13.3). Sometimes on CT the haematoma (if old) is isodense (of a similar density) to brain tissue and can be missed if careful evaluation is not performed. In such cases, MRI may be helpful.

Treatment

- A large SDH, particularly if there is reduced consciousness level or focal neurological signs or neurological progression, is a neurosurgical emergency.
- Small SDHs are managed conservatively and usually resolve over time.
- SDHs can be difficult to drain, particularly acutely, as the blood will be partly clotted.
- Neurosurgical teams often wait about a week until the haematoma has liquefied.
- SDH is drained through a burr hole, otherwise a full craniotomy is required to flush out the blood clot.
- A large trial of dexamethasone for chronic SDH, in combination with surgery if indicated, showed no benefit.
- In cases of recurrent or truly atraumatic SDHs, an underlying malformation, such as a dural arterial–venous fistula should be considered as these are often amenable to endovascular intervention.
- Endovascular middle meningeal artery embolization is being increasingly used to treat chronic (and recurrent) SDH either as an adjuvant treatment to open surgery or as an alternative.

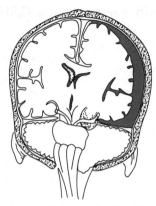

Fig. 13.2 Schematic diagram of the location of a subdural haemorrhage.

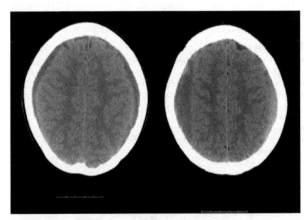

Fig. 13.3 This patient suffered bilateral subdural haemorrhages. The scan on the left is taken after about 1 week. The scan on the right is a month later. The right-sided subdural is larger and the left appears to have resolved; however, close inspection shows that it is still present but isodense. © Anthony Pereira.

Subarachnoid haemorrhage (SAH)

Introduction

SAH is where bleeding occurs into the subarachnoid space (see Fig. 13.4). It most often presents with sudden-onset headache and meningism but can cause focal symptoms, i.e. present as a stroke. This occurs when:
- there is a focal haematoma; this is most common for MCA aneurysms
- secondary vasospasm may result in focal ischaemia.
- Cortical spreading depression or depolarization due to focal convexity SAH.

SAH is generally divided into aneurysmal (aSAH around 85% of the total) and non-aneurysmal (naSAH) after computed tomography angiography (CTA) or digital subtraction angiography (DSA).

Owing to a high risk of early rebleeding, aSAH is a medical and neurosurgical emergency. Patients should be admitted and the diagnosis made either with CT scan and/or lumbar puncture.

aSAH is caused by Berry aneurysms or arteriovenous malformations

naSAH is caused by hypertension, trauma, cerebral amyloid angiopathy (CAA), or reversible cerebral vasoconstriction syndrome (RCVS)

The incidence of SAH is about 8 per 100 000 compared to ICH, which is just below 30 per 100 000.

It is proportionally commoner in younger stroke patients.

Site of haemorrhage

- Most haemorrhage is from aneurysms of the circle of Willis vessels, which arise intracranially
- Atraumatic, isolated convexity SAH is typically due to CAA
- SAH localized in the region of the midbrain is termed peri-mesencephalic SAH (non-aneurysmal, generally benign, believed to be due to deep vein rupture)
- A small proportion occurs in the spine
- Bleeding is into the subarachnoid space, which normally contains cerebrospinal fluid (CSF).

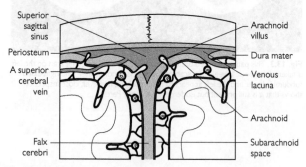

Fig. 13.4 The diagram shows the anatomy of the subarachnoid space. It is a 'potential' space lying between the arachnoid mater and the pia mater. The space is very narrow but blood vessels traverse it.

Risk factors

- Female gender (30% more common in women)
- Hypertension
- Excess alcohol consumption
- Smoking
- Diseases predisposing to berry aneurysms, such as polycystic kidney disease.

Berry (saccular) aneurysms

This is the most common pathology underlying SAH. However, berry aneurysms are found in 2% of asymptomatic individuals at postmortem. They:
• are thin-walled
• are saccular
• most commonly occur at arterial bifurcations (see Fig. 13.5).

Common sites of aneurysms are:
• posterior communicating artery (30%)
• anterior communicating artery (25%)
• middle cerebral artery (25%)
• 15% are multiple.

Most are asymptomatic. They cause symptoms either when they rupture or occasionally if they increase in size. A ruptured aneurysm resulting in SAH is a common cause of sudden death, particularly in the young.

Rupture rates depend on size and position of the aneurysm. The cumulative 5-year rupture rates for aneurysms in the anterior and posterior circulation are listed here:
• Anterior circulation: internal carotid artery, anterior communicating or anterior cerebral artery, middle cerebral artery:
  • <7 mm: 0%
  • 7–12 mm: 2.6%
  • 13–24 mm: 14.5%
  • >25 mm: 40%
• Posterior circulation: posterior cerebral and posterior communicating:
  • <7 mm: 2.5%
  • 7–12 mm: 14.5%
  • 13–24 mm: 18.4%
  • >25 mm: 50%

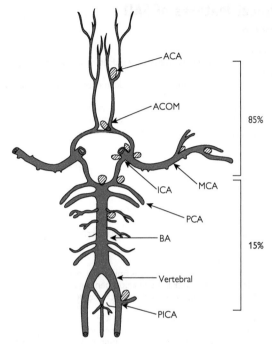

Fig. 13.5 Common sites of berry aneurysms. ACA, anterior cerebral artery; ACOM, anterior communicating artery; BA, berry aneurysm; ICA, internal carotid artery; MCA, middle cerebral artery; PCA, posterior cerebral artery; PICA, posterior interior cerebral artery.

Adapted from McCormick W. F. Vascular diseases. In: Rosenberg R. N., Grossman R. G., Crochet S. S. JR. et al. (eds), *The clinical neurosciences: neurology, neurosurgery, neuropathology, neuroradiology, neurobiology*, volume 3, pp. 35–83, Copyright (1983), with permission from Elsevier.

Clinical features of SAH

Symptoms

Headache
- The classic presentation is with a very sudden-onset (thunderclap) severe headache
- It is often occipital but any new very sudden-onset headache should be considered as a potential SAH
- Some patients with a SAH may have had a warning or so-called sentinel headache in the preceding days owing to a minor leak of blood.

Other frequent accompanying symptoms
- Nausea
- Vomiting
- Photophobia
- Neck stiffness.

Conscious level
- This may be reduced and is associated with worse prognosis
- SAH can present with sudden death
- A short period of loss of consciousness may occur at onset.

Signs
- Meningism—marked neck stiffness:
  - Kernig's sign—straight leg raising is limited and induces pain
  - Brudzinsky's sign—neck flexion induces bending of the legs
  - Interestingly, although flexion of the neck may be impossible, lateral rotation of the neck is unaffected
- Bilateral VI cranial nerve palsy from raised ICP
- Focal neurological signs—these are often not present but may occur depending on the site of bleeding, the presence of focal haematoma and secondary to complications such as vasospasm
- Fundoscopy may show subhyaloid haemorrhage.

Differential diagnoses
- Migraine
- Coital cephalgia
- Meningitis
- RCVS (Reversible cerebral vasoconstriction syndrome) (➔ see p. 354)
- Thunderclap headache without SAH:
  - This usually occurs without meningism or focal neurology
  - CT imaging and CSF examination are normal
  - It has a good outcome and low incidence of subsequent SAH.

Grading of SAH

There are several grading systems used to describe the severity of SAH. Two are given in Box 13.1: the Hunt and Hess grading and the World Federation of Neurological Surgeons grading system. Grading is a useful method to describe the severity of SAH and provides some indication of the likely outcome, which is worse with a higher grade.

Box 13.1 Grading systems for SAH

Hunt and Hess grades
- Grade I—asymptomatic, or minimal headache and slight nuchal rigidity
- Grade II—moderate to severe headache, nuchal rigidity, no neurological deficit except cranial nerve palsy
- Grade III—drowsiness, confusion or mild focal deficit
- Grade IV—stupor, moderate to severe hemiparesis, possibly early decerebrate rigidity, and vegetative disturbances
- Grade V—deep coma, decerebrate rigidity, moribund appearance.

World Federation of Neurological Surgeons

Grade	GCS score	Motor deficit
I	15	Absent
II	14–13	Absent
III	14–13	Present
IV	12–7	Present or absent
V	6–3	Present or absent

Investigation of SAH

Computed tomography

- Diagnosis can often be confirmed by an early CT
- This has become the first-line diagnostic test of choice and it often enables one to avoid lumbar puncture
- Sensitivity is 90% if performed within the first 24 hours
- Sensitivity is reduced to 50% by 72 hours as blood is reabsorbed
- CT may also identify the source of haemorrhage:
  - Anterior communicating artery aneurysm bleed produces blood at the front of the interhemispheric fissure
  - Middle cerebral artery aneurysm produces blood in the Sylvian fissure
  - Internal carotid artery bleeding produces blood in the suprasellar cistern on one side
  - Posterior communicating artery aneurysm produces blood in the suprasellar and prepontine cisterns
  - Basilar artery aneurysm produces blood in the basal cisterns.

Lumbar puncture

- Indicated if diagnosis is in doubt, i.e. if CT has given equivocal results, lumbar puncture is indicated
- Opening pressure may be raised
- Uniform blood-staining of CSF is seen. If it has been a traumatic or 'bloody' tap, the number of red cells will decline as time goes on. This can be seen if three serial samples are taken and the depth of blood staining visualized when they are held up to light
- The ratio of white cells to red cells will be 1:500, the same as in peripheral blood. A higher proportion of white cells may indicate a different diagnosis
- Xanthochromia (a yellow tinge to the fluid) appears as CSF blood haemolyses. It remains present for about 2 weeks
- Spectrophotometry of CSF for bilirubin quantitation to check for xanthochromia is the recommended method of analysis and should be done on the final bottle of CSF collected.

Cerebral angiography

- This is essential in all cases in which intervention might be possible to determine whether there is an underlying aneurysm and identify its site and size (see Fig. 13.6)
- CT angiography is good at identifying aneurysms and technology is continuing to improve but may miss very small aneurysms (3 mm or smaller). It is non-invasive and can be routinely performed as soon as SAH diagnosis is confirmed
- MRA can identify larger aneurysms but may miss those 3–5 mm in diameter or less
- The gold standard is intra-arterial DSA, which is necessary if CTA and MRA are negative.

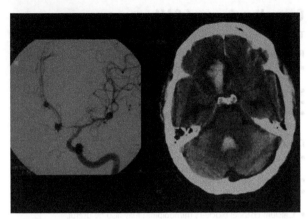

Fig. 13.6 A left anterior communicating artery aneurysm which caused intracerebral haemorrhage which can be seen both in the right frontal region. Blood is also visible on CT in the fourth ventricle. The aneurysm is visible on the angiogram. © Hugh Markus.

Complications of SAH

The major complications are as follows.

Rebleeding

- Risk of rebleed is 4% at 24 hours, 25% at 2 weeks, and 60% at 6 months if no measures are taken to prevent it
- The mean time for rebleeding is about 10 days
- Rebleeding is associated with an 80% mortality or poor outcome
- This high risk is why early identification and treatment of aneurysms to prevent rebleeding is required.

Delayed cerebral ischaemia (DCI)

- Vasospasm resulting from blood in the CSF may produce a secondary ischaemic neurological deficit
- It is most common after about 2 days and lasts up to 2 weeks
- Treatment is by maintaining cerebral perfusion with adequate hydration and adequate blood pressure
- Calcium channel blockers (nimodipine) may also be useful.
- Magnesium, statins, and prednisolone have shown not to help.

Hydrocephalus

- Results from impaired CSF reabsorption through arachnoid villi owing to blockage by blood in the CSF
- Ten per cent of patients will require CSF diversion or shunting.

Seizures

- Ten per cent of patients may suffer seizures
- The risk is higher the more severe the neurological deficit
- Seizures most frequently occur during the acute episode but can also occur months or more after the SAH.

Cardiac abnormalities

- ST elevation on the ECG is often seen and may mimic changes seen in acute myocardial infarction.

Syndrome of inappropriate ADH secretion (SIADH)

- This is caused by continued secretion of arginine vasopression (ADH) despite normal or increased plasma volume, causing salt wasting in the kidney
- The plasma sodium concentration drops. It can drop to 120 mmol/L or lower. This is accompanied by serum hypo-osmolality and high urine osmolality
- The key to management is to understand that hyponatraemia results from an excess of water rather than a deficiency of sodium.
- It is diagnosed by sending a simultaneous blood and urine sample to calculate the respective osmolalities
- Treatment is fluid restriction
- Vasopresson-2 receptor antagonists (e.g. conivaptan or tolvaptan) can be given
- SIADH normally abates spontaneously with these measures.

Management of SAH: medical

The patient should be admitted to hospital and transferred to a neuroscience centre.

General measures

- Maintain airway, breathing, circulation
- Intubate and ventilate if necessary
- Oxygen if needed
- Serum glucose—use sliding scale infusion of insulin if necessary
- Treat fever
- Consider antiemetics for nausea or vomiting
- Treat seizures
- Watch for SIADH by monitoring serum sodium, and treat if it occurs with fluid restriction
- Elevate the head of the bed 30° to facilitate intracranial venous drainage
- Maintain euvolaemia (central venous pressure, 5–8 mmHg).

Treatment of raised intracranial pressure

- This is a common complication
- ICP monitoring may be necessary
- Intubation with hyperventilation can reduce ICP via reducing carbon dioxide concentrations (induces vasoconstriction)
- Osmotic agents such as mannitol can reduce ICP by as much as 50% within 30 minutes. The effect peaks at about 90 minutes, and lasts 4 hours
- Loop diuretics such as furosemide
- Steroids probably do not work.

Cerebral vasospasm

- Nimodipine (dose 60 mg given every 4 hours) is usually given prophylactically. This was associated with a reduction of one poor outcome for every eight patients treated with oral nimodipine. It may improve outcome by reducing vasospasm and/or have a neuroprotective effect
- If cerebral vasospasm is present, maintain hypervolaemia (CVP 8–12 mmHg, or pulmonary capillary wedge pressure (PCWP) 12–16 mmHg)
- Percutaneous transluminal angioplasty has been used to treat vasospasm but has not been proven to be beneficial in controlled trials
- Transcranial Doppler ultrasound can be performed on a regular basis to monitor for the development of vasospasm (seen as increases in velocity in basal intracerebral vessels).

Management of SAH: surgical and endovascular

- The early risk of recurrent bleeding can be reduced by surgical clipping of the aneurysm
- Therefore, it is essential to identify any underlying aneurysm on angiography (see Investigation of SAH, ➲ p. 384)
- Endovascular treatment of aneurysms, with embolization with platinum coils, has become the first-line treatment
- The ISAT (International Subarachnoid Aneurysm Trial) showed that endovascular treatment resulted in better outcome compared with surgery (see Fig. 13.7)
- Of 1063 patients allocated to endovascular treatment, 23 (5%) were dead or dependent at 1 year, compared to 30 (9%) of 1055 patients allocated to neurosurgery. The early survival advantage was maintained for up to 7 years.

Timing of intervention

- Treatment to secure a ruptured aneurysm should ideally be undertaken within 48 hours of symptom onset.
- There is an increased risk of complications after this time due to vasospasm, which is maximal at 5–7 days. Some authorities wait until 10 days if surgery cannot be performed within the first 3 days. However, patients may die as a result of rebleeding during this period.

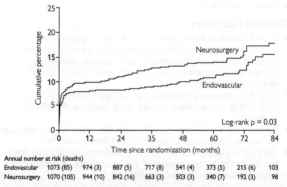

Fig. 13.7 Survival curves for patients treated with neurosurgery and endovascular treatment in the ISAT trial. It can be seen that patients treated with endovascular therapy had better survival, with the curves separating early.

Reproduced from *Lancet*, 366(9488), Molyneux AM, Kerr RSC, Yu L-M, *et al*. For the International Subarachnoid Aneurysm Trial (ISAT) of neurosurgical clipping versus endovascular coiling in 2143 patients with ruptured intracranial aneurysms: a randomized comparison of effects on survival, dependency, seizures, rebleeding, subgroups, and aneurysm occlusion, pp. 809–817, (2005), with permission from Elsevier.

Indication for surgery versus endovascular treatment

Generally endovascular treatment is preferred if it is technically feasible. In certain circumstances surgery may be considered preferable.

Indications for surgery in patients with SAH

- For Hunt and Hess/WFNS grades 4–5 (i.e. severe), the outcome is poor with or without surgical intervention.
- Large and giant aneurysms.
- Wide-necked aneurysms.
- Vessels emanating from the aneurysm dome.
- Mass effect or haematoma associated with the aneurysm.
- Recurrent aneurysm after coil embolization clotting. This appears to be a safer procedure and is more appealing and acceptable to patients. However, there is a 5% failure rate and, if not completely obliterated, the aneurysm may reform.

Asymptomatic aneurysms

These can be found:
- incidentally on neuroimaging performed for another cause
- in patients who have another symptomatic aneurysm
- when family members are screened.

Risk of rupture of asymptomatic intracranial aneurysm

Aneurysm size is the major predictor of risk of rupture. Other factors include increasing size, and the radiological appearance of secondary pouches (due to degeneration) within the aneurysm wall. The best data on risk related to aneurysm size is from the prospective studies ISUIA study cohort of 1692 patients with a mean follow-up of 4.1 years (see Tables 13.1 and 13.2).

Table 13.1 Risk of haemorrhage over the next 5 years for posterior aneurysms (posterior communicating/posterior circulation)

Size of aneurysm	No SAH (%)	History of SAH (%)
<7 mm	2.5	3.4
7–12 mm	14.5	14.5
13–24 mm	18.4	18.4
>24 mm	50	50

Table 13.2 Risk of haemorrhage over the next 5 years for anterior aneurysms (ACA/MCA/ICA)

Size of aneurysm	No SAH (%)	History of SAH (%)
<7 mm	0	1.5
7–12 mm	2.5	2.5
13–24 mm	14.5	14.5
>24 mm	40	40

Screening for intracranial aneurysms

There is an increased risk of aneurysms in family members where one member has already been diagnosed with a berry aneurysm. If they have more than one first-degree relative, their risk is much higher but is still only 10%.

In a cohort study, some individuals with a positive family history of SAH (two or more first-degree relatives who had SAH or unruptured intracranial aneurysms) were screened and followed up over 20 years. Aneurysms were found in 51 (11%) of 458 individuals at first screening, in 21 (8%) of 261 at second screening, in seven (5%) of 128 at third screening, and three (5%) of 63 at fourth screening. Five (3%) of 188 individuals without a history of aneurysms and with two negative screens had a *de novo* aneurysm in a follow-up screen. History of previous aneurysms was the only significant risk factor for aneurysms at follow-up screening.

When considering whether to screen, one must consider the following:
- The risk to the patient of intra-arterial angiography to detect an aneurysm
- Both MRA and CTA can miss small aneurysms (<5 mm for MRA, <2–3 mm for CT)
- Not all aneurysms will rupture
- Aneurysms found will probably require treatment with associated risks
- Some aneurysms found will be untreatable.

Screening should be considered in:
- individuals with two or more first-degree relatives with aneurysms/SAH
- patients with autosomal dominant polycystic kidney disease.

Aneurysms are very rare in childhood. Therefore, screening is usually started in adult life.

The benefit of screening is reduced in older patients in whom the lifetime risk of aneurysm rupture is less—therefore screening is recommended up to the age of 70 years.

In our practice:
- We tend not to advise treatment for aneurysms found to be <7 mm in diameter. However, we normally repeat imaging at yearly intervals for a couple of years to determine if the aneurysm is enlarging
- In older patients the benefit of treatment is less, especially if there are additional comorbidities that limit life expectancy
- For aneurysms >7 mm we consider treatment if it is technically possible with low risk
- The risk of treating asymptomatic aneurysms depends on many factors, including the aneurysm itself and the patient, but as ballpark figures:
  - neurosurgical clipping has a mortality of 2–3% and causes permanent morbidity in another 11%
  - endovascular treatment has a mortality of 0.5–1% and causes permanent morbidity in another 7%.

Intracerebral haemorrhage (ICH)

- About 20% of all stroke is due to ICH depending on geographical region (UK typically 12-13% - northern China 50%). In the Global Burden of Disease study published in 2021, around 28% of all stroke is ICH but ICH is responsible for almost 50% of stroke mortality at 12 months.
- ICH occurs when blood leaks spontaneously into the brain parenchyma, resulting in a focal haematoma. Secondary leakage of blood into the subarachnoid space may also occur
- Blood leaks into the brain at arterial pressure and may continue for a prolonged period. Early haematoma growth occurs in 18–38% of patients scanned within 3 hours of ICH
- Mortality is higher after cerebral haemorrhage than after ischaemic stroke and half the fatalities occur within the first 48 hours.

The following list of causes is a bit simplistic as different causes and risk factors interact. For example, in a patient with cerebral small-vessel disease and white matter hyperintensities who bleeds on warfarin and is also hypertensive, all three factors are contributing. Nevertheless, the classification forms a useful list to work through when assessing a patient with ICH.

Detailed descriptions of specific causes are given later in the chapter along with any specific treatments required for that cause.

Causes of intracerebral haemorrhage

Cerebral haemorrhage may be caused by:
- abnormal cerebral vessels
- abnormalities in blood.

These interact with risk factors which increase the risk of bleeding whatever the underlying causes.

Abnormal blood vessels
- Cerebral small-vessel disease:
  - Hypertension with lipohyalinosis
- Cerebral amyloid angiopathy
- Vascular malformations:
  - Arteriovenous malformations
  - Saccular aneurysms
  - Cavernous haemangiomas (cavernomas).
- Cerebral tumours
- Cerebral venous thrombosis
- Moyamoya disease and syndrome
- Septic and mycotic aneurysms
- Cerebral vasculitis
- Reversible cerebral vasoconstriction syndrome.

Abnormalities in the blood
- Systemic bleeding tendency:
  - Haemophilia
  - Leukaemia
  - Thrombocytopenia.
- Drug therapy:
  - Anticoagulants

- Antiplatelet agents
- Thrombolytic agents.

Other causes
- Haemorrhagic transformation of a cerebral infarct
- Illicit drugs:
  - Methamphetamine
  - Cocaine.
- Hyperperfusion syndrome post carotid endarterectomy
- Trauma.

Major risk factors for intracerebral haemorrhage
- Hypertension
- Age
- Alcohol excess
- White matter hyperintensities on brain imaging.

Clinical features and investigation of ICH

Clinical features

Like ischaemic stroke, ICH presents with the sudden onset of a focal neurological deficit. Prior to the wide availability of brain CT, scales were developed to try to separate ischaemia from cerebral haemorrhage on clinical grounds. Although some features may suggest haemorrhage (e.g. headache at onset or very early symptoms/sign progression), it is impossible to distinguish cerebral haemorrhage from ischaemic stroke reliably on clinical grounds. ICH presents like any other form of stroke with sudden-onset neurological deficit.

> Therefore, the important message is that it is impossible clinically to differentiate ICH from ischaemic stroke. Urgent brain imaging is essential in all cases of suspected stroke.

Nevertheless, there are certain clinical features which suggest ICH:
- If blood leaks into the subarachnoid space, a severe headache, which may come on very suddenly, may occur. Other features of meningism may also be present (vomiting, neck stiffness)
- Headache is also more common in ICH, even in the absence of subarachnoid blood. However, it can also occur with cerebral infarcts and may be absent in ICH
- Clinical worsening early after onset is well described in ICH
- Seizures are more common with ICH, but can also occur with infarcts.

The focal signs accompanying ICH depend on the location of the haematoma and are indistinguishable from those caused by infarction.

Investigation of ICH

General tests

These will only rarely identify specific causes of haemorrhage but should be performed. They may include the following:
- An urgent INR in anyone suspected of being on warfarin.
- Coagulation system screen when indicated. Direct oral anticoagulants (DOACs) have largely replaced warfarin for stroke prevention in patients with atrial fibrillation (AF). Effective reversal agents are available for DOACs. Think about the possibility that patients with ICH (or ischaemic stroke for thrombolysis) might be taking these drugs and importantly, and the time of the last dose. DOACs fall into two classes, direct thrombin inhibitors (dabigatran) and factor Xa inhibitors (rivaroxaban, apixaban, and edoxaban). They are difficult to test for reliably.
- APTT may be prolonged in patients taking either class of drug.
- PT is not prolonged by thrombin inhibitors but may be prolonged by Xa inhibitors.
- TT may be prolonged by thrombin inhibitors but not by Xa inhibitors.

- Anti-factor Xa assays are useful for measuring the actions of Xa inhibitors but are not routinely available.
- Blood tests for FBC (particularly platelets).
- Testing for illicit drugs should be performed if this is suspected.

However, the key to identifying ICH and determining the underlying causes is brain imaging, see Brain imaging in ICH, p. 396.

Brain imaging in ICH

CT is most widely used but MRI also has good sensitivity and adds additional information.

CT

- Blood appears as high signal
- CT has a high sensitivity for fresh blood
- Usually the hyperdense appearance lasts a few weeks but for small haemorrhages it can be shorter
- Once the blood has been resorbed (over a few weeks), a hypodense area remains and it is impossible on CT to tell whether an old stroke was an infarct or a haemorrhage
- In contrast, MRI can differentiate old haematomas from old infarcts
- CTA can demonstrate ongoing extravasation into the haematoma (the 'spot sign'). The 'spot sign' has been mainly used in clinical trials to predict ICH at risk of expansion for inclusion into interventional studies.

MRI

- MRI has a similar sensitivity to CT in diagnosing haemorrhage, as long as the appropriate sequences are done
- Interpreting the scan can be more difficult than for CT
- The time course of symptoms needs to be known when reviewing the scan (see Table 13.3):
  - Within minutes, blood is low density on T1 imaging and bright on T2
  - This remains between hours and a few days
  - Between days and weeks, it becomes high signal on T1 and low on T2
  - After weeks, it becomes high signal on T1 and high on T2 with a dark rim
- Blood sensitive sequences (gradient echo (T2*) or susceptibility-weighted imaging (SWI) sequences) should be performed as these are most sensitive to both recent and old haemorrhage
- Gradient echo and SWI are very sensitive to haemosiderin from the breakdown of blood products, which appear as areas of signal loss (black), and this persists for years after haemorrhage. This allows:
  - detection of old haemorrhage at other sites
  - determination of whether an old stroke is due to haemorrhage or infarctions (note infarcts which have undergone haemorrhagic infarction will show haemosiderin)
  - detection of cerebral microbleeds.
- More modern machines use SWI, which is very sensitive to blood and improves on the T2* imaging effect.

Other clues from imaging

- Imaging reveals the location of haemorrhage, which may give useful clues as to the cause, particularly whether it is lobar or subcortical
- Clues to the cause may be seen, including:
  - abnormal vessels around an arteriovenous malformation (AVM)
  - evidence of cerebral venous thrombosis (filling defects and venous sinus thrombus)
  - congestion of pial vessels suggesting a dural fistula.

Table 13.3 Evolution of the MR appearance of haemorrhage over time

Phase	Time	Haemoglobin	T1	T2
Hyperacute	<24 hours	Oxyhaemoglobin (intracellular)	Iso or hypo	Hyper
Acute	1–3 days	Deoxyhaemoglobin (intracellular)	Iso or hypo	Hypo
Early subacute	>3 days	Methaemoglobin	Hyper	Hypo
Late subacute	>7 days	Methaemoglobin (extracellular)	Hyper	Hyper
Chronic	>14 days	Haemosiderin (extracellular)	Iso or hypo	Hypo

Patterns of haemorrhage

Imaging allows division of haemorrhage into different types according to brain regions affected. This is useful in determining the underlying causes, as different causes tend to be prevalent in different locations:

- Lobar (cortical) haemorrhage
- Subcortical haemorrhage.

Scans should also be classified as to whether secondary haemorrhage into the subarachnoid space/intraventricular system has occurred.

In some cases, multiple ICHs are seen. More common causes of these include the following:

- Cerebral amyloid angiopathy (MRI may show evidence of previous bleeding, cerebral microbleeds, or old parenchymal haemorrhages or superficial cortical siderosis) as well as white matter hyperintensities and enlarged perivascular spaces.
- Certain metastatic tumours:
  - Melanoma
  - Bronchogenic carcinoma
  - Renal carcinoma
  - Choriocarcinoma
- Cerebral venous thrombosis
- Haematological disorders (including diffuse intravascular coagulation and leukaemia)
- Cerebral vasculitis
- Thrombolytic and other anticoagulant therapy
- Head injury.

Investigation of underlying cause

- Once the patient has recovered from ICH, it is important to look for the underlying cause
- Often in the acute phase there is too much blood around and it is impossible to identify an underlying cause unless a large lesion such as a tumour is present

- Occasionally acute investigation is performed if a lesion with a high early recurrent bleeding risk is suspected, e.g. cerebral aneurysm with a small ICH
- Therefore, usually one should wait until the blood has been resorbed; normally 6–8 weeks but it may take up to 3 months
- Imaging is then performed with CT with contrast, or MRI
- MRI is more likely to detect underlying causes than CT, and if gradient echo or SWI is included, it may identify other old bleeds and other features of CAA; this is particularly helpful in diagnosing amyloid angiopathy
- Therefore it can be useful to perform an acute MRI in cases where the pattern of ICH fits with CAA (i.e. is cortical or lobar). If this shows characteristic features of CAA, such as superficial siderosis or cortical microbleeds, then further interval imaging is not necessary.
- MRA and CTA may also show underlying vascular malformations
- In a proportion of cases, it is necessary to progress to intra-arterial angiography to look for an underlying lesion. Practice varies as to how many patients undergo this. The yield is highest for cortical haemorrhages in younger individuals (<50 years) without a history or MR changes of hypertension. However, small sub-cortical AVMs can still be detected on DSA in ICH patients with no other seeming cause for ICH and normal MRI, and the decision to proceed with DSA needs to be individualized.
- In the acute phase always think of cerebral venous thrombosis and if the pattern of ICH fits with this then do an urgent CTA or MRA (➲ see Chapter 12).

Treatment of ICH

This includes:
- emergency department 'care bundle' approach
- acute stroke unit care
- neurosurgery
- treatment of complications
- treatment of the underlying cause.

The emergency 'care bundle' approach

- Suspected stroke is a medical emergency and needs urgent brain imaging to confirm the diagnosis. As soon as ICH is confirmed in this scenario, although time critical reperfusion therapy is no longer indicated, there are 'time is brain' interventions that can improve outcome. Many of these work through improving haemostasis.
- 1 in 3 ICH patients exhibit haematoma expansion in the first 3 hours after onset. In INTERACT 1 as every 1 mL of haematoma expansion from baseline in the first 24 hours, was associated with a 5% increase in risk of death and severe disability.
- The care bundle successfully tested in INTERACT 3 comprised lowering systolic BP <140 mmHg within 1 hr of arrival to hospital, treating Blood Sugar Levels (BSL) <6.1–7.8 mmol/L (7.8–10.0 mmol/L in diabetics), actively lowering any raised temperature <37.5, and reversal of INR if ≥1.5
- BP rises acutely in ICH. Reducing it might reduce further haemorrhage risk but could reduce perfusion to compromised tissue. Evidence suggests acute treatment is safe and may reduce haematoma expansion and improve clinical outcome, In INTERACT4 blood pressure lowering was associated with improved outcome.
- A useful target systolic BP is130–140 mmHg. The choice of agent depends upon local hospital protocol but will likely need to be given intravenously with close monitoring, in order to be effective. Agents used include labetolol, nicardipine, hydralazine, and clevidipine. In INTERACT 4 the intravenous alpha blocker urapidil was successfully used but this is not widely available outside China. We would caution use of GTN as it appeared to worsen ICH in the RIGHT-2 trial.
- Any provoking disorder of blood clotting or coagulation requires **immediate** reversal in ED
- platelet transfusion if platelet count <50
- reversal of warfarin INR >1.4 with prothrombin complex concentrate (PPC)
- reversal agent for Dabigatran (idarucizumab)
- reversal agent for apixaban, rivaroxaban, and edoxaban (Andexanet)

Platelet transfusions should not routinely be given to ICH patients taking antiplatelet therapy (PATCH trial, 2016) but may be needed ahead of neurosurgical intervention

- Drugs that can cause bleeding should be stopped or avoided, e.g. aspirin and clopidogrel and non-steroidal anti-inflammatory agents

Trials of homeostatic agents such as tranexamic acid (TXA) and recombinant factor VII have not been shown to improve outcome. Further trials of these agents are ongoing.

Acute stroke unit care

- The benefits of acute stroke unit care are proven to extend to ICH patients and not just those with ischaemic stroke.
- Acute assessment of swallow and management plan for the appropriate route for nutrition, hydration and medication should be continuously in view of the high chance of haematoma expansion and early clinical deterioration.
- Temperature management—keep core temperature below 38°C.
- VTE prophylaxis, ideally with intermittent pneumatic compression
- Control BP.
- Bladder and bowel dysfunction is more common after ICH.
- There is no role for prophylactic antiepileptic drugs.
- Do Not Resuscitate Orders should not be routinely placed on ICH. They should be part of informed clinical decision-making taking into consideration advanced care directives.

Neurosurgery

- The aim of surgery for intracerebral haemorrhage is to reduce the volume of haemorrhage, prevent rebleeding, and remove blood products and mass effect, so that tissue damage is reduced.
- Surgery can be considered in three scenarios:
- Supratentorial ICH
- Posterior fossa ICH
- Intraventricular haemorrhage (IVH)

Supratentorial ICH

- The first neurosurgical controlled clinical trial in ICH was performed in 1961 at Atkinson Morley Hospital in Wimbledon, UK, by Wylie McKissock. The result was negative. Subsequent trials, the largest of which was supratentorial lobar intracerebral haematomas (STICH), have been neutral or negative.
- More recent ICH trials have used minimally invasive surgical approaches. The MISTIE III study overall showed no benefit in clinical outcome using minimally invasive catheter-based evacuation but in those patients that achieved technical success (residual ICH volume of <15 mL), there was a trend to favourable functional outcome compared to conservative medical therapy.
- The ENRICH trial randomized 300 patients with lobar or anterior basal ganglia haematoma (volume 30–80 mL) within 24 hours of onset to minimally invasive surgical evacuation or medical management. At 180 days, 45% of patients in the surgery group were independent compared to 26% in the medical group. The positive results were attributed to the effect of surgery for lobar ICH.
- A different approach to pre-emptive hemicraniectomy was tested in the SWITCH trial. 201 patients with severe deep or non-lobar, ICH (median GCS 10, NIHSS 18, 55 mL ICH volume), were randomized to best medical treatment alone or with surgery. Decompressive hemicraniectomy was performed on average 26 hours post onset. At 6 months, the surgically treated group showed a trend of less death and severe disability.

Posterior fossa ICH

- Although untested in RCTs cerebellar haemorrhage, should be considered for surgical evacuation. This can be life-threatening because the posterior fossa space is taken up by haematoma and brainstem compression occurs, causing coning and death.
- Patients may make remarkable recoveries from cerebellar lesions and early neurosurgery should be contemplated.
- Patients with large (>3 cm diameter) cerebellar haemorrhage, or those with brainstem compression or hydrocephalus related to their haemorrhage should be considered for decompressive surgery.

Intraventricular haemorrhage

- External ventricular drainage should be considered in patients with hydrocephalus contributing to an impaired conscious state.
- The efficacy and safety of intraventricular administration of rtPA is uncertain, but it is sometimes considered for clearance of EVDs and has a low complication rate.

Treatment of complications

- Raised ICP is common in ICH. There is no good evidence of how to manage it.
- Hyperventilation has been used to reduce ICP but will reduce cerebral blood flow. There is no trial evidence to support this approach.
- Osmotic agents such as mannitol and glycerol are also used but there is no good trial evidence supporting their use.

One should be vigilant for hydrocephalus which is common after ICH with intraventricular haemorrhage, and can be treated with external ventricular drainage.

Treatment of the underlying cause

- Small-vessel cerebrovascular disease is the main cause of ICH
- Follow-up brain imaging will define the underlying aetiology of ICH and guide secondary stroke prevention.
- ICH patients should have blood pressure lowered long term to the value of ≤ 130/80 mmHg.
- ICH patients should be counselled towards lifestyle risk factor modification including smoking cessation, cessation of illicit drug use and alcohol intake of ≤2 iu/day.
- Statins do not reduce the risk of recurrent ICH and should only be prescribed as preventative medicine in the context of concomitant atherosclerotic risk.
- Restarting antiplatelet or anticoagulant therapy is an individualized treatment decision. Many ICH patients are also at risk of ischaemic stroke, and between 15-30% of ICH patients have evidence of DWI lesions and marked small-vessel disease ischaemic changes.
- A small proportion – 2–3% of all ICH is due to a structural abnormality such as cerebral cavernous (CCM) or AVMs. Surgical excision or stereotactic radiotherapy (gamma knife treatment) are helpful to consider for such lesions that have bled at least once.
- Other rare causes such as CVT (\Rightarrow see p. 357), tumours and cerebral vasculitis (see p. 342) have specific treatments.

Prognosis of ICH

- This is much worse than that for ischaemic stroke
- Population-based studies report a 1-month mortality rate of about 40% compared with 10–20% for ischaemic stroke. After this the risk falls to 8% per annum (similar to that for ischaemic stroke)
- Factors associated with a worse prognosis include:
  - increasing age
  - early reduction in the level of consciousness
  - larger haematoma volume
  - intraventricular extension of ICH
  - anticoagulant therapy
  - secondary hydrocephalus.

Cerebral small-vessel disease

- Cerebral small-vessel disease (SVD) is the most common pathology underlying ICH
- There are two main types of SVD
- Sporadic SVD affects the subcortex, usually in hypertensive individuals, and causes deep ICH. Also sometimes called hypertensive SVD or subcortical SVD
- Cerebral amyloid angiopathy (see next section) usually causes lobar ICH
- Rarer causes of SVD include familial forms (e.g. CADASIL), post-radiotherapy SVD, and vasculitis.
- Pathological changes may relate to the haemorrhage:
- Sporadic SVD is covered in detail in Chapter 8.
- MRI features of sporadic SVD include white matter hyperintensities and cerebral microbleeds, both of which are associated with increased ICH risk.
- Treatment of blood pressure, to a systolic of 130 mmHg, is key in long-term management of SVD. This reduces the risk of further ICH, as well as the risk of ischaemic stroke and dementia.

Cerebral amyloid angiopathy (CAA)

Pathology

- Cerebral amyloid (Aβ) is a misfolded protein generated by neurons in the brain.
- The amyloid seen in CAA (Aβ 40) is closely related to the amyloid seen in Alzheimer's disease (Aβ 42) but is different from systemic amyloidosis.
- CAA is a 'protein elimination failure angiopathy' with deposition of Aβ (predominantly Aβ 40—not Aβ 42) in the cerebral vessels mapping to the intramural perivascular drainage pathways.
- This perivascular transport system allows interstitial fluid and solutes to drain in and out of the brain via the basement membranes of capillaries and between smooth muscle cells in the tunica media of small arteries. The process is thought to be driven by vessel pulsations, which diminish with Aβ deposition and increasing age (as arteriosclerosis) increases vessel stiffness.
- ApoE ε4 influences the composition and function of the small-vessel basement membrane to increase Aβ deposition, further impairing Aβ clearance.
- Ageing and possession of ApoE ε4 reduce enzymatic degradation of cerebral Aβ via numerous proteolytic pathways and reduces clearance by perivascular macrophages, astrocytes, and microglia.
- Aβ 40 accumulation in CAA then occurs characteristically in the media and adventitia of small and medium-sized vessels, arterioles, and capillaries of the cerebral cortex, subcortex, and leptomeninges.
- Imaging changes seen in CAA are consequently typically lobar, seen especially in the occipital lobe, as well as the parietal, frontal and temporal lobes, while deep structures such as the basal ganglia and hippocampus are often spared.
- CAA predisposes to ICH through three main mechanisms:
  - physical disruption of microvascular architecture causing fibrinoid necrosis, focal vessel wall fragmentation, and microaneurysm formation
  - Aβ presence also induces a significant inflammatory response resulting in degradation of the extracellular membrane, disruption to the blood–brain barrier (BBB) and therefore increased risk of ICH
  - Impaired dynamic cerebral autoregulation and reduction in the protective buffer mechanism against fluctuations in systemic blood pressure.

Epidemiology

- Amyloid angiopathy becomes increasingly common with age and may occur in over half of unselected postmortems in those aged over 90 years but is now recognized as a major cause of lobar ICH in those over 50 years.
- Most cases are sporadic, although there are a few familial forms but these are very rare:
  - Dutch familial amyloid: autosomal dominant, mutations are in the beta-amyloid precursor protein and therefore the abnormal protein is a beta protein similar to that seen in sporadic CAA and Alzheimer's disease

- Icelandic amyloid: autosomal dominant, the abnormal protein is antigenically different, being the cystatin C protein.

Clinical features

CAA can present with the following:
- Intracerebral haemorrhage—usually lobar.
- Cognitive impairment.
- Nontraumatic acute convexity subarachnoid haemorrhage).
- Transient focal neurological episodes (TFNEs) or 'amyloid spells'. These are transient, progressive neurological symptoms (e.g. progressive sensory, motor or speech disturbance) that move at a similar rate to migraine aura. They are thought to be caused by spreading cortical depolarization. Often, imaging shows small, acute convexity subarachnoid bleeding, or cortical superficial siderosis.
- TFNEs are usually self-limiting and are diagnosed clinically. Secondary stroke prevention, including antiplatelets is usually not required. If stubborn and distressing, antiepileptic medication can be helpful. We often use levetiracetam as first line and then either topiramate or lamotrigine as second line, depending on the individual patient.

Brain imaging appearances

- ICH—this is usually lobar or in the grey–white matter boundary.
- On gradient echo MRI or SWI (see Figs 13.8 and 13.9), old larger haemorrhages and/or microbleeds are seen, particularly in the cortex and at the grey-white matter boundary.
- SWI or gradient echo imaging may show superficial siderosis- this is seen as low density along the cortical sulci caused by previous leakage of blood into the subarachnoid space.
- White matter hyperintensities on MRI or leukoaraiosis on CT may be seen.
- Enlarged perivascular spaces are common.

Diagnosis

- This is suggested by multiple cortical haemorrhages, particularly in an older person.
- The presence of multiple microbleeds in the typical location in a patient with cortical haemorrhage strongly supports the diagnosis.
- Definitive diagnosis requires brain biopsy—the amyloid can be diagnosed with biopsy as a characteristic apple-green birefringence under polarized light after Congo red staining.
- In clinical practice, biopsy is rarely performed as a probable diagnosis can be made based on MRI appearances, and making a definite diagnosis will not alter management.
- The Boston criteria have been developed to help with *in vivo* diagnosis, and validated (Table 13.5) against pathological diagnosis, and have reasonable sensitivity and specificity. These were updated in 2022 to version 2.0. The age of onset has been reduced to 50 years and the pathological importance of expanded perivascular spaces in the region of the centrum semi-ovale is emphasized as well as the association of convexity sub-arachnoid haemorrhage (cSAH).
- CT diagnostic criteria (especially useful in those patients unable to undergo MRI) have been developed by the Edinburgh group and are listed in Table 13.4.

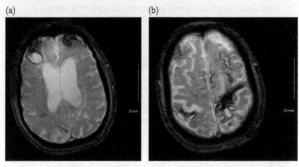

Fig. 13.8 Imaging appearances of CAA on MRI. In the upper scan, a right frontal ICH can be seen. There are also cerebral microbleeds best seen in the left parietal region. In the lower image high signal can be seen along a number of cortical sulci. This is superficial siderosis (copyright: Hugh Markus).

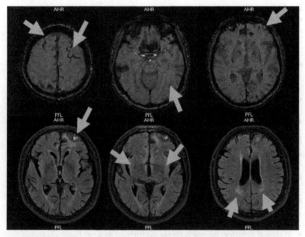

Fig. 13.9 MRI scans from a patient presenting with recurrent TFNEs of transient R-sided weakness with probable amyloid angiopathy according to Boston 2.0 Criteria. Sequences are from left top row: are SWI and bottom T2, FLAIR. The SWI sequences show cortical superficial siderosis, lobar cerebral microbleeds, and an acute haemorrhage present in the left frontal lobe. The T2FLAIR sequences also show the acute bleed as well as enlarged perivascular spaces and deep white matter ischaemic changes in the posterior periventricular region © Geoffrey Cloud.

Table 13.4 The Edinburgh CT and genetic diagnostic criteria for lobar ICH associated with CAA

High-probability CAA	Lobar ICH showing subarachnoid haemorrhage on CT and either finger-like projections from the ICH on CT or possession of at least 1 ApoE ε4 allele
Intermediate probability CAA	Lobar ICH showing either subarachnoid haemorrhage on CT or possession of at least 1 ApoE ε4 allele
Low-probability CAA: rule-out criteria	Lobar ICH showing neither subarachnoid haemorrhage on CT nor possession of at least 1 ApoE ε4 allele

ApoE indicates apolipoprotein E; CAA, cerebral amyloid angiopathy; CT, computed tomography; and ICH, intracerebral haemorrhage.

Adapted from Rodrigues et al. (2018) Lancet Neurol **17**:232–240.

Table 13.5 Boston 2.0 criteria for diagnosis of CAA *(in those presenting symptomatically with spontaneous tICH, TFNEs, cSAH, or CI/dementia)*

Definite CAA	Full postmortem examination demonstrating severe CAA with vasculopathy and absence of other diagnostic lesion
Probable CAA with supporting pathology	Clinical data and pathologic tissue (evacuated hematoma or cortical biopsy) demonstrating: some degree of CAA in specimen and absence of other diagnostic lesion
Probable CAA clinical data and MRI demonstrating	• Age ≥50 years • ≥2 of the following strictly lobar haemorrhagic lesions on T2*-weighted MRI, in any combination: ICH, CMB, cSS/cSAH foci OR • 1 lobar haemorrhagic lesion + 1 white matter feature (severe CSO-PVS or WMH-MS) • Absence of any deep haemorrhagic lesions (ICH, CMB) on T2-weighted MRI • Absence of other cause of haemorrhagic lesions • Haemorrhagic lesion in cerebellum not counted as either lobar or deep haemorrhagic lesion
Possible CAA Clinical data and MRI demonstrating:	• Age ≥50 years • Absence of other cause of haemorrhage • 1 strictly lobar haemorrhagic lesion on T2*-weighted MRI: ICH, CMB, cSS/cSAH focus OR • 1 white matter feature (Severe CSO-PVS or WMH-MS) • Absence of any deep haemorrhagic lesions (ICH, CMB) on T2*-weighted MRI • Absence of other cause of haemorrhagic lesions

Abbreviations: CAA, cerebral amyloid angiopathy; MRI, magnetic resonance imaging; ICH, intracerebral haemorrhage; TFNE, transient focal neurologic episodes, CI, cognitive impairment; CMB, cerebral microbleed; cSS, cortical superficial siderosis; cSAH, convexity subarachnoid haemorrhage; CSO-PVS, visible perivascular spaces in the centrum semiovale; WMH-MS, white matter hyperintensities in a multispot pattern.

Unusual types of CAA

CAA-related inflammation (CAA-ri)

- This is an autoimmune reaction to Aβ deposits causing severe perivascular inflammation (and so not causing damage to the vessel well itself and hence does not tend to cause ICH).
- CAA-ri is a rare form of CAA.
- It presents with severe headache, recurrent seizures as well as accelerated cognitive impairment or even coma but not lobar ICH.
- A systematic review reported the following frequency of symptoms:
  - Cognitive decline 48%
  - Seizures 32%
  - Headaches 32%
  - Motor weakness 16%
  - Aphasia 14%
  - Visual disturbance including neglect 13%.
- The onset is often insidious with symptoms of >30 days' duration at presentation in 60%.
- It has a characteristic appearance on MRI with asymmetric confluent FLAIR signal. It may be enhanced with contrast.
- Cerebral microbleeds are usually present (83%) and may be most frequent in the vicinity of the FLAIR high signal lesions.
- CSF usually shows a raised protein (83%), may show a raised white cell count (44%), and oligoclonal band can be present (17%).
- There are no trials of treatment but it is usually treated with prednisolone (e.g. methylprednisolone 1 g/day for 5/7) followed by oral prednisolone and/or immunosuppressive agents such as cyclophosphamide or mycophenolate.
- Brain biopsy should be considered if the diagnosis is not clear on MRI. to exclude other diagnoses as CAA-ri is usually very steroid responsive.
- A review of those who received steroid and/or immunosuppressives reported the following outcomes: asymptomatic 23%, mild disability 32%, moderate or severe disability 16%, dead 29%.
- Two pathological subtypes have been described on pathology, but in a quarter, both pathologies are present:
  - CAA_ related inflammation (CAA-ri)
  - Amyloid β-related angiitis (ABRA).
- ABRA is part of the CAA-ri spectrum where Aβ deposition causes transmural granulomatous inflammation.
- 70% with ABRA have an ApoE e4/e4 genotype.

Iatrogenic CAA (iCAA)

- CAA type disease has been recently seen in young individuals with a history of cadaveric duramater grafting in childhood or neurosurgery using other cadaveric central nervous system (CNS) material including human growth hormone injections.
- While rare and currently poorly understood, there is suggestion of a prion-like exposure in childhood with an incubation of 3–4 decades before clinical presentation with CAA symptoms, including ICH (Fig 13.10).

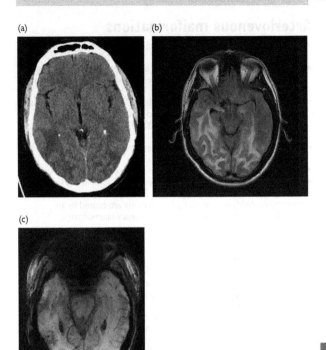

Fig. 13.10 CAA-related inflammation. A man in his 60s presented with headache and tonic-clonic seizures. CSF showed elevated protein (2.2 g/L), increased white cells (52 lymphocytes) and oligoclonal bands. (a) CT showed low density in the parieto-occipital regions worse on the right. (b) FLAIR MRI showed extensive T2-high signal. (c) SWI MRI showed cerebral microbleeds. A brain biopsy confirmed amyloid deposition, and showed inflammatory changes. ©Hugh Markus

Arteriovenous malformations

- AVMs are caused by an abnormal communication between arteries and veins
- One or more feeding arteries supplies blood directly into a draining vein, without a capillary network between the two. The vein is therefore exposed to high (arterial) BP
- The cause of rupture may be because high-pressure blood is continually pumped into the venous system. Associated aneurysms may also be found on the feeding vessel in about 20% of AVMs and these can rupture
- Most are probably congenital malformations but some can be acquired, e.g. dural fistulas occurring after trauma
- About 1% of intracranial haemorrhages are associated with an AVM
- These are more usually lobar rather than subcortical haemorrhages, although can be subcortical depending on the site of the AVM
- Sometimes AVMs may be multiple, and rarely are caused by an underlying systemic disorder such as hereditary haemorrhagic telangiectasia
- AVMs are associated with epilepsy, independent of ICH.

Dural AVMs or fistulas

- These are a specific type of AVM. In a dural AVM the arteries are derived from the dural and meningeal branches of the external carotid artery, and drainage is most commonly into the dural sinuses, most often the transverse and sigmoid
- They can occur secondary to blockage of drainage of a venous sinus after cerebral venous thrombosis or can be due to other causes such as neoplasia. They also occur secondary to trauma
- They can cause pulsatile tinnitus if the fistula is near the temporal bone
- Although rare, they are an important cause of ICH particularly in the young as they require specific treatment. Treatment can be surgical or endovascular. Fistulas are anatomically heterogenous, so treatment needs to be tailored to the individual case.

Diagnosis of AVMs

- The tangled vessels may be seen on routine brain CT (particularly with contrast) or MRI (flow voids in the vessels) (see Fig. 13.11)
- They can often be well seen on CTA or MRA
- Small AVMs and dural fistulas may require an intra-arterial angiogram to diagnose; this will also be necessary for larger AVMs to plan treatment
- It may be impossible to visualize an AVM following cerebral haemorrhage owing to its being obscured by a haematoma. Therefore, further imaging is often delayed for 2–3 months.

Prognosis

- The risk of rebleeding in AVMs is about 2–3% per annum
- This increases to as high as 7% if there is an associated aneurysm on a feeding vessel
- The risk appears to be higher in the first few months after a bleed.

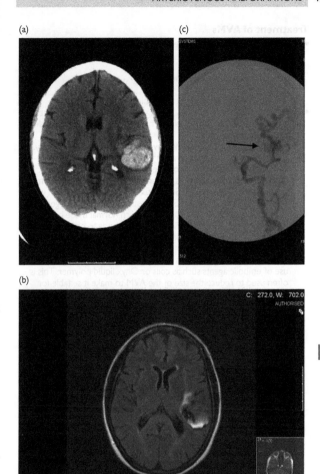

(a)

(c)

(b)

Fig. 13.11 An AVM presenting with an ICH. This patient presented to the acute stroke unit. (a) The initial CT showed a left-sided cortical haemorrhage; (b) MR in the subacute stage showed a resolving haemorrhage as well as flow voids owing to dilated vessels; (c) an intra-arterial angiogram shows an AVM (arrowed). © Hugh Markus.

Treatment of AVMs
- There are the following treatment options:
  - Do nothing—conservative
  - Surgical excision
  - Stereotactic radiotherapy (radiosurgery)
  - Endovascular embolization
  - Very large AVMs may not be amenable for surgery.
- There are no randomized trials looking at what is the best treatment approach for AVMs that have bled. The following is a possible guideline until evidence is available:
  - Superficial or large aneurysms may be amenable to neurosurgery. Successful brain AVM obliteration was achieved in 96% (range, 0–100%) of patients after microsurgery.
  - Small AVMs in eloquent sites or smaller than 3 cm in diameter may be treated by radiosurgery. Successful brain AVM obliteration was achieved in 38% (range, 0–75%) after stereotactic radiosurgery. Larger lesions are not suitable as too much normal tissue has to be included in the radiation field. Radiation leads to obliteration of vessels but this takes some time and therefore the reduction is bleeding risk is delayed.
  - Endovascular treatment aims to occlude the feeding vessels by the use of embolic agents such as coils or Onyx liquid polymer. This is often used to reduce the size of the AVM to make it suitable for surgery or radiosurgery.
  - The ARUBA trial demonstrated conservative therapy (incidence of death or symptomatic stroke 3.4 per 100 patient-years) was better than surgical therapy (12.3 per 100 patient-years) for unruptured AVMs with up to 5-year follow-up.

Cavernous malformations

- Cerebral cavernous malformations (CCM) are small (mm to a few cm), thin-walled vascular malformations, lined by endothelium without muscular or elastic layers and with no intervening brain tissues. They may be single, multiple, and are sometimes calcified
- Usually sporadic and of unknown aetiology
- Present asymptomatically in 0.5% of postmortems and MRIs
- Rare familial variants exist. CCM1 and CCM2 are caused by mutations in the *KRIT1* (~55%), *MGC4607* (~10%) and *PDCD10* (~10%) genes. The underlying genes of other familial cases (~15%) are not yet known. These familial forms are associated with multiple cavernomas
- Occur in hemispheric white matter or cortex in one-half, posterior fossa (most commonly the brainstem) in one-third, and basal ganglia or thalamus in one-sixth
- They may be associated with ICH, but more commonly blood leaks out, slowly causing a ring of haemosiderin deposition.

Imaging

Easily diagnosed on MRI (see Fig. 13.12):
- On T2-MRI: mixed signal intensity core, with surrounding rim of decreased signal intensity corresponding to haemosiderin
- The surrounding haemosiderin is better seen on gradient echo MRI which is the most sensitive technique for their detection. Gradient echo MRI may show multiple cavernomas
- Imaging studies have shown they may grow, or regress, and may occur *de novo* in familial cases
- No abnormalities are seen on angiography.

Clinical features

- Cerebral haemorrhage—these are usually small and, depending on the site, may not cause much in the way of symptoms
- Local compressive symptoms—these occur for some brainstem cavernomas which compress the surrounding tightly packed brainstem nuclei and tracts. Chronic leakage and gradual expansion may occur
- Epileptic seizures
- Asymptomatic— the most common clinical picture is an incidental finding on brain imaging.

Treatment

- Usually no treatment is required.
- The risk of recurrent haemorrhage is highest in the first year after symptomatic ICH presentation (up to 20%) but then declines (5 % at 5 years).
- CCMs in the brainstem have the worst prognosis in terms of disability and mortality.
- Occasionally, surgical excision is performed, particularly if compressive symptoms are occurring, although excision of brainstem cavernomas can have high surgical risk.

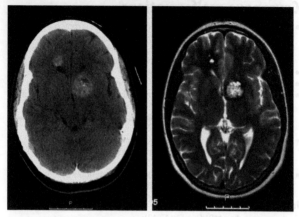

Fig. 13.12 A left thalamic cavernoma can be seen on CT on the left and on T2-weighted MRI on the right. On MRI a typical dark ring can be seen corresponding to haemosiderin deposition caused by bleeding. A second right frontal lesion can also be seen. © Hugh Markus.

- Stereotactic 'gamma knife' radiation has also been used, although there is no controlled trial data to support its use.
- Brainstem cavernoma lesions sometimes bleed and expand very slowly, causing brainstem compression. Surgical treatment is very hazardous with risk of permanent damage to the brainstem.

Other vascular abnormalities causing ICH

Cerebral venous thrombosis

- This is an important cause of haemorrhage and is often diagnosed late
- As haemorrhage occurs from the veins (low pressure), it is often not as devastating as in an arterial haemorrhage, and its onset is slower
- Often, the ICH is preceded by ischaemic symptoms with focal deficits, seizures, or encephalopathy without imaging evidence of haemorrhage, which may occur hours or days later
- Occasionally, ICH can be the first presentation
- It can be more difficult to diagnose and, if untreated, may progress
- The diagnosis can be suspected by the location and pattern of haemorrhage, which will depend on the site of the thrombosis:
  - Superior sagittal sinus thrombosis, in the parasagittal region, often bilateral
  - Transverse sinus tends to cause haemorrhage in the temporal lobes
  - Cerebral convexity with leakage from a cortical vein
  - Straight sinus causing bilateral thalamic oedema
- More details on this topic are given in ➲ Chapter 12.

Moyamoya disease and syndrome

- This is a rare condition affecting children and young adults. Stenosis or occlusion occurs in childhood in the basal intracerebral arteries. This is followed by new vessel formation to try to bypass the obstruction. These new vessels are fragile and can leak
- The syndrome can be primary (of unknown cause but more common in individuals from East Asia) or secondary to other causes of basal cerebral artery occlusion (e.g. sickle cell disease)
- More details are given on ➲ p. 338.

Vasculitis

- CNS vasculitis, either primary or as part of systemic vasculitis, can occasionally cause haemorrhage (➲ see Chapter 11)
- It can cause the combination of separate infarcts and haemorrhage, and is also a cause of multiple haemorrhages.

Septic arteritis and mycotic aneurysms

- Infective endocarditis is complicated by ICH in 5% of cases.
- This can occur due to:
  - acute pyogenic necrosis of the arterial wall caused by virulent organisms such as *Staphylococcus aureus*
  - mycotic aneurysms which can rupture; this may occur later, including while on antibiotic therapy and with less virulent organisms.

Haemostatic factors causing ICH

Antithrombotic medication is associated with ICH. It may not cause the ICH is likely to make ICH worse.

Anticoagulation treatment

- Historically, treatment with warfarin increases the risk of ICH 8–10-fold.
- The risk of haemorrhage is related to the degree of anticoagulation (INR).
- ICH risk with anticoagulation is markedly increased in the presence of white matter hyperintensities on MRI or leukoaraiosis on CT, as shown in data from the SPIRIT trial.
- DOACs (predominantly the Xa inhibitor drugs) have largely replaced warfarin for stroke prevention in AF and prevention of recurrent VTE in developed countries and account for about 80% of oral anticoagulant prescriptions. RCTs show DOACs have 50% less risk of intracranial bleeding than warfarin. However risk of ICH is still increased, and ICH accounts for 17% of major bleeding complications in patients taking Xa inhibitor DOACs.
- In the US 'Get With the Guidelines' study from 2013 to 2018 of 219,701 ICH patients—9202 (4.2%) occurred on Xa inhibitors and 21,430 (9.8%) on warfarin.
- ICHs in patients on anticoagulants are, on average, larger than those in patients not on anticoagulants and carry a higher mortality.
- A blood-fluid level is often seen on brain imaging in up to 80% of oral anticoagulant-associated ICH.

Antiplatelet agents

- The absolute risk of haemorrhage from aspirin is low: about 1 per 1000 extra ICH per 3–5 years of treatment on aspirin.
- Most major aspirin-related bleeding is gastrointestinal not ICH.

Thrombolytic agents

- ICH can be associated with thrombolysis for stroke or MI
- When thrombolysis is given for acute ischaemic stroke, the haemorrhagic transformation usually occurs at the site of the infarct unless there is underlying structural blood vessel disease such as CAA
- For other thrombolysis, most commonly MI, haemorrhage may occur at any site in the brain.

Systemic bleeding tendency

- Disorders such as haemophilia are rare causes of ICH. In such disorders, ICH may be provoked by minor trauma
- ICH is a well-recognized complication of acute myeloid leukaemia, occurring in about 20% of cases. It is rare in lymphatic leukaemia
- Disseminated intravascular coagulation can be complicated by ICH which may be multifocal
- Thrombocytopenia can be complicated by ICH, but this will usually only occur if the platelet count is below 20×10^9/L.

Haemorrhagic transformation of a cerebral infarct

- Haemorrhagic transformation is a common complication of cerebral infarction (see Fig. 13.13). It occurs because of blood–brain barrier disruption secondary to the ischaemia
- It is most common a few days after the infarct
- It is usually minor but can sometimes cause massive haemorrhage with space-occupying effects and secondary oedema
- Risk factors include thrombolysis and hypertension
- Symptomatic parenchymal haemorrhage occurs in about 0.6% of stroke not treated with thrombolysis
- Thrombolysis with alteplase for myocardial infarction is associated with an approximately 0.5% risk of ICH
- Thrombolysis with alteplase for stroke is associated with an approximately 3–6% risk of symptomatic haemorrhage, depending on the definition used.

(a)   (b)

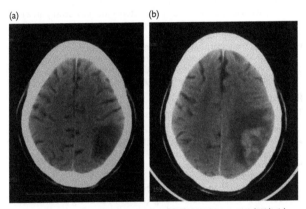

Fig. 13.13 Haemorrhagic transformation on CT. This patient presented with right homonymous hemianopia and dysphasia. (a) A scan on day 1 shows a left parietal infarct; (b) on day 15, she deteriorated with worsening dysphasia. A repeat scan showed haemorrhage within the infarct. © Hugh Markus.

Other specific causes of ICH

Cerebral tumours

- Bleeding into cerebral tumours may account for up to 5% of ICH
- Often the diagnosis is easy if the patient has a known cerebral tumour or an extracranial malignancy
- Some secondary (metastatic) tumours have a particular tendency to bleed such as:
  - malignant melanoma
  - choriocarcinoma
  - renal cell carcinoma
  - breast and lung metastases have a lower tendency to bleed individually but as they are very common they are relatively frequent causes of ICH-related tumours
- Primary tumours tend not to bleed, but glioblastoma multiforme is the exception and can bleed
- Clues to an underlying tumour on imaging include:
  - a disproportionate amount of oedema or mass effect
  - nodular enhancement of surrounding tissue with IV contrast
  - irregular patchy appearance of haematoma with low-density area in the centre on CT suggesting necrotic tissue
  - multiple haemorrhages
- Therefore, the underlying tumour can often be suspected on the original brain imaging. However, it cannot be excluded and therefore, repeat imaging (CT or preferably MRI) is required for all ICH cases when the haematoma has resolved (usually at about 3 months).

Illicit drugs

There are two classes of drugs that cause ICH.

Amphetamines

- These cause haemorrhage from minutes to a few hours after administration
- Contributing factors include:
  - a hypertensive surge
  - drug-induced fibrinoid necrosis in small and medium-sized vessels—seen angiographically as 'beading' (areas of narrowing and dilatation and occlusion) and associated with chronic use.
- Underlying vascular abnormalities (e.g. aneurysm, AVM) are often found, suggesting that amphetamines increase the risk of bleeding from these.

Cocaine

- Cocaine haemorrhages occur soon after ingestion
- They are more common with crack cocaine
- Most common in the white matter and may be multifocal
- As for amphetamines, an underlying vascular malformation is often present. Haemodynamic factors may be important. Otherwise at postmortem, blood vessels are usually normal
- For more details on stroke caused by illicit drugs, see ⊃ Chapter 11.

Hyperperfusion syndrome

- This is a rare but a well-recognized complication of carotid endarterectomy, and carotid stenting, affecting <1% of cases
- The haemorrhage usually occurs within a week of the operation, with haemorrhages and oedema in the carotid artery territory distal to the endarterectomy
- It can also cause seizures
- It is more likely to occur in hypertensive individuals with haemodynamic compromise to the cerebral circulation and a poor collateral supply
- There is some evidence that careful control of BP postoperatively, avoiding hypertension and fluctuations, can reduce the risk of this syndrome.

Reversible cerebral vasoconstriction syndrome (RCVS)

- RCVS is characterized by severe (often thunderclap) headaches and neurological symptoms. ICH can be a feature
- Imaging (CTA, MRA, or formal angiography) shows a 'string and beads' appearance of the cerebral arteries. It resolves spontaneously in 1 to 3 months.

Ducros described a series of 67 patients:
- 43 were female
- RCVS was spontaneous in 37%
- RCVS was secondary in 63% (postpartum and exposure to vasoactive substances, e.g. cannabis, selective serotonin-recapture inhibitors and nasal decongestants)
- The presentation was:
  - multiple thunderclap headaches or headache (94%)
  - cortical SAH (22%)
  - ICH (6%)
  - seizures (3%)
  - reversible posterior leucoencephalopathy (9%)
  - TIAs (16%)
  - cerebral infarction (4%)

For more details on RCVS ➔ see Chapter 11.

Further reading

Global impact of ICH

Parry-Jones AR, Krishnamurthi R, Ziai WC, et al. (2025) World Stroke Organization (WSO): Global intracerebral hemorrhage factsheet 2025. *Int J Stroke* **6**, 17474930241307876.

Berry (saccular) aneurysms

Deshmukh AS, Priola SM, Katsanos AH, et al. (2024). The management of intracranial aneurysms: current trends and future directions. *Neurol Int* **16**(1), 74–94.

Management of SAH: medical

Lawton MT, Vates GE (2017). Subarachnoid hemorrhage. *N Engl J Med* **377**, 257–266.

Asymptomatic aneurysms
Risk of rupture of asymptomatic intracranial aneurysm

Wiebers DO, Whisnant JP, Huston J, et al. (2003). Unruptured intracranial aneurysms: natural history, clinical outcome, and risks of surgical and endovascular treatment. *Lancet* **362**, 103–110.

Screening for intracranial aneurysms

Bor AS, Rinkel GJ, van Norden J, et al. (2014). Long-term, serial screening for intracranial aneurysms in individuals with a family history of aneurysmal subarachnoid haemorrhage: a cohort study. *Lancet Neurol* **13**, 385–392.

Brown RDJr, Broderick JP (2014). Unruptured intracranial aneurysms: epidemiology, natural history, management options, and familial screening. *Lancet Neurol* **13**, 393–404.

Brain imaging in ICH

Du FZ, Jiang R, Gu M, He C, Guan J (2014). The accuracy of spot sign in predicting hematoma expansion after intracerebral hemorrhage: a systematic review and meta-analysis. *PLoS One* **9**, e115777.

Treatment of ICH

Parry-Jones AR, Moullaali TJ, Ziai WC (2020). Treatment of intracerebral hemorrhage: from specific interventions to bundles of care. *Int J Stroke* **15**:945–953.

Parry-Jones AR, Järhult SJ, Kreitzer N, et al. (2024). Acute care bundles should be used for patients with intracerebral haemorrhage: an expert consensus statement. *Eur Stroke J* **9**, 295–302.

Ma J, Hu X, Song L, et al. INTERACT3 Investigators (2023). The third Intensive Care Bundle with Blood Pressure Reduction in Acute Cerebral Haemorrhage Trial (INTERACT3): an international, stepped wedge cluster randomised controlled trial. *Lancet* **402**, 27–40.

Medical treatment to reduce haematoma size

McGurgan IJ, Ziai WC, Werring DJ, et al. (2021) Acute intracerebral haemorrhage: diagnosis and management. *Pract Neurol* **21**, 128–136.

Baharoglu MI, Cordonnier C, Salman RA, et al. (2016). Platelet transfusion versus standard care after acute stroke due to spontaneous cerebral haemorrhage associated with antiplatelet therapy (PATCH): a randomised, open-label, phase 3 trial. *Lancet* **387**, 2605–2613.

Li G, Lin Y, Yang J, et al. INTERACT4 Investigators (2024). Intensive ambulance-delivered blood-pressure reduction in hyperacute stroke. *N Engl J Med* **390**, 1862–1872.

Seiffge DJ, Anderson CS (2024). Treatment for intracerebral hemorrhage: dawn of a new era. *Int J Stroke* **19**, 482–489.

Sarhan K, Mohamed RG, Elmahdi RR, et al. (2025). Efficacy and safety of andexanet alfa versus four factor prothrombin complex concentrate for emergent reversal of factor Xa inhibitor associated intracranial hemorrhage: a systematic review and meta-analysis. *Neurocrit Care* **42**(2), 701–714.

Surgery for ICH

Mendelow AD, Gregson BA, Rowan EN, et al. STICH II Investigators (2013). Early surgery versus initial conservative treatment in patients with spontaneous supratentorial lobar intracerebral haematomas (STICH II): a randomised trial. *Lancet* **382**, 397–408.

Kellner CP, Schupper AJ, Mocco J (2021). Surgical evacuation of intracerebral hemorrhage: the potential importance of timing. *Stroke* **52**, 3391–3398.

Pradilla G, Ratcliff JJ, Hall AJ, et al. ENRICH Trial Investigators (2024). Trial of early minimally invasive removal of intracerebral hemorrhage. *N Engl J Med* **390**, 1277–1289.

Treatment of complications

Khan NR (2014). Fibrinolysis for intraventricular hemorrhage: an updated meta-analysis and systematic review of the literature. *Stroke* **45**, 2662–2669.

Cerebral amyloid angiopathy

Banerjee G, Samra K, Adams ME, et al. (2022) Iatrogenic cerebral amyloid angiopathy: an emerging clinical phenomenon. *JNNP* jnnp-2022-328792.

Charidimou A, Boulouis G, Frosch MP, et al. (2022). The Boston criteria version 2.0 for cerebral amyloid angiopathy: a multicentre, retrospective, MRI-neuropathology diagnostic accuracy study. *Lancet Neurol* **21**, 714–725.

Corovic A, Kelly S, Markus HS (2018). Cerebral amyloid angiopathy associated with inflammation: a systematic review of clinical and imaging features and outcome. *Int J Stroke* **13**, 257–267.

Kozberg MG, Perosa V, Gurol ME, van Veluw SJ (2021). A practical approach to the management of cerebral amyloid angiopathy. *Int J Stroke* **16**(4), 356–369.

Rodrigues MA, Samarasekera N, Lerpiniere C, et al. (2018). The Edinburgh CT and genetic diagnostic criteria for lobar intracerebral haemorrhage associated with cerebral amyloid angiopathy: model development and diagnostic test accuracy study. *Lancet Neurol* **17**, 232–240.

Arteriovenous and cavernous malformations

Al-Shahi Salman R, Hall JM, Horne MA, et al. (2012). Scottish Audit of Intracranial Vascular Malformations (SAIVMs) collaborators. Untreated clinical course of cerebral cavernous malformations: a prospective, population-based cohort study. *Lancet Neurol* **11**, 217–224.

Mohr JP, Overbey JR, Hartmann A, et al. ARUBA co-investigators (2020). Medical management with interventional therapy versus medical management alone for unruptured brain arteriovenous malformations (ARUBA): final follow-up of a multicentre, non-blinded, randomised controlled trial. *Lancet Neuro* **19**, 573–581.

van Beijnum J, van der Worp HB, Buis DR, et al. (2011). Treatment of brain arteriovenous malformations: a systematic review and meta-analysis. *JAMA* **306**, 2011–2019.

Haemorrhagic transformation of a cerebral infarct

Trouillas T, von Kummer R (2006). Classification and pathogenesis of cerebral hemorrhages after thrombolysis in ischemic stroke. *Stroke* **37**, 556–561.

Other specific causes of ICH

Ducros A, Boukobza M, Porcher R, et al. (2007). The clinical and radiological spectrum of reversible cerebral vasoconstriction syndrome. A prospective series of 67 patients. *Brain* **130**, 3091–3101.

Miller TR, Shivashankar R, Mossa-Basha M, Gandhi D (2015). Reversible cerebral vasoconstriction syndrome, Part 1: epidemiology, pathogenesis, and clinical course. *AJNR Am J Neuroradiol* **36**, 1392–1399.

Miller TR, Shivashankar R, Mossa-Basha M, Gandhi D (2015). Reversible cerebral vasoconstriction syndrome, Part 2: diagnostic work-up, imaging evaluation, and differential diagnosis. *AJNR Am J Neuroradiol* **36**, 1580–1588.

Recovery
and rehabilitation

Introduction

Life is never the same after stroke. The processes that can help go into picking up the pieces and returning to a pre-stroke life and lifestyle are outlined in this chapter.

Rehabilitation is an active, participatory process to minimize the neurological impairment resulting from stroke translating into disability and handicap.

Rehabilitation interventions are designed to:
- reduce impairment (*restorative*)
- help people adapt to impairment (*compensatory*).

Rehabilitation requires a multiprofessional team of healthcare workers and patient-centred goals.

For many affected by stroke, *vocational rehabilitation* may be appropriate. Returning to employment or an alternative meaningful occupation is always a major challenge after stroke. Returning to work is not only fundamental to psychosocial well-being for many but has significant financial implications. Vocational rehabilitation is designed specifically to maximize the potential for a successful return to work. It frequently involves a collaboration between health and social services and independent and voluntary organizations.

The 5 'R's of rehabilitation
- Realization of potential—to help the patient improve so their recovery plateaus close to their best anticipated function
- Re-enablement—to maximize functional independence
- Resettlement—to provide safe and confident transfer of care
- Role fulfilment—to re-establish personal status and autonomy
- Readjustment—to adapt to and accept a new lifestyle after stroke.

Basic science of stroke recovery

After stroke, early recovery of function is thought to be due to reperfusion of hypoxic brain or reduction in vasogenic oedema associated with ischaemic brain tissue. All subsequent recovery is thought to be related to the brain's ability to compensate and remodel after injury, termed 'neuronal plasticity'. Dead brain tissue does not regenerate or re-grow but the remaining brain is not 'hard wired'.

Mechanisms underlying neuronal plasticity may include:

• change in balance of excitation and inhibition: 'unmasking' of connections and neuronal pathways
• strengthening or weakening of existing synapses: long-term potentiation or depression of key pathways
• change in neuronal membrane excitability
• anatomical changes, such as sprouting new axons/synaptic connections.

The way in which these mechanisms are implemented is thought to influence functional outcome. The ability to utilize or recruit adjacent areas of undamaged cortex is thought to be associated with good outcome, using contralateral pathways and cortical 'maps' is less good and using deep short connections leads to the least good outcome.

A key aspect of neuronal plasticity, with important implications for rehabilitation, is that the modifications in neuronal networks are use-dependent. Animal experimental studies and clinical trials in humans using functional imaging have shown that forced use and functional training contribute to improved function. On the other hand, techniques that promote non-use may inhibit recovery. Therefore, repetitive 'task-specific' training and 'dose' is a key element of many rehabilitation strategies. There is currently a huge interest in using assistive technologies—such as robots, virtual reality, or other computer-based technologies to implement this. While these approaches are exciting, they are yet to be validated and proven in randomized controlled trials (RCTs) in stroke.

Natural history of stroke recovery

The rate of recovery is influenced by site, size of lesion, age, concomitant brain disease, and other systemic physical and psychological comorbidities.

The greatest rate of recovery is within the first 3–4 months after stroke and it is within this window that therapy intervention is thought to have the biggest impact. Functional change often continues beyond this stage, so each patient should be taken as an individual case when considering the spectrum of outcomes after stroke. Patients with marked aphasia for example, typically demonstrate limited early recovery but after 3 months, provided they can tolerate high-intensity (e.g. 6 hours/day) therapy, they can make significant and sustained improvement in specialist comprehensive aphasia programmes.

It is currently accepted that:

• approximately 35% (one in three) of survivors with leg paralysis do not regain useful function and about 25% of all stroke survivors are unable to walk independently
• 6 months after stroke, 65% (two of three) of those with upper limb weakness cannot use their affected hand in normal functional tasks.

While acute treatment is targeted at reducing the extent of brain injury from stroke, rehabilitation has much to do to improve these statistics.

Good prognostic features:
• Absence of coma
• Early motor recovery, especially thumb and foot
• Continence.

Poor prognostic features:
• Coma
• Older age
• Incontinence
• Marked communication deficits
• Cognitive impairment
• Spatial neglect
• No leg movement at 2 weeks
• Flaccid upper limb with no selective finger movement at 4 weeks.

Another aspect to consider is the fact that skeletal muscle mass naturally diminishes in a paretic limb (in the order of 20%) and is replaced by intramuscular fat resulting in reduced muscle 'quality'. Resistance training in a paretic limb can counter this.

Cardiovascular fitness also dramatically falls away after stroke and exercise with a combination of cardiovascular and strength training has been shown to improve stroke recovery in chronic stroke patients.

Trials have shown that coordinated stroke unit care saves lives and improves outcome, but the evidence base for the efficacy of specific components of stroke rehabilitation is scant with respect to RCT data.

Trial design is difficult as stroke is so heterogeneous in terms of sub-type and natural history, where physical deficits recover spontaneously and variably over time. For example, a weak arm may be part of a large hemispheric cortical infarct, a small subcortical lacune, or a brainstem lesion affecting the corticospinal pathway; all of these recover differently.

As well as stroke type, the rate of recovery is dependent on comorbidity which influences neuronal plasticity.

Furthermore, many interventions are difficult to 'control', e.g. what is placebo physiotherapy?

As a result, most evidence on therapy intervention comes from case-controlled series. In the UK and Ireland National Clinical Guideline for Stroke, the evidence base for the majority of rehabilitation and therapy is Grade 'D' or 'consensus', based on expert committee reports, opinions, and/or experience of respected authorities.

The multidisciplinary stroke team

- Members of the multiprofessional stroke team and their roles in the stroke recovery process are covered here.
- All are involved in goal setting and discharge planning.
- A functional and cohesive multidisciplinary/professional team (MDT) is essential for comprehensive and successful stroke care.

Nursing

Nursing staff have a pivotal role in inpatient stroke rehabilitation as they are the only members of the MDT who are with the patient 24 hours a day. Rehabilitation should be a 24/7 process with all members of staff working together with the patient to achieve agreed goals and promote recovery.

Nursing staff have important roles in many areas of stroke care, including:
- medication administration including monitoring and titrating analgesia and re-enforcing stroke secondary prevention plans
- practising transfers
- supervising mobility
- promoting continence
- being vigilant for signs of breakdown in skin integrity
- identifying disturbance of mood
- supervising patients' nutritional intake and monitoring their weight
- liaising with carers and families outside office hours and managing their expectations of recovery, as well as facilitating transfer of care back to the community.

Medical team

The diagnosis of stroke is made by doctors, as is the management of secondary prevention, early complications, and recovery.

In the acute stages of stroke, different specialties will contribute to care, including the stroke physician/neurologist/ radiologist/cardiologist, and vascular surgeon.

Later on, medical input is from the primary care physician with the help of hospital- or community-based rehabilitation medicine.

Physiotherapy

This is 'physical', often 'hands-on' therapy, which predominantly aids motor recovery (mobility and upper limb function).

With all therapies, but especially physiotherapy, there is a 30% or more placebo component.

Also, it is difficult to separate spontaneous recovery from the effects of therapy.

Physiotherapists use different approaches:
- Bobath—here the ethos is to maintain symmetry and correct adverse compensations such as 'pushing' with the good side. It is fundamentally a 'hands-on' approach
- Carr and Shepherd—this approach uses a motor relearning programme. Patients are given repeated functional movement pattern exercises, e.g. bending and stretching the arm. This improves strength and specific functional movements but not all the movements used

in normal life. It is less 'hands-on', making it difficult for patients with cognitive or low arousal states to participate
• Neurofacilitation—here abnormal muscle tone is inhibited through weightbearing, sustained stretch, and more normal movement promoted by trying to recruit paretic muscle activity through functional strength training in 'conventional' physiotherapy.

Traditionally, the Bobath approach has influenced UK physiotherapy practice more than any other. Most physiotherapists use a combination based on their experience and the individual needs of the patient of:
• 'conventional' physiotherapy approaches (usually a combination of those listed earlier)
• assistive devices, e.g. treadmill retraining
• novel approaches, e.g. constraint therapy, 'robot training', mirror imagery
• functional electrical stimulation (FES)
• use of orthoses.

Potential promoters of plasticity by physical therapy include:
• repetition ('dose')
• functional goal-directed activity
• attention during learning
• electrical stimulation
• immobilization.

Occupational therapy

Occupational therapists (OTs) work closely with physiotherapists but particularly are involved in the following:
• Seating
• Functional assessment of personal care, including transfers (e.g. bed-to-chair), washing, dressing, using the toilet, working in the kitchen, and other high-level assessments such as fitness to drive and vocational assessment
• Training motor and sensory function (e.g. 'errorless learning', a technique particularly helpful in managing dyspraxia)
• Provision of splints, static, or dynamic, for the affected upper limb
• Training compensatory skills
• Training cognitive function
• Advice and instruction over assisted devices, from adaptive cutlery to the appropriate use of rails, wheelchairs, and hoists
• Education of primary caregiver and family. The pre-discharge home visit is part of this, as well as advising over assisted devices and adaptations.

Speech and language therapy (SLT) or speech pathology

This therapist has a number of major roles in the assessment and treatment of stroke patients:
• Swallow (dysphagia) assessment in complex cases or in those patients who fail an initial bedside swallow
• Assessment and treatment of patients with speech/communication disorders, including:
  • dysarthria

- aphasia
- cognitive communication disorder
- They also serve as facilitators and advocates for those with communication problems in a wide range of issues.

Dietician

Dieticians assess nutritional status and prescribe regimens of enteral nutrition for those who cannot swallow. They also help in establishing percutaneous endoscopic gastrostomy (PEG) feeding in patients who have longer-term feeding problems.

- It is estimated that between 8% and 18% of acute stroke patients are malnourished on admission
- Nutritional status can be judged by anthropometric factors, including body mass index, skinfold thickness, and biochemical markers such as serum albumin
- Stroke patients are at high risk of worsening malnutrition
- The number of malnourished patients increases significantly during the first week after stroke
- Stroke size, location, and severity have no effect on resting energy expenditure, but infection will increase energy requirements
- Dysphagia will also result in decreased intake, as will functional deficits such as weakness, sensory, and visual disturbance
- Texture-modified diets often have a relatively low nutritional content and low patient tolerability
- In the FOOD trial, early tube feeding was associated with a non-significant reduction in risk of death of 5.8% (95% CI –0.8 to 12.5, $P = 0.09$)
- Stroke patients are at risk of a metabolic and multiorgan crisis called 're-feeding syndrome' if they are given enteral feed:
  - After 10 days or more of no nutritional intake
  - Are depleted in potassium, phosphate, and magnesium pre-feeding
  - Have unintentional weight loss of >15% of usual body weight in the previous 3–6 months.

In patients at risk of re-feeding syndrome, enteral feeding usually starts at a low rate—10 mL/hour, increasing up to 120 mL/hour as tolerated. The calorie delivery would typically start at 10 kcal/kg/day, increasing slowly to meet full requirements by the end of the first week. Thiamine 200–300 mg is given daily for the first 10 days and daily measures of potassium, magnesium, and phosphate to guide oral/enteral or IV supplements are required. After a week of enteral feeding, the risk of metabolic crisis is rare and feeding can be increased as normal.

Pharmacist

Pharmacists have an increasingly extended role in the stroke MDT. As well as general medicines management (including appropriate antibiotic prescribing and venous thromboembolism (VTE) management), we use prescribing pharmacists on ward rounds and in outpatient anticoagulation clinic settings. There are four principles of optimal medicine management, which are worth mentioning here:

- Aim to understand the patient's experience
- Evidence-based choice of medicines
- Ensure medicines are as safe as possible
- Making medicines optimization part of routine practice

Clinical psychology/neuropsychology

Psychologists help with the following:

- *Diagnosis*—detecting the presence and nature of cognitive impairment, and diagnosing mood disorder
- *Management and goal planning*—neuropsychological assessment provides an analysis of an individual's cognitive function and outlines areas of strengths and weakness, providing a descriptive basis for rehabilitation goal planning. Clinical psychology can also help provide insight and techniques to help with psychological adjustment issues after stroke for patients, carers, and family members
- *Monitoring change/evaluation*—the individual's performance on the neuropsychological tests provides baseline data against which their degree of recovery can be measured. It can also be an important form of feedback for families and carers
- *Aiding assessments of capacity*

Domains of cognitive testing include:

- overall intellectual ability
- attention and concentration
- speed of processing information
- memory and learning
- language and communication
- visuospatial and spatial–constructional skills
- 'executive functions', including complex abstract reasoning, planning, organization, and flexibility of thinking.

Social work

- Social work teams work with multidisciplinary colleagues to assist patients and carers in adjusting to and managing the impact of stroke
- They work in partnership with a client and their social network to promote independence and provide care in the community
- This involves assessment of individual need, care planning, implementing a care plan, monitoring, and review
- There is also a separate assessment of the needs of the carer
- Social workers assess the psychosocial impact of stroke and issues around welfare and benefits
- Patients may have a 'continuing care assessment', after which social services will instigate an appropriate care package and, if necessary, help facilitate day centre, respite or long-term care, applications for re-housing, and access to voluntary based resources
- Social workers play a key part in managing safeguarding issues.

Common problems after stroke

Seating

Mobilization and seating is a cornerstone of early stroke care aimed to:
- maximize:
  - function
  - comfort
- minimize:
  - development of deformities
  - development of tissue trauma
- improve:
  - self-esteem
  - eating, swallowing, digestive function
  - visual, cognitive, and perceptual ability
  - cardiovascular efficiency
  - functional symmetry and balance
- decrease:
  - risk of chest infection
  - effects of abnormal reflexes and muscle tone.

The timing of seating a stroke patient needs to be assessed on an individual basis. Effective seating should:
- control alignment
- provide an appropriate and stable base
- relieve stress on loaded structures.

Four types of seating commonly used outside of a standard hospital armchair include the following:
1. Standard wheelchairs—used for mobility, transfers, patients with poor exercise tolerance, outdoor use.
2. Standard wheelchairs with adaptations—used *for patients with:*
   - good head and trunk control
   - poor pelvic stability
   - one-sided weakness—hemiplegia, pusher syndrome
   - perceptual problems in addition to hemiplegia.
3. Recliner wheelchairs—used for patients with:
   - perceptual problems in addition to hemiplegia
   - good head control
   - moderate trunk control
   - poor pelvic stability.
4. Tilt-in-space wheelchairs—used for patients with:
   - poor head and trunk control
   - compromised haemodynamic status
   - overactivity in non-hemiplegic side
   - dense hemiplegia
   - decreased alertness and arousal.

Weakness

Predictors of motor recovery
- Early, selective movement across joints is a good prognostic marker
- Early thumb movement is a good indicator of future useful hand function.

Patterns of recovery
- In middle cerebral artery (MCA) territory stroke, leg weakness recovers before the arm because the cortical area controlling leg function is in the vascular territory of the anterior cerebral artery
- Subcortical strokes affecting the arm may recover distal function early; this is attributed to preserved hand cortex
- Cortical infarcts typically recover better proximally; late selective finger movement is associated with poor dexterity
- Striatocapsular infarcts may show cortical signs which recover rapidly but hemiparesis is longer term. They usually result from embolic proximal trunk MCA occlusions, which rapidly re-canalize. Transient widespread MCA hypoperfusion occurs but there is only permanent infarction in the striatal region supplied by the perforating arteries, which have no collateral supply. This pattern is often seen following thrombolysis.

When to start mobilization after stroke?

- The AVERT trial, published in 2015, randomized 2104 acute stroke patients between usual stroke unit care alone or very early mobilization in addition to usual care
- Fewer patients in the very early mobilization group had a favourable outcome than those in the usual care group ($n = 480$ (46%) vs. $n = 525$ (50%); adjusted OR 0.73, 95% CI 0.59–0.90; $P = 0.004$)
- It was concluded that a very early mobilization protocol was associated with a reduction in the odds of a favourable outcome at 3 months. The investigators concluded that despite early mobilization after stroke being recommended in many clinical practice guidelines worldwide, the AVERT findings should affect clinical practice by refining present guidelines
- When considering the results of the AVERT study it is important to remember that the usual care arm of the trial saw patients sit out of bed within 24 hours of stroke and the trial results should not put a stop to this routine of acute stroke care. However, AVERT does suggest caution in forcibly mobilizing patients very early after stroke.
- Timing of mobilization after stroke requires knowledge of the underlying stroke pathophysiology and natural history. For example, patients with haemodynamic stroke symptoms due to acute internal carotid artery (ICA) occlusion are poor candidates for early mobilization—even if they have only mild deficits. Similarly, patients with large core infarcts or hematoma volumes will predictably deteriorate acutely due to oedema effects before they start to spontaneously improve, and early mobilization can cause harm in such scenarios.

Communication

Communication problems are common after stroke—up to 70% of stroke patients have altered speech at the time of presentation and persistent problems are a major adverse factor in rehabilitation.

The major types of speech and language disorders after stroke are listed in this section. They frequently coexist, and correct interpretation of brain imaging can help guide treatment and predict recovery. Dysarthria is a disorder of speech and articulation; aphasia/dysphasia is a disorder of language. They are often confused if adequate examination is not performed (see ➜ Speech and language, p. 108).

- *Dysarthria* or slurred speech is common after stroke
- *Anarthria* is severe dysarthria where no intelligible sound is made
- *Aphasia/dysphasia* is a disorder of language comprehension and/or production
- *Dysphonia* is a marked reduction in voice with preserved language and articulation (e.g. due to vocal cord palsy).

Dysarthria

- Occurs owing to motor weakness of muscles involved in speech or brain areas involved in control of articulation (e.g. cerebellum)
- Exacerbated by non-stroke factors, e.g. dry mouth, ill-fitting dentures
- Treatment includes facial muscle exercise and education around breaking sentences and words into discrete intelligible blocks
- Give dysarthric patients time to articulate and never pretend to understand when you haven't—this leads to frustration for the patient. Alternative lines of communication may be available—writing, gesture, or using assistive devices such as a sign-writer.

Aphasia/dysphasia

The terms aphasia and dysphasia are used interchangeably, which can cause confusion. Aphasia really means loss of speech owing to a disorder of language rather than articulation, and dysphasia is the same disorder without complete loss. However, in some countries (including the UK) aphasia is now the preferred terminology for a primary disorder of language and we have used it in this book.

Aphasia can comprise:

- poor understanding of language (*receptive* component)
- poor verbalization of language—reduced verbal fluency, paraphrasic syntax, grammatical, and naming/nominal errors (*expressive* component).

While aphasia is nearly always made up of these two components, it is not unusual for one component to dominate. Global aphasia is where there is no apparent understanding or language output. Usually, it is a mixture of receptive and expressive language problems, characterized by poor verbal fluency, naming or nominal difficulties, paraphrasic, syntax, and semantic errors with speech.

Features of aphasia
- Aphasia is caused by dominant hemisphere stroke (usually left hemisphere but remember to determine handedness) and can be isolated as part of a branch MCA cortical stroke or more often associated with hemiparesis if the stroke is extensive. It can also be part of a subcortical stroke, e.g. thalamic aphasia
- Between 20% and 40% or one in three of all acute stroke patients present with primary language disturbance or aphasia
- Approximately 80% of aphasic patients have persistent language problems at 1 year
- Aphasia is strongly associated with post-stroke depression
- The relationship between stroke type, location, and aphasia recovery is complex and needs to be considered on an individual basis. Young age and good early comprehension are positive prognostic indicators
- The ability to reorganize language within the dominant hemisphere (especially the left temporal area) seems to be associated with better recovery
- It may be associated with the inability to read (dyslexia) and write (dysgraphia).

Aphasia treatment
- Patients with predominant receptive problems, rather than expressive problems, are far more challenging to treat
- There is little RCT data but some suggestion that SLT may improve outcome. Interventions include melodic intervention therapy (MIT), lexical semantic therapy, and other focused techniques to develop verbal output and understanding. Computer programs are sometimes helpful and computer tablet-based 'Apps' for aphasia treatment and facilitation of communication are becoming increasingly popular
- An RCT (ACT NoW) in 170 stroke patients compared enhanced, agreed best practice, communication therapy specific to aphasia or dysarthria, offered by speech and language therapists according to participants' needs for up to 4 months, with continuity from hospital to community with similarly resourced social contact (without communication therapy) from employed visitors. Specific communication therapy had no added benefit beyond that of everyday communication in the first 4 months after stroke
- In contrast, there is a suggestion from meta-analysis of SLT intervention, that 'dose' of therapy is also important with 100 hours being suggested as the minimum useful dose. The timing of such intervention needs to be individualized as aphasic patients can make considerable recovery late after stroke and not all aphasic patient can 'cope' with intensive communication therapy acutely after stroke
- It is suggested the minimum effective SLT intervention is thought to be 2 hours a week, with improved outcomes demonstrated if the intensity is increased to 9 hours a week
- More data from RCTs is required
- There is growing interest in brain stimulation as adjunctive aphasia treatment—especially with transcranial direct current stimulation

(tDCS), in the sub-acute phase of recovery, but for now such treatment should be considered experimental
• It is possible that biological treatment that increases brain acetylcholine levels may help conventional SLT treatment. Piracetam may help experimentally but there is no demonstrable long-term effect of any pharmacological intervention for aphasia that is RCT proven to date.

Cognitive communication disorder (CCD)

This is poorly understood and under-recognized. CCD may be more prominent in right hemisphere stroke.

There are no typical features of aphasia, but:
• altered non-verbal communication, e.g. monotone voice, flat facial expression, reduced eye contact
• verbose and tangential output with poor self-monitoring
• reduced awareness of the listener
• associated with other signs of cognitive impairment, such as altered attention, affect, and neglect.

Neuropsychiatric symptoms post-stroke

The most common neuropsychiatric outcomes of stroke are depression, anxiety, fatigue, and apathy, which each occur in at least 30% of patients and have a substantial overlap of prevalence and symptoms.

Emotional lability, psychosis, and mania are less common but distressing and difficult to manage.

Low mood and post-stroke depression

Depression is extremely common after stroke and often exists with other mood disorders such as anxiety. The diagnosis is frequently missed. Treatment can have a dramatic effect on recovery and quality of life.

- Up to 70% of stroke patients experience low mood after stroke and 25–30% show significant post-stroke depression (PSD)
- The later the symptoms present after stroke onset, the worse depression is likely to be
- Early emotionalism may be considered a 'normal/expected' accompaniment to stroke and usually resolves spontaneously
- Previous history of major depression is associated with developing PSD
- The cognitive effects of stroke may mimic PSD, making the diagnosis difficult
- On the stroke unit, one can use a questionnaire tool such as the Hospital Anxiety and Depression Scale (HADS), or the Beck Depression Inventory, GDS, HAMDS, or PHQ9 (see ➲ Appendix 2: Useful stroke scales, p. 561)
- The Visual Analogue Self-esteem Scale (VASES) can be helpful to assess mood in some aphasic patients
- Patients with PSD have worse functional outcome, slower recovery, and increased mortality, so timely detection and intervention is important
- One should consider whether somatic symptoms such as psychomotor retardation, fatigue, sleep, and appetite disturbances are related to mood and not to the physical symptoms of stroke
- We recommend that all patients are screened for mood disorders within 6 weeks of a stroke.

In the recent DSM-5 Major Depressive Episode criteria, to qualify for a major depressive disorder, you need to have been experiencing your symptoms almost every day for at least 2 weeks, and they must be more intense than the normal fluctuations in mood we all experience in our daily lives. You need to have at least five of the criteria in section A to qualify, and one of these five has to be either a depressed mood or loss of interest or pleasure in activities:

- A.
  1. Depressed mood most of the day, almost every day, indicated by your own subjective report or by the report of others. This mood might be characterized by sadness, emptiness, or hopelessness
  2. Markedly diminished interest or pleasure in all or almost all activities most of the day nearly every day
  3. Significant weight loss when not dieting or weight gain
  4. Inability to sleep or oversleeping nearly every day
  5. Psychomotor agitation or retardation nearly every day
  6. Fatigue or loss of energy nearly every day
  7. Feelings of worthlessness or excessive or inappropriate guilt (which may be delusional) nearly every day
  8. Diminished ability to think or concentrate, or indecisiveness, nearly every day

9. Recurrent thoughts of death (not just fear of dying), recurrent suicidal ideation without a specific plan, or a suicide attempt or a specific plan for committing suicide
- B. Symptoms cause clinically significant distress or impairment in social, occupational, or other important areas of functioning
- C. The episode is not due to the effects of a substance or to a medical condition
- D. The occurrence is not better explained by schizoaffective disorder, schizophrenia, schizophreniform disorder, delusional disorder, or other specified and unspecified schizophrenia spectrum and other psychotic disorders
- E. There has never been a manic episode or a hypomanic episode.

Treatment of PSD

- Prompt identification and treatment improve outcome. Explain it is a very common complication of stroke and responds to treatment. Warn stroke patients it may occur and what to watch out for. This reduces the stigma often attached to the diagnosis
- *Non-pharmacological*: counselling motivational interviewing, cognitive behavioural therapy, problem-solving therapy, or acceptance and commitment therapy are often underused and helpful
- *Pharmacological:* little RCT evidence but:
  - symptoms need to be present continually for at least 2 weeks to be significant and warrant drug treatment
  - most classes of antidepressants seem safe post-stroke
  - anticholinergic side effects should be avoided (dry mouth, constipation, confusion, and worsening cognitive impairment)
  - SSRIs: citalopram, sertraline, and fluoxetine are commonly used.
  - If there is no improvement after 6 weeks with SSRI, consider a dose increase or venlafaxine. The minimum treatment period should be 6 months and at least 4 months after any beneficial effect is noted.
  - If possible, use in conjunction with psychological therapies and counselling as outlined earlier.

It has also been suggested that fluoxetine might reduce neurological disability after stroke, but large trials have failed to confirm this hypothesis.

SSRIs have been shown to increase the risk of seizures and bone (hip) fractures after stroke, so it is important to consider the non-pharmacological interventions and review the need to continue on an individualized basis.

Other neuropsychiatric symptoms post-stroke

Post-stroke apathy

- Apathy is a disorder of motivation.
- It occurs in about one-third of patients post-stroke.
- At least as common as PSD and probably the most frequent neuropsychiatric complication of stroke.
- Apathy can be defined as a quantitative reduction in goal-directed behaviour (GDB) occurring in the cognitive/behavioural, emotional, or social domains of an individual's life. Reductions are relative to an individual's previous level of functioning.
- Post-stroke patients with apathy suffer from greater functional impairment and demonstrate slower recovery times.
- Can be difficult to distinguish from depression after stroke but the two are distinct syndromes with a different biological basis.
- Negative emotionality is a key characteristic of depression that distinguishes it from apathy. Depressed patients may present with pessimism and hopelessness, while those with apathy show a lack of emotional distress.
- Apathy is traditionally described as the result of damage to specific brain structures related to GDB such as the basal ganglia and prefrontal cortex. If this lesion-deficit view of apathy was true, one would expect a clear relationship between lesion location and apathy. However, no common localizations across stroke studies have been found, suggesting that relationships between structural damage and functional deficits are more complex than initially thought. More recently, it has been suggested apathy in cerebrovascular disease is the product of damage to brain networks underlying GDB.
- Apathy may be during the history and examination of an observed loss of motivation. Informant histories may also reveal symptoms of apathy, such as loss of interest in previous activities and hobbies or doing little when left alone, which can be valuable as patients may underplay symptoms. Apathy assessments can be supplemented with questionnaires such as the apathy evaluation scale.
- Antidepressant drugs do not help apathetic symptoms.

Post-stroke emotionalism

- Emotionalism following stroke is a common yet under-researched disorder of emotional expression typically involving recurrent uncontrollable episodes of crying and occasionally laughter.
- Also called pathological laughter or crying, emotional incontinence, involuntary emotional expression disorder, and emotional lability.
- Most common after bilateral anterior frontal cortical lesions, or subcortical disease leading to white matter tract disruption and bilateral frontal cortical disconnection. Pathways related to serotonin production have also been implicated.
- Occurs in about 1 in 5 stroke patients.
- It can be extremely distressing for both patient and family/carers

- Crying alone can be mistaken for depression, although it can coexist with depression.
- There is some evidence that emotional lability can be helped with SSRIs and it is often worth a therapeutic trial for a couple of months but stop if no benefit is seen. A Cochrane review found evidence that antidepressants helped, but no particular drug was superior.

Anxiety

- For patients to meet diagnostic criteria for a generalized anxiety disorder, anxiety symptoms that are out of proportion to the actual threat or danger the situation poses must be present for 6 months, plus at least three of the following: feeling wound-up, tense, or restless; fatigue; difficulty concentrating; irritability; substantial muscle tension; and difficulty sleeping
- A systematic review of 4706 patients indicated that 24% of stroke patients had anxiety symptoms, and 18% had an anxiety disorder in the first 5 years after stroke.
- Anxiety is commonly seen in association with depression

Psychosis and psychotic symptoms

- Psychosis refers to disorders involving a severe distortion in thought content. The most prominent symptoms of psychosis include delusions and hallucinations
- Delusions are fixed beliefs that are not amenable to change in light of conflicting evidence. Hallucinations are abnormal perceptions that are not experienced by others.
- Isolated psychotic symptoms can also be due to causes other than stroke, including delirium, dementia, or use of psychoactive drugs.

Acute psychotic states may develop unexpectedly in acute stroke patients. Causes include:
- acute organic reactions
- severe depression
- acute paranoid psychosis
- exacerbation of pre-existing schizophrenia or mania.

Clues to the cause may be obtained from the history including:
- past psychiatric problems and dementia
- medication history (cimetidine, anticholinergics)
- drug history, including alcohol, cannabis, cocaine
- drug withdrawal (e.g. benzodiazepines, barbiturates)
- underlying systemic disease (e.g. cardiac, renal, hepatic failure)
- infection.

Management
- It is important to try to manage patients using a calm approach in a well-lit, quiet place
- Management involves treatment of the underlying cause and withdrawal or reduction of as many psychotropic drugs as possible
- Avoid hypnotics
- If sedation is required, small doses of olanzapine (5–10 mg, maximum 20 mg daily) or chlorpromazine (25–50 mg max four times a day) may be given orally.

Fatigue after stroke

- It is important to distinguish between normal fatigue (a state of general tiredness that develops acutely after overexertion and improves after rest), and pathological fatigue (constant weariness unrelated to previous exertion levels and not usually ameliorated by rest).
- The proportion of people with post-stroke fatigue (PSF) ranges from 23% to 75%.
- How to manage and prevent fatigue is ranked by stroke survivors and health professionals among the top 10 research priorities relating to life after stroke.
- Fatigue often persists in individual patients if it is present early after stroke.
- Five longitudinal studies ($n = 762$) investigated the course of PSF in individual patients and found that more than one-third of patients had fatigue at the initial assessment (usually within the first 3 months after stroke). Among patients with fatigue at the initial assessment, about two-thirds of them had fatigue at a later stage (usually over 1 year after stroke), with perhaps one-third of them recovering by this time. Among patients without fatigue at the initial assessment, fatigue developed in approximately 12–58% of them during the course of follow-up. These findings reveal three patterns of temporal course of fatigue after stroke, that is, persistent fatigue, recovered fatigue, and late-onset fatigue.
- Although depressive symptoms are associated with fatigue, antidepressants showed no effect on reducing fatigue after stroke.
- Psychosocial and behavioural factors may play an important role in triggering and maintaining fatigue symptoms. Although early fatigue may be triggered by biological factors, late fatigue may be more attributable to psychological and behavioural factors. A model for the pathogenesis of fatigue is shown in Fig. 14.1.
- No robust relationship with strokes in any particular location has been found.
- PSF is a complex symptom that is influenced by different factors, and there are interactions between these factors. Complex interventions targeting these psychobehavioural factors are effective in treating fatigue in other conditions and can be tried in stroke, although more data from trials is required to be sure of their benefit.
- Treat potentially reversible causes (e.g. anaemia, CPAP for obstructive sleep apnoea, or depression) and then for patients without a clinical mood disorder or reversible medical problem, the recommendation of graduated exercise and cognitive behavioural approaches such as activity scheduling could be considered.
- The centrally acting stimulant Modafinil—used in narcolepsy—was found to have benefit in a phase 2 study. It is now being tested in the phase 3 MIDAS study.

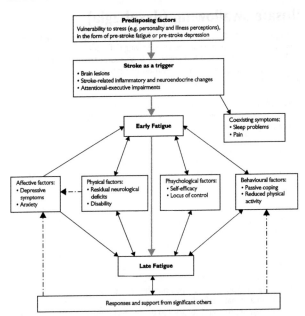

Fig. 14.1 A conceptual model of post-stroke fatigue. The unidirectional arrows indicate a causal direction; the bidirectional arrows indicate an unknown direction of the association; the dotted arrows indicate potential interactions between factors. Other symptoms may coexist with and maintain symptoms of fatigue.

Unsafe swallowing (dysphagia)

Forty per cent of acute stroke patients have altered swallow or dysphagia—
20% will go on to have prolonged swallowing difficulties.

- A bedside swallow test is mandatory in all acute stroke patients (see
  Fig. 14.2). This generally involves trials of sips/teaspoons of water
- Patients with severe facial weakness are at particularly high risk of
  unsafe swallow and lung aspiration
- Oropharyngeal weakness, poor coordination, and other comorbidity
  such as poor dentition worsen swallowing problems
- Dysphagia will result in decreased oral intake, a problem magnified by
  functional deficits such as weakness, and sensory and visual disturbances
- Patients with large cortical strokes predictably deteriorate clinically over
  the ensuing 4–7 days owing to worsening brain oedema. These patients
  become drowsy and may no longer be alert enough to swallow safely.
  Therefore, swallowing should be screened repeatedly even if the initial
  screen was successful.

For patients with an unsafe swallow, most stroke units instigate early enteral
nutrition using nasogastric (NG) feeding within the first 24–48 hours.

Early feeding in the FOOD trial showed a (non-significant) trend towards improved functional outcome and reduced mortality. The same trial
showed no evidence to suggest routine PEG feeding was better than NG
feeding. In the first 3–4 weeks, NG feeding should be the preferred route
unless there are strong practical reasons for PEG.

Where patients repeatedly pull out the NG tube, placement with a 'nasal
bridle' is an alternative. Such tubes have a bridle 'tape', which is looped behind the nasal septum and secured to the feeding tube. If the patient pulls on
the tube it will be uncomfortable and deter further pulling but remain *in situ*.
With significant force, the bridle will stretch and the NG tube will loosen
and still come out but without nasal septum injury.

Most units consider PEG or Radiological Inserted Gastrostomy (RIG)
tube at 4–6 weeks if there has been no improvement in swallow and patients are likely to rely on enteral nutrition in the medium term (few patients
fail to regain any swallow by 6 months after stroke). Percutaneous endoscopic jejunostomy (PEJ) tubes are rarely indicated after stroke.

Management involves graded reintroduction of oral intake with trials of
varied consistencies of diet and fluid supervised by SLT, nursing staff, and
dietician. Exercises for facial weakness, tongue base movement, laryngeal
elevation, and sensory stimulation with ice may also help.

Trials of prophylactic antibiotics in dysphagic stroke patients have not
been proven to reduce the incidence of (aspiration) pneumonia and should
not be routinely prescribed.

Flow chart for nutritional management of acute stroke patients

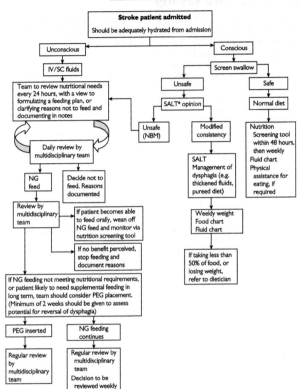

Fig. 14.2 Algorithm of swallowing assessment from St George's acute stroke unit.

Courtesy of Helen Mann.

Indications for videofluoroscopy to assess swallowing

A videofluoroscopy swallow study (also known as a dysphagia barium swallow) is a dynamic X-ray taken while swallowing a bolus containing X-ray contrast (see Fig. 14.3). Usually, videofluoroscopy will only be carried out after a bedside evaluation of swallowing to give an objective view of the pharyngeal stage of swallowing. It was considered the gold standard for dysphagia assessment but there is variability in the interpretation of the procedure.

In terms of management, it allows:
• visualization of structure and function of the oral, pharyngeal, and upper oesophageal stages of the swallow
• specific recommendations for food/fluid consistencies and non-oral feeding
• trialling of therapy.

Indications for videofluoroscopy include:
• unclear signs on bedside evaluation
• silent aspiration suspected or seen on previous videofluoroscopy
• to establish a baseline of swallowing function with progressive disorders (this may be relevant in patients with previous stroke and pre-existing swallow problems or patients with extensive subcortical cerebrovascular disease)
• known or suspected dysphagia of structural origin
• to try therapeutic manoeuvres, e.g. supraglottic swallow, Mendelssohn's manoeuvre.

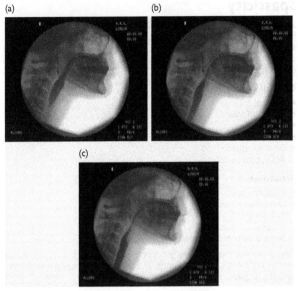

Fig. 14.3 Videofluoroscopy showing passage of liquid bolus without aspiration. © Geoffrey Cloud.

Spasticity

Symptoms relating to spasticity are present in up to 60% of strokes. Spasticity is excessive, inappropriate, and involuntary muscle activity resulting in stiffness, loss of movement, and pain. At worst it produces fixed deformity known as contracture, chronic pain, and can lead to development of pressure sores.

Clinical characteristics

- High tone
- Hyper-reflexia
- Flexor spasms
- Clasp knife reaction
- Extensor spasms
- Associated reactions.

Treatments

- Physiotherapy
- Drug treatments:
  - Systemic
  - Local
- Surgical treatments (rarely).

Drug treatment should generally not be used in isolation but in combination with physiotherapy, active splinting, and positioning. Drugs are either systemic or targeted/focal.

Systemic treatment of spasticity: drugs

Baclofen
- Structurally related to gamma aminobutyric acid (GABA)
- GABA agonist, acts presynaptically on $GABA_B$ with inhibitory effect
- Starting dose 5 mg twice daily, increasing gradually up to a maximum of 100 mg in divided doses
- Side effects include drowsiness, hallucinations, confusion, and generalized weakness
- There has been a single small RCT of intrathecal baclofen (ITB) compared to best medical management in 60 stroke survivors with severe spasticity (SISTERS). ITB has been previously studied in multiple sclerosis and cerebral palsy and interest in treating severe and refractory spasticity after stroke with ITB has grown from positive small case series from the USA and Europe. SISTERS showed ITB reduced spasticity but at the cost of adverse events related to ITB pump insertion and titration of ITB.
- Abrupt withdrawal can cause severe ill effects (severe spasticity, high fever, rhabdomyolysis, multiorgan failure, acute confusional state and seizures), and patients must be counselled towards this so they do not run out of medication—oral or ITB and do not stop treatment without supervision

Tizanidine
- Alpha-2-adrenergic receptor agonist
- Inhibitory effect on spinal interneurons

- Some anti-nociceptive action on spasticity-related pain
- Less muscle weakness than baclofen (and diazepam)
- Side effects: drowsiness
- Main trials in multiple sclerosis patients.

Dantrolene
- Acts directly on contractile apparatus of muscles
- Inhibits release of intramuscular calcium
- Can cause irreversible liver damage
- No central nervous system (CNS) action and therefore can be used in combination with other centrally acting agents
- Useful if baclofen causes excessive drowsiness
- More useful in spinal causes of spasticity
- Start at 25 mg once daily and increase slowly to maximum dose of 400 mg daily. Stop if no benefit demonstrable within 6 weeks
- Side effects: nausea, vomiting, and muscle weakness.

Diazepam
- Increases GABA-mediated inhibition by increasing affinity of the receptors
- More helpful in spinal causes
- May cause CNS depression and drowsiness, respiratory depression, paradoxical anxiety, and hallucinations
- Risk of addiction
- Start at low-dose 2 mg twice daily and increase to maximum of typically 60 mg in divided doses.

Clonidine
- Central alpha-2-agonist (like tizanidine) and antihypertensive
- Mechanism of action not understood
- Helpful in reducing flexor spasms.

Other drugs used predominately in spasticity of traumatic spinal origin but on occasion trialled on stroke patients include gabapentin, vigabatrin, tetrazepam, orphenadrine, and cannabinoids.

Focal treatment of spasticity: botulinum toxin

Introduction
- Since 1817, when Justinus Kerner first described food-borne botulism, the Gram-negative anaerobic bacterium *Clostridium botulinum* has been known to produce a potent neurotoxin resulting in muscle paralysis by blockade of neuromuscular transmission
- When injected directly into a muscle, it causes chemical denervation of peripheral cholinergic nerve endings and local paralysis, an effect which has been shown to have therapeutic use for treating dystonia and spasticity
- Nerve sprouting and muscle reinnervation lead to functional recovery and reversal of effect within 2–4 months.

Subtypes
- There are seven immunologically distinct serotypes of botulinum toxin labelled A–G

- Only A is in routine clinical use currently and is produced commercially in purified form as either Dysport® (Ipsen) or Botox® (Allergan)
- A vial of Dysport® contains 500 units, and a vial of Botox® 100 units. Botox is considered 3–4 times more potent per unit than Dysport®
- A commercial preparation of botulinum toxin B (NeuroBloc®) has recently been licensed.

Advantages over other spasticity treatments

- Unlike systemic antispasticity drugs, which are non-selective and commonly associated with generalized weakness and functional loss, botulinum toxin is targeted therapy
- Unlike chemical neurolysis with alcohol or phenol, botulinum toxin injection does not cause skin sensory loss or dysaesthesia.

Disadvantages over other spasticity treatments

- Expensive.

Indications in post-stroke spasticity

- In randomized studies, botulinum toxin injection in the post-stroke spastic upper and lower limb has been shown to reduce spasticity and improve function
- Best results are gained with concomitant physical therapy, which may involve the use of splints/orthoses
- The decision to inject a muscle with botulinum toxin after stroke should always be made together with a neurophysiotherapist and ideally be attached to the aim of achieving a functional goal, e.g. being able to put a spastic arm through a garment sleeve. It should rarely be considered in the first 3 months after stroke. Injection may also give some short-term relief from the pain associated with chronic post-stroke spasticity and reduce the carer burden
- Treatment should be individualized and reviewed as part of a rehabilitation programme
- It is contraindicated in myasthenia gravis, Lambert–Eaton syndrome and other neuromuscular disorders, pregnancy, and with the use of aminoglycoside antibiotics.

Administration

- Both should be reconstituted in a small (2 mL) volume of saline (reconstituting in water makes for a painful injection)
- The motor endplate zone of the muscle to be injected should be identified using conventional electromyography (EMG) surface anatomy landmarks. Where this is difficult, EMG guidance should be used. A needle appropriate to the size of the muscle to be injected (size 10–12 G) should be used
- The suggested dose for injections of muscles commonly treated after stroke is available, and injection regimens are available in 'Spasticity in adults: management using botulinum toxin', National Guidelines 2018 (RCP). These guidelines include suggested dose ranges for OnabotulinumtoxinA (BOTOX®), AbobotulinumtoxinA (Dysport®), and IncobotulinumtoxinA (Xeomin®). See ℜ https://www.rcp.ac.uk/improving-care/resources/spasticity-in-adults-management-using-botulinum-toxin/

- The peak effect usually occurs 4 weeks after injection. Physiotherapy review is recommended within 7–14 days after injection
- Treatments may be safely repeated at intervals of 12 weeks but a total dose of 1500 units of Dysport® or equivalent should not be exceeded in any one treatment.

Side effects

- The most common local side effect is weakness, which is usually mild and transient. Pain at the injection site and local irritation are reported in less than 5% of cases
- More systemic flu-like symptoms, anaphylaxis, and excessive fatigue are rare
- Occasionally, antibody formation can occur which makes repeated injection ineffective. Higher and more frequent doses increase the chance of immunoresistance and non-responsiveness

Surgical treatments for spasticity

Surgical treatment is rarely used. It may be a last resort to enable proper seating, fitting of orthoses, or enable appropriate hygiene. Examples include adductor tenotomies or obturator neurectomies.

Hemiplegic shoulder pain

- The shoulder is a shallow 'ball and socket' type joint with a relatively small surface area of articulation, which makes for a wide range of movement but poor joint stability
- The 'rotator cuff' comprises muscles and tendons around the joint, which act as a lever for elevation during abduction
- Weakness of the rotator cuff can cause subluxation of the humeral head, impingement, and inflammation in the joint and tendon insertions of the rotator cuff muscles.

Hemiplegic shoulder pain (HSP) is common (9–40% of hemiplegic stroke) and typically occurs 2–3 months after stroke onset. It may be classified into four groups:

- Joint pain caused by misaligned joint producing sharp pain on movement (active or passive). This is a frequent complication of a flaccid arm
- Overactive or spastic muscle pain—deep pulling pain on movement. Can be associated with adhesive capsulitis
- Diffuse pain from altered sensation from stroke—constant ache around shoulder
- Reflex sympathetic dystrophy pain—diffusely involving the whole limb and shoulder together. May be associated with vasomotor changes (sweating and altered coloration), trophic changes, and oedema.

HSP is associated with motor loss, sensory loss, and low mood. Shoulder X-rays are of little use in management.

Prevention and treatment

- HSP can be prevented by attention to handling and position, especially in those with flaccid arms early in stroke recovery. Slings or supports may be useful in reducing subluxation and tension in the shoulder capsule. Wearing a support device may promote immobility and possible contracture formation. Such devices, therefore, need to be worn as part of a regimen in conjunction with active therapy treatment. Pillows to support the shoulder and maintain alignment while seated are standard. Elevation of the arm supported on a pillow may also prevent dependent oedema. Positions that avoid patterns of spasticity are key. The Bexhill armrest on wheelchairs is commonly used to facilitate this
- FES has shown some success in maintaining tone and reducing atrophy of rotator cuff muscle groups, so reducing the incidence of subluxation acutely. The effects tend to be short-lived, however, and benefits disappear on discontinuation of treatment
- Local steroid joint injection may help adhesive capsulitis
- Transcutaneous electrical nerve stimulation (TENS) may relieve pain to enable passive movement around the joint and improve functional range for purposes of dressing and hygiene
- Drug therapy may require only simple analgesics or specific anti-spasticity medication such as botulinum toxin injection or baclofen.

Central post-stroke pain syndrome

Central post-stroke pain syndrome (CPSP) is pain of central neurogenic origin. It is unusual after stroke but when it occurs it can be extremely distressing and difficult to treat.

- It occurs in approximately 4–8% of patients with stroke
- At least half have moderate to severe pain
- More common in older stroke patients (those over 80 years) and is, therefore, likely to be under-reported
- CPSP syndrome typically develops between 4 and 8 weeks after stroke but can develop over a year after stroke
- Classically associated with thalamic lesions—previously known as 'thalamic pain'. It is now appreciated that it can also occur with extra-thalamic strokes, and only around 60% cases have thalamic involvement
- The mechanism of CPSP is poorly understood. Strokes involving either the thalamic nuclei (particularly ventrocaudal and ventroposterior inferior nuclei) or the spinothalamic cortical pathway may cause alterations in thalamocortical processing and altered sensory perception.

CPSP syndrome has several distinct characteristic forms:

- Muscle pain—typically cramping
- Dysaesthesia—unpleasant, delayed onset after stimulus, burning
- Hyperaesthesia—heightened response to trivial stimuli
- Allodynia—present in up to 60% of CPSP patients, this is the interpretation of non-painful stimuli such as thermal or light touch as being painful or the location of the pain in an area remote from that being stimulated
- Shooting pain—intermittent and localized, usually
- Circulatory pain—pins and needles, insect bites, walking on broken glass
- Peristaltic/visceral pain—fullness of bladder, dysuria with urinary urge, abdominal bloating.

Treatment

- Low-dose tricyclic antidepressant drugs, amitriptyline 10–25 mg once daily (remember these are not antidepressant doses, however)
- Antiepileptic drugs (AEDs)—lamotrigine (doses of at least 200 mg/day required) has more evidence than carbamazepine. Gabapentin/pregabalin may be the best of this class
- A meta-analysis concluded evidence only for amitriptyline and lamotrigine, but there is emerging evidence for gabapentin and pregabalin
- IV drugs such as lidocaine, propofol, and ketamine have shown efficacy for short-term control of CPSP, but their application and potential side effects make them unsuitable for long-term treatment
- Opiates can help in acute exacerbations but are not recommended for chronic pain management
- Non-pharmacological—there is experimental work with deep brain stimulation for the most refractory and debilitated cases.

Post-stroke epilepsy

- Seizures can occur at the time of stroke or in the recovery phase. The implication and treatment of the two are quite different
- More common with cortical, versus subcortical, strokes
- Cerebrovascular disease (which may be previously asymptomatic) is the most common cause of late-onset epilepsy. A first fit in a person aged over 65 years is likely to be due to underlying cerebrovascular disease and such patients are at increased risk of developing stroke
- Remember, a diagnosis of epilepsy should only be made if there are repeated unprovoked seizures. A single seizure is not epilepsy
- Seizures are more common if there is pre-existing dementia and there is some evidence that post-stroke seizures may increase the risk of subsequent dementia.

Seizures during the acute phase (within 7 days of stroke)

- The reported frequency of seizures during the first days of stroke ranges from 2% to 23%, depending on study designs. The true risk is probably at the lower end of the range
- Likely to be partial with or without secondary generalization. Status epilepticus is rare
- Haemorrhagic stroke is associated with seizure activity more than ischaemic stroke
- There is some controversy as to whether they are more common with cardioembolic stroke.

Late seizures after stroke (after 7 days of stroke)

- Late seizures have been reported in between 3% and 67% of strokes in different series. The true incidence is again probably at the lower end
- Most seizures occur within the first year of stroke
- It is unusual to develop seizures more than 2 years after stroke onset
- Perhaps half will have recurrent seizures (epilepsy).
- A patient with a single late post-stroke seizure, is now diagnosed with epilepsy according to the International League Against Epilepsy (ILAE) definition

Treatment of seizures

Seizures at stroke onset

- A seizure at stroke presentation does not generally warrant regular AED medication
- Nor does it merit IV benzodiazepine therapy at the time of seizure to terminate it. It usually self-terminates and IV benzodiazepines can lead to unnecessary respiratory depression and are only required for continuing seizures (status epilepticus)
- For those who present with prolonged and generalized seizures, usually in the context of large and haemorrhagic infarcts or primary intracerebral bleeding, anticonvulsants should be started, such as intravenous levetiracetum.

Seizures occurring after the acute stroke presentation
- For seizures not associated with the immediate stroke presentation, it needs to be ascertained whether they were 'provoked', e.g. due to intercurrent metabolic disturbance, severe infection, or change in medication, which may lower seizure threshold or new stroke episode
- For unprovoked seizures, an individual risk:benefit assessment needs to be carried out—risk of further potentially harmful seizures against risk of side effects and drug interactions caused by AEDs
- Bear in mind that even small, short-lived partial seizures can cause considerable anxiety and morbidity in older people living alone and having suffered the consequences of a previous stroke.

Choice of antiepileptic drug
- There is no good quality trial data evaluating AEDs in post-stroke epilepsy. Therefore, there is no evidence that one AED is superior in this setting and the choice of agent will be influenced by age, concomitant medication, and comorbidity
- It has been suggested that phenytoin is not the most appropriate choice in stroke patients because of its potential harmful impact on functional recovery and bone health
- Common first-line choices include levetiracetam and lamotrigine. Side effect profile and potential drug interactions with stroke secondary prevention medication need to be considered, and AED choice individualized
- There are no data on whether prophylactic AEDs can prevent seizure onset.

Lifestyle and seizures
- It is important to warn of lifestyle risks, e.g. danger of drowning in bathwater
- Warn of the risk of driving and inform of local regulations. These differ in different countries. For example, in the UK driving is forbidden until free of seizures for 1 year (although occasionally, an exception may be made for provoked seizures).

Neglect and inattention

- Defined as a disorder of 'attention' and often described in behavioural terms
- Normal attention is reliant on intact sensory registration, and neglect can occur in any sensory modality (tactile, auditory, visual)
- Visual and spatial inattention are the most frequently recognized after stroke
- Right-sided brain lesions typically result in the most severe neglect
- Left-sided stroke with right-sided inattention is probably less common and is poorly understood—principally as it often coexists with marked language disorder in patients with left hemispheric stroke. It also appears to resolve rapidly in many cases.

Neglect behaviours

- *Extinction*—simultaneous stimuli to left and right result in failure to recognize the stimulus on the neglected side
- *Allaesthesia*—mislocation of stimulus
- *Anosognosia*—lack of awareness of the problem
- Decreased spontaneous movement of side demonstrating neglect:
  - *Hypokinesia*—delayed movements
  - *Hypometria*—decreased amplitude of the movement
  - *Akinesia*—no movement.

The implications for patients with inattention in daily living can be numerous. Examples of these may include reading, writing, drawing, walking, driving, socializing, and with activities of personal care. Patients with neglect have poor or slow recovery because of loss of awareness, and tend to have difficulty relearning to dress, walk, and care for themselves. A lack of awareness can undermine participation in the rehabilitation process.

Treatment

- Sitting or addressing patients from the neglected side, scanning, and auditory feedback are thought to be ineffective
- Environmental modifications
- Prisms
- A half field patch (for patients with no hemianopia)
- Cognitive strategies
- Limb activation treatment (grading position, trunk rotation, other adaptive approaches).

Apraxia and abnormal perception

Praxis is the ability to use the limbs and body in skilled tasks in order to function. It has three stages—ideation, motor planning, and execution.

Dyspraxia is a form of developmental coordination disorder diagnosis often made in children.

Apraxia is an acquired disorder of the execution of learned movement which cannot be accounted for by weakness, incoordination, sensory loss, incomprehension, or inattention to command.

It can be categorized clinically into:

1. *Ideational*:
   • Incorrect object use (e.g. using a toothbrush to comb hair)
   • Incorrect order of elements of activity
   • Sections of the sequence omitted
   • Two or more elements of an activity blended
   • Overshooting of action
   • After interruption, unable to continue an action
   • Perseveration.

2. *Ideomotor*:
   • Spatial orientation errors
   • Initiation and timing mistakes
   • Poor distal differentiation
   • View body part as object
   • Verbalization instead of action
   • Gestural enhancement
   • Fragmentary responses.

The type of deficit can be related to location of stroke. Ideational araxia tends to be caused by lesions in the left posterior parietal, occipital, and temporal lobes. Ideomotor is seen more in left frontal lobe strokes. Apraxia is also seen in right hemisphere stroke but equivalent lesions on the right do not necessarily produce apraxic symptoms.

Treatment is based on principles of 'errorless learning' and needs to be structured, goal-based, and functional.

Hemianopia (visual field loss)

This is common in stroke. Patients are often unaware of homonymous hemianopia.

Examination for and determination of the site of lesion causing hemianopia is described on ➔ p. 118. Usually accurate assessment can be obtained on bedside examination, but full visual field testing may be necessary, particularly for partial defects and where assessment for driving or other vocational activities is required.

Hemianopia causes problems such as being unaware of things on one side, bumping into things on one side (especially when walking through doorways), and reading difficulty.

Bilateral occipital lobe stroke can cause 'cortical blindness'. Up to 10% of such patients deny their visual difficulties (Anton's syndrome).

• *Orthoptists* specialize in eye movement disorders
• *Ophthalmologists* specialize in medical disorders of the eye
• *Optometrists or opticians* generally practice in High Street locations and deal with disorders of vision correctable with spectacles.

Management

• Functional assessment and counselling (especially with respect to driving)
• Head posture and movement
• Lighting
• Mirrors
• Prisms
• Stimulation—computer-based training (visual restitution training; VRT) for an hour a day for 6 months can improve the visual field typically by 5°. VRT is still not widely available and awaits further validation.

Hemianopic alexia

• Characterized by reduced reading ability after hemianopic stroke and thought to relate to reduced compensatory eye movements (left-to-right scanning in English speakers with hemianopia encroaching on their right foveal or parafoveal visual field)
• Can be helped by training eye movements by reading moving text (♾ see http://www.readright.ucl.ac.uk)

Pressure sores

These are a disaster on a stroke unit and are almost always avoidable with appropriate assessment and management. However, a number of patients present to acute stroke services after a 'long lie' on the floor as a consequence of the acute stroke, and every stroke unit will see pressure sores. They are traditionally graded from 1 to 4 (see Fig. 14.5).

The Waterlow score (Fig. 14.4) can be used to triage those most at risk and stratify the need for low air flow ripple mattress, soft mattress, or normal mattress with regular turning.

Common sites are bony prominences such as heels, sacrum, pelvic prominences, and over kyphotic spines. They can be caused by ill-fitting anti-embolism (TED) stockings or even periods as short as 30 minutes immobilized on a hard surface in X-ray.

Vigilance is required as, once established, they are a considerable cause of morbidity (principally through pain) and are associated with poor stroke recovery. Treatment often takes months and may even require surgical intervention.

WATERLOW PRESSURE ULCER PREVENTION/TREATMENT POLICY

RING SCORES IN TABLE, ADD TOTAL MORE THAN 1 SCORE/CATEGORY CAN BE USED

BUILD/WEIGHT FOR HEIGHT		SKIN TYPE VISUAL RISK AREAS		SEX AGE		MALNUTRITION SCREENING TOOL (MST) (Nutrition Vol.15, No.6 1999 – Australia)		
AVERAGE BMI = 20-24.9	0	HEALTHY	0	MALE	1	A – HAS PATIENT LOST		B – WEIGHT LOSS SCORE
ABOVE AVERAGE BMI = 25-29.9	1	TISSUE PAPER	1	FEMALE	2	WEIGHT RECENTLY?		0.5-5kg = 1
OBESE BMI > 30	2	DRY	1	14-49	1	YES – GO TO B		5-10kg = 2
		OEDEMATOUS	1	50-64	2	NO – GO TO C		10-15kg = 3
BELOW AVERAGE BMI < 20	3	CLAMMY, PYREXIA	1	65-74	3	UNSURE – GO TO C		>15kg = 4
BMI = Wt(Kg)/Ht (m)²		DISCOLOURED GRADE 1	2	75-80	4	AND		Unsure = 2
		BROKEN/SPOTS GRADE 2-4	3	81+	5	C – PATIENT EATING POORLY OR LACK OF APPETITE 'NO' = 0; 'YES' SCORE = 1		NUTRITION SCORE If > 2, refer for nutrition assessment/intervention

CONTINENCE		MOBILITY		SPECIAL RISKS			
COMPLETE/ CATHETERIZED	0	FULLY	0	TISSUE MALNUTRITION		NEUROLOGICAL DEFICIT	
URINE INCONT.	1	RESTLESS/FIDGETY	1	TERMINAL CACHEXIA	8	DIABETES, MS, CVA	4-6
FAECAL INCONT.	2	APATHETIC	2	MULTIPLE ORGAN FAILURE	8	MOTOR/SENSORY	4-6
URINARY + FAECAL INCONTINENCE	3	RESTRICTED	3	SINGLE ORGAN FAILURE (RESP., RENAL, CARDIAC)	5	PARAPLEGIA (MAX OF 6)	4-6
		BEDBOUND e.g. TRACTION	4	PERIPHERAL VASCULAR DISEASE	5	MAJOR SURGERY or TRAUMA	
		CHAIRBOUND e.g. WHEELCHAIR	5	ANAEMIA (Hb< 8)	2	ORTHOPAEDIC/SPINAL	5
				SMOKING	1	ON TABLE > 2 HR#	5
						ON TABLE > 6 HR#	8

SCORE
10+ AT RISK
15+ HIGH RISK
20+ VERY HIGH RISK

MEDICATION – CYTOTOXICS, LONG-TERM/HIGH-DOSE STEROIDS, ANTI-INFLAMMATORY   MAX OF 4

Scores can be discounted after 48 hours, provided patient is recovering normally

©J Waterlow 1985 Revised 2005*
Obtainable from the Nook, Stoke Road, Henlade TAUNTON TA3 5LX
* The 2005 revision incorporates the research undertaken by Queensland Health.

www.judy-waterlow.co.uk

Fig. 14.4 The Waterlow pressure score scale. © J. Waterlow 1985, revised 2005.

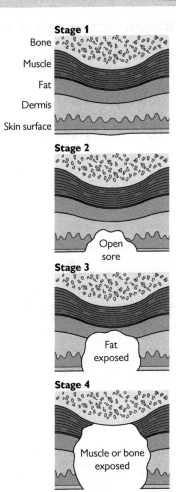

Fig. 14.5 The four stages of bed sores. Stage 1: discolouration of intact skin not affected by light finger pressure (non-blanching erythema). This may be difficult to identify in darkly pigmented skin. Stage 2: partial thickness skin loss or damage involving the epidermis and/or dermis. The pressure ulcer is superficial and presents clinically as an abrasion, blister, or shallow crater. Stage 3: full-thickness skin loss involving damage of subcutaneous tissue but not extending to the underlying fascia. The pressure ulcer presents clinically as a deep crater with or without undermining of the adjacent tissue. Stage 4: full-thickness skin loss with extensive destruction and necrosis extending to underlying tissue.

Urinary incontinence or retention

- Occurs in 40–60% of patients admitted to hospital following stroke
- Pre-stroke incontinence prevalence is 2.5–17%
- Twenty-five per cent of stroke patients have urinary incontinence at discharge and 15% are still incontinent at 1 year
- Incontinence is associated with any stroke lesion except for the occipital lobe. Anteromedial region (ACA territory) and frontal lobe are frequently associated with urinary incontinence. The micturition centre is located in the pons
- Strokes with cortical and subcortical involvement (i.e. large volume strokes) are five times more likely to be associated with incontinence than lacunar infarcts, suggesting that the size of the stroke may be more important than location. The extent of cortical damage is likely to affect levels of arousal and awareness, which are more likely to lead to incontinent state.

Prognostic significance

- Urinary incontinence is a key indicator of mortality after stroke. Of stroke patients with urinary incontinence, 52% are dead at 6 months compared with 7% of continent stroke survivors. Urinary incontinence 30 days after stroke is associated with almost four times the 1-year mortality compared with continent stroke survivors and two times increased mortality within 5 years
- Early urinary incontinence after stroke is a strong predictor of severe/ moderate disability at 3 months: in one study, the OR was 5.4 (95% CI 3.3–9.0). It is associated with poor functional outcomes, immobility, and increased likelihood of discharge to an institutionalized care home
- It may also predict recovery of limb strength and activities of daily living
- The presence of continence is a better predictor of recovery at 4 weeks than almost any other predictive scoring
- Urinary incontinence after stroke is also associated with falls:
  - Incontinence is associated with 2.3 times (1.3–4.1) relative risk of falls
  - Twenty per cent of falls occurred during visits to the toilet or bathroom
  - Other factors: cognitive impairment, heart disease, previous fall.

Causes

Mechanisms of urinary incontinence after stroke are unclear. Few studies have performed urodynamic examinations in stroke patients. Simple bladder scanning is of benefit in establishing the cause of incontinence if urodynamic studies are not practicable.

No specific type of incontinence is associated with stroke—a number of different types can occur:

- Detrusor hyperreflexia is the commonest lesion, in 50–82%. This is thought to be caused by disruption of neuromicturition pathways causing urge incontinence
- Acontractile bladder in 17–25%. This may be caused by concurrent neuropathy or medication use, resulting in overflow-type incontinence
- Outflow tract obstruction (exclude faecal impaction, which is a common cause)

- Incontinence owing to stroke-related cognitive and language deficits, with normal bladder function, is common. A new subtype of post-stroke incontinence, 'impaired awareness urge incontinence' (AI-UI) has been described. This group of patients, often with parietal lobe damage, have little urge to urinate and frequently no sense of full bladder or leakage and, as such, tend to fail to recognize and report their incontinence. Bladder training is usually unsuccessful in such cases.

Management of urinary incontinence or retention

- Exclude exacerbating/precipitating features, particularly urinary tract infections, drugs (e.g. diuretics), faecal impaction (see Fig. 14.6)
- Comprehensive assessment is paramount. Portable bladder scanners can give useful estimates of post-voiding residual volume (PVR) at the bedside. A PVR of greater than 50–100 cm^3 may indicate the need for further urodynamic studies
- Importance of lower urinary tract symptoms, rather than 'incontinence'
- Mobility
- Dexterity
- Environment
- Scheduled voiding/bladder retraining
- Drugs (anticholinergics are the mainstay)
- Botulinum toxin intravesical injection (for detrusor instability)
- Pads and continence aids (female urinal, penile pouch, convenes)
- Non-implanted electrical stimulation (e.g. tibial and parasacral TENS) have been reported to be helpful adjunctive treatment but convincing RCTs are lacking in post-stroke patients
- Catheterization as a last resort
- Approaches used include behavioural interventions, such as timed voiding and pelvic floor muscle training, professional input interventions (e.g. structured assessment and management by continence nurse advisors), and drug therapy (e.g. meclofenoxate, oxybutynin, or oestrogen)

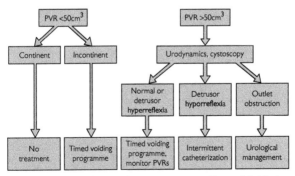

Fig. 14.6 Management of post-stroke urinary incontinence. First, exclude infection and other exacerbating factors. PVR, post-voiding residual volume.

- A Cochrane review concluded that good quality trial data is not available, but there is suggestive evidence that professional input through structured assessment and management of care and specialist continence nursing may reduce urinary incontinence and related symptoms after stroke
- Where long-term catheterization is the only solution (and this should be considered a last resort), it is better for suprapubic insertion as opposed to urethral, regardless of gender. Long-term urethral catheters are associated with local pressure sores and can erode the bladder neck sphincter leading to troublesome on going bypassing of a catheter.

Bowel management

Bowel incontinence

New-onset faecal incontinence after stroke is very common: 56% acutely, 30% at 7–10 days, and 11% at 3 months. Older patients, women, and those with severe strokes are most at risk. The impact of faecal incontinence is always devastating:
- Social taboo
- Poor self-image
- Depression
- Tissue viability
- Carer stress
- Reduced rehabilitation participation.

Comprehensive assessment requires:
- bowel history
- medication review
- diet/fluid intake
- mobility
- current bowel movement status
- abdominal exam
- rectal exam (by a trained person).

Incontinence is more likely when stool is loose, commonly caused by:
- drugs—proton pump inhibitors, antibiotics, laxatives, NSAIDs, antihypertensives, and potassium supplements
- artificial feeding (NG/PEG)
- infection (*Clostridium difficile*).

Functional bowel incontinence may be caused by impairments in mobility, dexterity, communication, and vision, and be improved with:
- communication aids (call bell/picture cards)
- regular toileting programme (in line with normal bowel habits)
- simple, bold signage.

Bowel urgency
- Bladder training has been found to be useful with urgency or frequency of micturition, and similar training may help bowel incontinence
- Patients distressed by faecal incontinence may become hypervigilant and hypersensitive, and any bowel sensation may be interpreted as urgency. This may then result in anxiety or panic if a toilet is not readily available. A vicious circle can then develop as anxiety is a known bowel stimulant
- A progressive programme of urge resistance is recommended
- Smoking cessation may be useful in patients with urgency.

Management of ongoing bowel incontinence
- Skin care (repeated wiping can spread digestive enzymes and bacteria contained within the stool and cause local skin irritation)
- Difficult to find any product that reliably disguises bowel leakage and smell
- Pads

- Faecal collectors
- Anal plugs.

Bowel programmes, e.g. daily codeine phosphate with twice-weekly enemas, resulted in 75% of nursing home patients achieving bowel continence.

Use of loperamide 2 mg up to three times per day according to symptoms can be a last resort.

Trans-anal or rectal irrigation is a way of emptying the lower bowel and can be used in more mobile patients to manage chronic constipation and faecal incontinence.

There has been a single small but positive trial of TENS for post-stroke faecal incontinence.

Constipation

Constipation is a common problem in older people and is particularly common after stroke. Constipation is present in up to 60% of stroke patients in rehabilitation wards.

The cost of prescribed laxatives to the NHS is £48 million (and a further over-the-counter cost estimated at £27 million).

Constipation can be defined by Rome II criteria by two or more of the following:
- Fewer than three bowel movements per week
- Hard stool or sense of incomplete emptying in 25% of bowel movements
- Excessive straining in 25% of bowel movements
- Necessity of digital manipulation to facilitate evacuation.

Objective recording of bowel opening is key. The Bristol Stool chart can be helpful.

Studies show that 65% of older people reporting constipation had their bowels open at least once a day, and 25% of people have no symptoms of constipation but feel that a regular stool is necessary. One man's constipation is another man's diarrhoea!

Poor evidence base underlies treatment of constipation after stroke.

Predisposing factors for acquired constipation are:
- drugs
- tricyclic antidepressants
- opiates
- anticonvulsants
- drugs for Parkinson's disease
- beta blockers, diuretics
- anticholinergic drugs
- diet/dehydration
- immobility.

Constipation can be behaviourally induced by deliberately ignoring the urge to defecate due to embarrassment in acute debilitating stroke, where toileting independence has been lost.

Constipation can result in faecal impaction with overflow incontinence.

Faecal impaction may result in urinary retention as impaction may impinge on bladder neck emptying (as well as cause external compression of deep pelvic veins).

Constipation invariably causes abdominal discomfort and distension and commonly increases confusion.

Treatment of constipation
- Keep a bedside stool chart (e.g. Bristol Stool chart)
- Review current medication
- Consider metabolic disorder (hypothyroidism, hypokalaemia, hypercalcaemia)
- Review diet, fluid intake
- Bulk-forming agents
- Macrogols (NG and PEG compatible but require special care when used with thickening agents in dysphagic patients)
- Glycerol suppositories may be used to soften stool
- If there is no result after 2 days, consider the use of an enema
- If problems remain, consider adding in senna for 1 week (overuse or misuse of senna can cause water, sodium, and potassium depletion)
- Education (what constitutes normal bowel habit, correction of misperceptions, misuse of laxatives)
- Individuals should have the opportunity to attempt defecation within half an hour of breakfast. Comfort and privacy are required
- Positioning correctly to facilitate bowel opening—it is far easier sitting forward than lying back.

Driving after stroke

It is important to make patients aware of the driving regulations post-stroke and transient ischaemic attack (TIA) in their country.

In the UK, all patients with a Group 1 licence (car, moped, or motorcycle) who experience a stroke episode (including TIA or amaurosis fugax) should not drive for 1 month. The current UK rules are as follows.

Stroke:
- Must not drive for 1 month.
- May resume driving after this period if the clinical recovery is satisfactory. There is no need to notify the Driver Vehicle Licensing Authority (DVLA) unless there is residual neurological deficit 1 month after the episode; in particular, visual field defects, cognitive defects, and impaired limb function. Minor limb weakness alone will not require notification unless restriction to certain types of vehicle or vehicles with adapted controls is needed. Adaptations may be able to overcome severe physical impairment. Seizures occurring at the time of a stroke/TIA or in the ensuing 24 hours may be treated as provoked for licensing purposes in the absence of any previous seizure history or cerebral pathology.

TIAs:
- Must not drive for 1 month
- *Single* TIA: no need to notify DVLA
- *Multiple* TIAs over a short period will require 3 months free from further attacks before resuming driving, and DVLA should be notified.

If they have neurological deficit at 1 month that may impair driving ability, they are obliged to inform the DVLA and need a medical assessment of their fitness to drive before attempting to drive again.

Holders of light goods vehicle (LGV) or passenger-carrying vehicle (PCV) licences should notify the DVLA of any stroke episode and should not drive such vehicles until after further medical enquiry. The rules are:
- Licence refused or revoked for 1 year following a stroke or TIA. Can be considered for licensing after this period provided that there is no debarring residual impairment likely to affect safe driving and there are no other significant risk factors. Licensing may be subject to satisfactory medical report, including exercise electrocardiograph (ECG) testing. Where there is imaging evidence of less than 50% carotid artery stenosis and no previous history of cardiovascular disease Group 2 licensing may be allowed without the need for functional cardiac assessment. However, if there are recurrent TIAs or strokes, functional cardiac testing will still be required.

All patients should inform their insurers of their change in health circumstances.

Persistent limb disability following a stroke may not prevent a patient from holding a driving licence again. Adaptations to a vehicle and/or restriction to automatic types of vehicle may help to overcome driving difficulties even with quite complex disabilities.

The law requires adaptations or restrictions to certain types of vehicles to be noted on the licence. Therefore, in the UK the DVLA should be notified if adaptations are necessary.

In the UK, a series of charity funded mobility centres offer assessment of driving ability and potential for driving adapted vehicles, e.g.

℘ https://www.qef.org.uk/service/mobility/driving-assessment/

Such assessments can be helpful for restoring driving confidence as well as provide practical information for the DVLA about the ability to return to safe driving. They generally involve 'classroom' tests of driving attributes, including reading, processing, and reaction time and assessment in a driving simulator, followed by driving a dual-controlled car in a closed environment before, if able, venturing out into open traffic. The outcome will provide the stroke survivor with a clear indication of their ability to drive safely with or without car adaptations.

Flying after stroke

- There is no absolute medical bar on flying after a stroke and no central UK guidance.
- Each airline has its own rules about whom it allows on its planes.
- British Airways suggests that, providing symptoms are stable or improving, air travel is possible 3 days after stroke but wish to be notified in advance if a stroke episode has occurred within the last 10 days.
- The UK Civil Aviation Authority repeats this advice—suggesting to wait at least 10 days after a stroke to fly, but if you are recovered and well, you can fly at 3 days after TIA or minor stroke.
- The oxygen pressure during flight is lower than that at sea level, so there is a theoretical risk of harm to someone who has suffered a recent stroke.
- Most advise not flying for a fortnight after the stroke unless it is imperative. After that, there is no medical reason why an otherwise fit stroke patient shouldn't fly.
- Patients with physical disability should notify the airline that they will need extra help at the airport or on the plane. They should also inform their insurers.

Measuring outcome and progress

Goal planning

This is a central ethos in neurorehabilitation, particularly in recovery from complex neurological deficits associated with stroke. After a period of multidisciplinary assessment, the patient, their carer, and family are engaged in a process of setting relevant goals over an agreed time period. Long-term goals are then broken down into 'stepping stone' goals that are reviewed and reassessed at regular intervals. For example, a long-term goal may be to achieve independent transfers from bed-to-chair at 3 months. In this case, these would be the interim 'stepping stone' goals: obtaining independent sitting balance, then assisted sliding board transfers, then assisted pivot transfers, and then independent standing transfers. Goals need to be specific for individual patients and measurable.

Remember SMART goals:

- **S**pecific
- **M**easurable
- **A**chievable
- **R**elevant
- **T**ime-limited.

Goals achieved is a valid and individualized outcome measure.

Goal attainment scaling tool

The goal attainment scaling (GAS) tool was developed for 'goal-driven management mentoring' in the 1960s and has been used in industry, relationship counselling, and recently neurorehabilitation.

GAS can judge progress against goals set jointly between the MDT and the patient, as part of a case management process. To do this, the expected outcome needs to be defined when identifying goals. The MDT and patient need to agree what would constitute 'more than expected' or 'less than expected' outcomes. A time for review of achievement of the goal is set when completing the form.

The expected outcome is defined as the result that could reasonably be expected to be achieved within a given time; it is scored as '0'. These outcomes are tailored to each individual. GAS involves identifying descriptors, preferably behavioural, to provide evidence that the goal has been achieved.

The first step is identifying high-priority goal areas. Write the first in the box labelled 'Goal 1' and add others as appropriate for the patient's needs and period of neurorehabilitation.

The next step is to identify possible outcomes in each chosen goal area. Outcomes should be specific and, where possible, expressed as a behavioural statement or something that is observable. Examples of a completed form are shown in Table 14.1.

Start with the most likely outcome. This is what you would reasonably expect to occur within the time agreed and indicates success. This is recorded as 0. Then describe what would be considered a higher or better outcome (+1) and an even higher or better outcome (+2). Then do the same for lower levels of success (−1) and (−2). An example is shown in Table 14.1. At the end of the agreed time frame the level of achievement is reviewed. If the team and patient are setting realistic goals for the timeframe available, you would expect most outcomes to be the 0 result.

Advantages of GAS

- Cheap
- Goals can be completely individualized
- Goals can be changed or abandoned if circumstances change.

Disadvantages of GAS

- Bias (make goals overly easy to attain, problems with multiple 'raters')
- Assumption that outcomes can be determined in advance (crystal ball gazing)
- Staff will need training in using the approach
- There is an additional time commitment involved in developing the outcome levels, though this is less of an impact if such discussion is part of routine practice
- Expected outcomes need to be set at a realistic level for the client's needs and circumstances, and the time period set for review, or results will be distorted
- Research has shown that a maximum of five goals is likely to be manageable at any one time and that most people would be working on two goals in any one period of time.

Table 14.1 GAS form

Level of expected outcome	Goal 1: Decision-making	Goal 2: Self-esteem	Goal 3: Isolation
Review date:			
Much more than expected (+2)	Makes plans, follows through, modifies if needed, and reaches goal	Expresses realistic positive feelings about self	Actively participates in group or social activities
More than expected (+1)	Makes plans, follows through without assistance unless plan needs changing	Expresses more positive than negative feelings about self	Attends activities, sometimes initiates contact with others
Most likely outcome (0)	Makes plans and follows through with assistance/ reminders	Expresses equally both positive and negative feelings about self	Leaves house and attends community centre. Responds if approached
Less than expected outcome (−1)	Makes plans but does not take any action to follow through	Expresses more negative than positive feelings about self	Leaves house occasionally, no social contact
Much less than expected (−2)	Can consider alternatives but doesn't decide on a plan	Expresses only negative feelings about self	Spends most of time in house except for formal appointments

When measuring goal attainment, the box which matches the outcome achieved is marked and the scores for each goal are added. This total is the GAS and again is an individualized outcome measure.

Reproduced from *Community Mental Health Journal*, 4(6), Kiresuk TJ, Sherman RE, Goal attainment scaling: a general method for evaluating comprehensive community mental health programs, pp. 443–453, Copyright (1967), With kind permission from Springer Science and Business Media.

Discharge planning

Discharge planning is an active process that 'aims to reduce hospital length of stay and unplanned readmission to hospital and improve the coordination of services following discharge from hospital thereby bridging the gap between hospital and place of discharge'.

Frequently suggested advantages to discharge planning include:

- reduced readmission rates
- shortened length of stay
- preventing unsafe discharges
- improved patient/carer satisfaction.

However, the evidence for this is not robust.

Discharge planning should start at the earliest possible opportunity by ensuring a full history is taken at the time of stroke presentation, including the patient's previous level of functioning and social circumstance. Preparing for discharge includes the entire multidisciplinary stroke team and is a focus of MDT meetings. Where appropriate, a provisional expected date of discharge should be set at the earliest opportunity.

Throughout the recovery and rehabilitation process the patient should remain central to the process but carers and family need to be engaged particularly with discharge planning. A survey by Carers UK found that 43% of carers felt they had inadequate support when the person returned home. This should not be ignored given that voluntary carers provide a huge amount of support which would otherwise need to be provided by health service. For example, in England alone carers provide in the region of £2 billion of stroke care per year.

Admission to hospital is a vulnerable time for patients. As a result of stroke, patients frequently experience a loss of functional ability, and require either a temporary increase in support or rehabilitation or more prolonged support. For most patients the ideal situation is to return to their premorbid state so that they can function as they previously had done. Less than 50% do.

Stroke patients with irreversible loss of function may require additional support at home. This can be achieved by increased care services (via social services), aids or home modifications (via occupational therapy), community nursing, or via the patient's informal care network. Ultimately, a small proportion of patients who are no longer able to manage at home will require long-term placement into a residential home (providing 24-hour care) or a nursing home (if specific nursing needs are evident). Finding a suitable placement for patients is something that should be started only after discussion with the patient, relatives, and the rest of the MDT.

To bridge the transition to home and reduce length of stay in more expensive specialized hospitals, intermediate care has become popular in some countries. 'Packages' of multidisciplinary care lasting a few weeks can be tailored to meet specific needs of stroke patients who no longer need acute hospital stay. These may be delivered in community hospitals, or at home with support from early supported discharge teams.

On discharge into the community, the quality of transfer of care relies on multidisciplinary and multiagency handover and communication.

We provide patients with a Joint Health and Social care plan. This is a comprehensive document that should describe the current functional, emotional, and psychological state of the person in order to promote continuity of care when back at home and continued adjustment and stroke recovery.

The core of this is a carer's pack, with the following information:
- How to transfer the person in and out of bed, chair, toilet, etc.
- Equipment required for transfers and other care
- Positioning required over a 24-hour period, including the use of pillows and lap trays
- Guidance on positioning and supports
- Guidance on when and how to apply upper or lower limb splints and the duration of use
- Simple functional exercises for therapeutic reasons or stretches for the person to perform with or without assistance from their carer
- Guidance on mobility and the level of assistance required
- Guidance on personal and domestic activities of daily living
- Checklists of how to do specific tasks (e.g. how to get dressed or make a cup of tea)
- Advice on wheelchair use and local services
- Advice on continence
- Advice on medication and blister packs if needed
- Maintaining healthy skin and avoiding pressure problems
- Advice on the best way of communication, communication aid, and the best method for engaging the person.
- Advice on swallowing
- Contacts with social services and the case manager.

Causes of increased risk of 'failed' discharge/early readmission include:
- great age
- history of repeated unplanned admissions
- social isolation/living alone
- in receipt of care package prior to stroke
- lack of informal care network
- admitted patient being a carer
- marked loss of physical or mental function
- issues of neglect or abuse.

Role of carers and voluntary sector
- The presence of an immediate support network is an important factor in not only discharge planning but also adjustment to life after stroke
- Carer burden is well documented in stroke
- Voluntary sector organizations can provide financial, emotional, and practical help for both stroke patients and carers
- Post-stroke groups can help with regaining confidence after stroke. These are often facilitated by former users or patients and can improve measures of anxiety and depression and 'self-efficacy'.

Further reading

Basic science of stroke recovery and new approaches

Dawson J, Abdul-Rahim AH, Kimberley TJ (2024). Neurostimulation for treatment of post-stroke impairments. *Nat Rev Neurol* **20**, 259–268.

Grefkes C, Ward NS (2014). Cortical reorganization after stroke: how much and how functional? *Neuroscientist* **20**(1), 56–70.

Kane E, Ward NS (2021). Neurobiology of stroke recovery. In: Platz T (ed.). *Clinical Pathways in Stroke Rehabilitation: Evidence-based Clinical Practice Recommendations*, pp. 1–14. Cham: Springer.

Marín-Medina DS, Arenas-Vargas PA, Arias-Botero JC, Gómez-Vásquez M, Jaramillo-López MF, Gaspar-Toro JM (2024). New approaches to recovery after stroke. *Neurol Sci* **45**, 55–63.

Common problems after stroke

AVERT Trial Collaboration group (2015). Efficacy and safety of very early mobilisation within 24 h of stroke onset (AVERT): a randomised controlled trial. *Lancet* **386**, 46–55.

Bowen A, Hesketh A, Patchick E, *et al.* (2012). Clinical effectiveness, cost effectiveness and service users' perceptions of early, well-resourced communication therapy following a stroke, a randomised controlled trial (The ACT NoW Study). *Health Technol Assess* **16**, 1–160.

Brady MC, Kelly H, Godwin J, *et al.* (2016). Speech and language therapy for aphasia following stroke. *Cochrane Database Syst Rev* **6**, CD000425.

Elsner B, Kugler J, Pohl M, Mehrholz J (2019). Transcranial direct current stimulation (tDCS) for improving aphasia in adults with aphasia after stroke. *Cochrane Database Syst Rev* **5**, CD009760.

Francisco GE, Wissel J, Platz T, Li S (2021). Post-stroke spasticity. In: Platz T (ed.). *Clinical Pathways in Stroke Rehabilitation: Evidence-based Clinical Practice Recommendations*, pp. 149–174. Cham: Springer.

Neuropsychiatric symptoms post stroke

Hackett ML, Köhler S, O'Brien JT, Mead GE (2014). Neuropsychiatric outcomes of stroke. *Lancet Neurol* **13**, 525–534.

Other neuropsychiatric symptoms post stroke

Tay J, Morris RG, Markus HS (2021). Apathy after stroke: diagnosis, mechanisms, consequences, and treatment. *Int J Stroke* **16**, 510–518.

Legg LA, Rudberg A-S, Hua X, Wu S, *et al.* (2021). Selective serotonin reuptake inhibitors (SSRIs) for stroke recovery. *Cochrane Database Syst Rev* **11**, CD009286.

Hackett ML, Köhler S, O'Brien JT, Mead GE (2014). Neuropsychiatric outcomes of stroke. *Lancet Neurol* **13**, 525–534.

Broomfield NM, Blake J, Gracey F, Steverson T (2024). Post-stroke emotionalism: diagnosis, pathophysiology, and treatment. *Int J Stroke* **19**, 857–866.

Ignacio KHD, Muir RT, Diestro JDB, *et al.* (2024). Prevalence of depression and anxiety symptoms after stroke in young adults: a systematic review and meta-analysis. *J Stroke Cerebrovasc Dis* **33**, 107732.

Fatigue after stroke

Chu SH, Zhao X, Komber A, *et al.* (2023). Systematic review: pharmacological interventions for the treatment of post-stroke fatigue. *Int J Stroke* **18**, 1071–1083.

Kuppuswamy A, Billinger S, Coupland KG, *et al.* (2024). Mechanisms of post-stroke fatigue: a follow-up from the third stroke recovery and rehabilitation roundtable. *Neurorehabil Neural Repair* **38**, 52–61.

Spasticity

National RCP Guidelines (2018). *Spasticity in Adults: Management Using Botulinum Toxin*. Available online at https://www.rcp.ac.uk/improving-care/resources/spasticity-in-adults-management-using-botulinum-toxin/

Dysphagia therapy and enteral nutrition

Dennis MS, Lewis SC, Warlow C (2005). FOOD Trial Collaboration. Effect of timing and method of enteral tube feeding for dysphagic stroke patients (FOOD): a multicentre randomised controlled trial. *Lancet* **365**, 764–772.

Labeit B, Michou E, Trapl-Grundschober M, *et al.* (2024). Dysphagia after stroke: research advances in treatment interventions. *Lancet Neurol* **23**, 418–428.

Sakai K, Niimi M, Momosaki R, *et al.* (2024) Nutritional therapy for reducing disability and improving activities of daily living in people after stroke. *Cochrane Database Syst Rev* **8**, CD014852.

Hemiplegic shoulder pain

Coskun Benlidayi I, Basaran S (2014). Hemiplegic shoulder pain: a common clinical consequence of stroke. *Pract Neurol* **14**, 88–91.

de Sire A, Moggio L, Demeco A, *et al.* (2022). Efficacy of rehabilitative techniques in reducing hemiplegic shoulder pain in stroke: systematic review and meta-analysis. *Ann Phys Rehabil Med* **65**, 101602.

Turner-Stokes L, Jackson D (2002). Shoulder pain after stroke: a review of the evidence base to inform the development of an integrated care pathway. *Clin Rehabil* **16**, 276–298.

Central post-stroke pain syndrome

Asadauskas A, Stieger A, Luedi MM, Andereggen L (2024). Advancements in modern treatment approaches for central post-stroke pain: a narrative review. *J Clin Med* **13**, 5377.

Frese A, Husstedt IW, Ringelstein EB, Evers S (2006). Pharmacologic treatment of central post-stroke pain. *Clin J Pain* **22**, 252–260.

Harrison RA, Field TS (2015). Post stroke pain: identification, assessment, and therapy. *Cerebrovasc Dis* **39**, 190–201.

Hemianopia and hemianopic alexia

Elfeky A, D'Août K, Lawson R, *et al.* (2021). Biomechanical adaptation to post-stroke visual field loss: a systematic review. *Syst Rev* **10**, 84.

Ong YH, Brown MM, Robinson P, *et al.* (2012). Read-Right: a 'web app' that improves reading speeds in patients with hemianopia. *J Neurol* **259**, 2611–2515.

Urinary incontinence or retention

Cruz E, Miller C, Zhang W, *et al.* (2022). Does non-implanted electrical stimulation reduce post-stroke urinary or fecal incontinence? A systematic review with meta-analysis. *Int J Stroke* **17**, 378–388.

Patel M, Coshill C, Rudd AG, Wolfe CD (2001). Natural history and effects on 2 year outcomes of urinary incontinence after stroke. *Stroke* **32**, 122–127.

Pettersen R, Stien R, Wyller TB (2007). Post-stroke urinary incontinence with impaired awareness of the need to void: clinical and urodynamic features. *Br J Urol Int* **99**, 1073–1077.

Thomas LH, Coupe J, Cross LD, *et al.* (2019). Interventions for treating urinary incontinence after stroke in adults. *Cochrane Database Syst Rev* **2**, CD004462.

Bowel management

Harari D, Coshall C, Rudd AG, Wolfe CD (2003). New-onset fecal incontinence after stroke: prevalence, natural history, risk factors, and impact. *Stroke* **34**, 144–150.

Lewis SJ, Heaton KW (1997). Stool form scale as a useful guide to intestinal transit time. *Scand J Gastroenterol* **32**, 920–924.

Potter J, Wagg A (2005). Management of bowel problems in older people: an update. *Clin Med* **5**, 289–295.

Discharge planning

Gonçalves-Bradley DC, Lannin NA, *et al.* (2022) Discharge planning from hospital. *Cochrane Database of Systematic Reviews* **2**, CD000313.

Vascular cognitive impairment (VCI)

Vascular cognitive impairment: concepts

Cognitive impairment is one of the most devastating consequences of cerebrovascular disease. Traditionally the term most used was vascular dementia. However cerebrovascular disease can cause lesser degree of cognitive impairment which does not meet the criteria for dementia but are nevertheless disabling. This has led to the use of the term vascular cognitive impairment (VCI) to cover any type of cognitive impairment caused by cerebrovascular disease.

A wide variety of vascular pathologies can cause dementia. These range from an insidious, progressive accumulation of microvascular pathological changes often due to cerebral small-vessel disease to a single or multiple clinical stroke events affecting brain structures critical for cognition.

Useful terms

Vascular cognitive impairment (VCI) refers to cognitive impairment of any severity associated with cerebrovascular disease

Vascular dementia is the end of a continuum of severity of VCI and is reached when the individual meets the criteria for dementia.

Post-stroke cognitive impairment (PSCI) refers to cognitive impairment of any severity noted after a clinical stroke.

Poststroke dementia (PSD) is the end of a continuum of severity of PSCI and is reached when the individual meets the criteria for dementia.

The field of vascular dementia is challenging for the following reasons:

• It is a syndrome, not a specific disease, and can be caused by multiple pathologies
• The cognitive features of vascular disease affecting different parts of the brain differ markedly (e.g. the cognitive profile of dementia caused by multiple cortical infarcts is quite different from that caused by diffuse subcortical disease)
• Many different definitions of vascular dementia have been used
• Most of the definitions and screening tests used have been designed for Alzheimer's type 'cortical dementias' and describe the features of vascular dementia, particularly subcortical vascular dementia, less well
• Vascular pathology and Alzheimer's pathology frequently coexist. In elderly populations mixed dementia is more common than pure vascular dementia
• Assessing dementia can be difficult in patients with stroke, particularly those with communication problems.

Classification of VCI

It is most useful to classify VCI and vascular dementia according to the type of vascular damage as this determines the cognitive profile (see Box 15.1).

Frequently more than one subtype can coexist, and vascular disease may coexist with a wide variety of other dementias, not only Alzheimer's disease but also Lewy body dementia and other dementias.

Strategic infarcts

- Single infarcts in specific sites may result in cognitive impairment which may meet the criteria for 'dementia'. Whether they meet the criteria for dementia depends largely on the definition of dementia used (see ➲ Definitions of vascular dementia, p. 482). They cause 'dementia' by resulting in discrete 'disconnections' within complex neuronal pathways concerned with cognitive processes
- Usually other signs of stroke make the diagnosis clear
- Diagnosis of the lesion is often more useful than making a diagnosis of dementia
- The following lesions may produce specific cognitive disturbances:
  - Frontal lesions (anterior cerebral artery)—apathy and emotional blunting (usually when bilateral)
  - Medial temporal lobe lesions—severe amnesia (especially when bilateral)
  - Thalamic infarcts—disturbances of attention, memory, language, and abstract thinking
  - Caudate head infarcts—apathy, disinhibition, and affective symptoms.

Multiple cortical infarcts

Here the pattern of cognitive impairment depends upon the site of the lesion. Whether patients with such lesions develop dementia depends upon the infarct size, the total infarct volume, and the age of the patient.

Small-vessel (subcortical) dementia

This occurs because of multiple subcortical lacunar infarcts, usually accompanied by more diffuse ischaemic changes (leukoaraiosis) (see ➲ p. 205). Patients may or may not have clinical evidence of lacunar stroke. A typical cognitive profile occurs with predominant impairment of executive function, attention, and speed of information processing. In contrast, memory and visuospatial cognition are relatively preserved, at least early in the disease. This is now thought to be the most common pathology causing vascular dementia.

Hypoperfusion dementia

This is a rare cause of dementia, and the clinical picture will depend upon the mechanism. For example, patients with subcortical vascular disease and impaired autoregulation in the white matter may deteriorate markedly following a period of hypoperfusion which worsens white matter ischaemia. In contrast, patients with large extracranial vessel occlusion (carotid and vertebral) may suffer watershed infarction following hypoperfusion involving both cortical and subcortical watershed regions.

Dementia caused by cerebral haemorrhage

This encompasses both subcortical and cortical pathologies. Cerebral haemorrhage is a frequent feature of subcortical vascular disease coexisting with small-vessel disease. The other major pathology producing dementia and cerebral haemorrhage is amyloid angiopathy, characterized by multiple areas of lobar microbleeding seen on dark-blood sequence MRI such as gradient echo, or CAA (see ⮕ p. 404).

Box 15.1 Subtypes of vascular dementia
- Multiple large cortical infarcts
- Small-vessel dementia (subcortical dementia)
- Strategic infarct dementia
- Hypoperfusion dementia
- Dementia secondary to cerebral haemorrhage
  Mixed dementia (vascular disease with Alzheimer's disease).

Epidemiology

- Vascular dementia is the second most common cause of dementia after Alzheimer's disease
- Worldwide, around 50 million people live with dementia, and this number is projected to triple by 2050. It has been estimated that 20% of all dementia cases have a predominant cerebrovascular pathology, while perhaps another 20% of vascular diseases contribute to a mixed dementia picture.
- Therefore, the vascular contribution to dementia affects 20 million people currently and will increase markedly in the next few decades, particularly in lower- and middle-income countries.
- Recent forecasts predict that the number of people with dementia will triple from around 57 million currently to 153 million by 2050.
- The greatest increase will be in low-income and middle-income countries (LMICs)
- Rates increase exponentially with age
- Dementia is seen in up to 10–30% of subjects 3 months after stroke. However, this figure depends greatly on the definition of dementia used and the stroke population studied.
- A meta-analysis reported a risk of dementia after a first stroke of 10%, and after a recurrent stroke of 30%.

Definitions of vascular dementia

- A definition of dementia is important both clinically and for research studies.
- However, there have been problems with the definition of vascular dementia.
- Older definitions, such as those from the Diagnostic and Statistical Manual (DSM-IV) and International Classification of Disease (ICD-10), were largely developed with Alzheimer's pathology in mind and required the presence of memory impairment as an absolute requirement.
- This approach has been criticized because memory impairment, which is commonly (though not universally) seen early in the course of Alzheimer's disease, is much less often seen in patients with cerebrovascular disease.
- It is a particular problem for subcortical dementia, which presents predominantly with executive dysfunction rather than memory impairment.
- The definition used has a marked effect on the prevalence of vascular dementia as it would miss many cases where, despite marked cognitive impairment, it has been suggested that a definition of vascular dementia should not absolutely require the presence of memory impairment.
- DSM-5 takes account of this by requiring the presence of acquired significant impairments (independence lost) in one of more cognitive domains. These include self-control/management (executive functions) impairment) as well as other domains, such as memory, so that dementia can be diagnosed in the absence of significant impairment in memory.

DSM-5

DSM-5 uses the term vascular neurocognitive disorder rather than VCI, and use the term major neurocognitive disorder to correspond to dementia.

Under DSM-5, an individual diagnosed with **vascular neurocognitive disorder** (corresponding to VCI) needs to meet all the following criteria:
1. The clinical features are consistent with a vascular aetiology, as suggested by either of the following:
- Onset of the cognitive deficits is temporally related to one or more cerebrovascular events.
- Evidence for decline is prominent in complex attention (including processing speed) and fronto-executive function.
2. There is evidence of the presence of cerebrovascular disease from history, physical examination, and/or neuroimaging considered sufficient to account for the neurocognitive deficits.
3. The symptoms are not better explained by another brain disease or systemic disorder.

For the diagnosis to meet the criteria for **major neurocognitive disorder** (i.e. dementia) the individual diagnosed with vascular neurocognitive disorder needs to meet all of the following criteria:
1. Evidence of significant cognitive decline from a previous level of performance in one or more cognitive domains (complex attention,

executive function, learning and memory, language, perceptual-motor, or social cognition) based on:

- Concern of the individual, a knowledgeable informant, or the clinician that there has been a significant decline in cognitive function; and
- A substantial impairment in cognitive performance, preferably documented by standardized neuropsychological testing or, in its absence, another quantified clinical assessment.

2. The cognitive deficits interfere with independence in everyday activities (i.e. at a minimum, requiring assistance with complex instrumental activities of daily living such as paying bills or managing medications).

3. The cognitive deficits do not occur exclusively in the context of a delirium.

4. The cognitive deficits are not better explained by another mental disorder (e.g. major depressive disorder, schizophrenia).

Post-stroke dementia

- A 2023 Scientific Statement From the American Heart Association/ American Stroke Association in 2023 concluded that PSD rates in the first year after stroke range from 7.4% (95% CI, 4.8–10.0%) in population-based studies of first-ever stroke in which pre-stroke dementia was excluded, to 41.3% (95% CI, 29.6–53.1%) in hospital-based studies of recurrent stroke in which pre-stroke dementia was included.
- About 10% of patients have dementia before the first stroke; 10% develop new dementia soon after first stroke; and more than one-third have dementia after recurrent stroke.
- PSD is more common after intracerebral haemorrhage, particularly lobar ICH.
- Any degree of PSCI, including milder degrees occurs in up to 60% of survivors in the first year after stroke, with the highest rate seen shortly after stroke. Up to 20% of these individuals recover fully, with the highest rate of recovery seen shortly after stroke. However, improvement in cognitive impairment without return to prestroke levels is more frequent than complete recovery.
- Whether the stroke results in PSD depends on a complex interplay between the features of the stroke lesion itself and the brain resilience of the individual. Large lesions or lesions located at 'strategic' sites (e.g. left frontotemporal lobe, left thalamus, or right parietal lobe) are more prone to result in cognitive impairment.
- Brain resilience depends on multiple factors, including pre-existing brain diseases (e.g. AD and SVD), cognitive reserve (e.g. educational level), and other demographic or medical conditions (e.g. age, diabetes, and frailty).
- Even a small lesion located in a non-strategic region, or a transient ischaemic attack, may trigger poststroke cognitive impairment in someone with low brain resilience.
- Even after the cognitive decline associated with an acute stroke has settled, the long-term rate of cognitive decline over subsequent years is faster when compared to that in stroke-free individuals and such a decline occurs even in the absence of recurrent stroke. Stroke. It has been suggested that one factor driving this delayed-onset cognitive decline is that the stroke episode triggers the progression of pre-existing brain diseases (e.g. AD and SVD).
- Different trajectories of cognitive decline and improvement are seen following stroke, and in VCI more generally, and these are illustrated in Fig. 15.1.

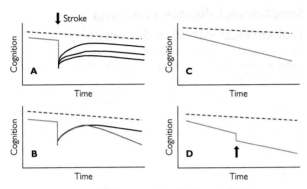

Fig. 15.1. Trajectories of different types of vascular dementia. In all figures, the dotted blue line represents cognitive decline with age in the absence of cerebrovascular disease: (A) Following a stroke cognition declines, and then recovers to a variable extent. The extent of the poststroke cognitive decline will depend both on the site and extent of the stroke, as well as brain resilience. Brain resilience depends on pre-existing brain diseases (e.g. AD and SVD), cognitive reserve (e.g. educational level and cognitive activity), and other demographic or medical conditions (e.g. age, diabetes, and frailty); (B) following stroke cognition can continue to decline in the longer term at a rate faster than that prestroke as illustrated by the red line; (C) cerebrovascular disease can result in gradual decline in cognition in the absence of stroke. This pattern is particularly seen with SVD; (D) other insults such as delirium and intercurrent infection (arrowed) can result in a decline in cognition which does not return to the pre-insult level.

Source: © Hugh Markus.

From: Mok V, Cai V, Markus HS. Vascular cognitive impairment and dementia: Mechanisms, treatment, and future directions. *Int J Stroke* 19, 838–856.

Small-vessel disease dementia (subcortical vascular dementia)

Subcortical vascular dementia results from ischaemia in the deep white matter and deep grey matter nuclei secondary to diffuse disease of the small perforating blood vessels supplying these regions.

It is an important cause of vascular dementia and VCI, and in treatment trials it accounted for more than half of cases of vascular dementia.

The true burden is likely to be underestimated because the major cognitive features are executive dysfunction and impairment of information processing speed. These deficits are not well identified by the screening tools often used (such as the MMSE), which were designed to detect impairments due to 'cortical' dementias such as Alzheimer's.

Causes

- Sporadic small-vessel disease (90% hypertensive)
- Monogenic forms of small-vessel disease (CADASIL and others)
- Small-vessel vasculitis (very rare)
- Other rare causes.

The vast majority of cases are caused by hypertensive small-vessel disease. In only approximately 10% of cases of sporadic small-vessel disease is hypertension not present. Diabetes and elevated serum homocysteine have also been identified as risk factors for small-vessel disease.

Radiological features

A combination of lacunar infarction (often multiple) and leukoaraiosis is usually seen. Leukoaraiosis is seen as periventricular and deep white matter with a low signal on CT or much better seen as high signal on T2-weighted or FLAIR MRI—white matter hyperintensities. Other common features include diffuse cerebral atrophy, multiple subcortical microbleeds on gradient echo or SWI MRI, and enlarged peri-vascular spaces. Diffuse damage throughout the white matter can be seen on diffusion tensor imaging (DTI), but is primarily used as a research technique.

Mechanism of dementia

Disruption of cortical–subcortical and cortical–cortical white matter tracts, with an ensuing 'disconnection' syndrome, is believed to play a central role. This could occur due to both lacunar infarcts and diffuse white matter disease (which have both been shown to disrupt white matter tracts using DTI tractography).

Diffuse atrophy is also a feature and correlates with cognitive impairment, although whether this is secondary to white matter tract disruption remains to be determined.

Clinical features

Some or all of the following features may be present. Clinical lacunar stroke is not essential for the diagnosis, although neuroimaging evidence of small-vessel disease is.

- Lacunar stroke
- Subcortical cognitive impairment

- Parkinsonian features
- Gait apraxia
- Depression
- Apathy
- Emotional lability.

Cognitive profile

There is a characteristic cognitive profile with major deficits seen in:
- attention
- speed of information processing
- executive function.

Such functions, predominantly served by frontostriatal–thalamic circuits, which are most disrupted by subcortical vascular change, are not well detected on current screening and assessment instruments for dementia. For example, there can be significant cognitive deficit despite an MMSE that is normal or slightly impaired.

Other bedside tests are more useful to screen for this deficit, including:
- verbal fluency
- trail making or maze tests
- clock drawing
- reverse digit span
- short cognitive batteries more sensitive to the deficit seen in VCI due to small-vessel disease have been developed; e.g. the Brief Memory and Executive Test (BMET) takes about 10 minutes to administer and has been shown to perform better than the MMSE and the MOCA. The BMET is freely downloadable from ℞ http://www.bmet.info.

Other clinical features

- Bradyphrenia, a slowing of mental agility, may be a marked feature in subcortical dementia. The patient may be slow to remember a list of items but will eventually respond correctly, in contrast to patients with cortical dementia who tend to remember immediately or not at all
- Depression is common. Recent evidence suggests that many white matter diseases disrupting subcortical–cortical circuits predispose to depression. It is a major predictor of poor quality of life in patients with VCI due to small-vessel disease
- Apathy—this is a common feature of VCI due to small-vessel disease and can be greatly disabling to the patient and their family
- Confusional episodes may occur, particularly in the later stages. Marked deterioration can occur in response to systemic disorders (e.g. infection or following a seizure)
- Gait apraxia with poor gait ignition ('stuttering standing start'), wide base, and small steps (*march a petit pas*). Occasionally, patients present with an extrapyramidal, seemingly Parkinsonian, syndrome, but this is non-DOPA responsive and there is a lack of tremor
- In advanced cases, other features include pseudobulbar palsy, emotional lability, extensor plantar responses, and urinary incontinence
- Chronic hypertension is usually present, but it is important to note that in the later stages of the disease, blood pressure measurements may

decline to the normal range. Therefore, taking a premorbid history of hypertension is important.

Overlap with Alzheimer's disease

Increasing evidence has shown that Alzheimer's and vascular pathology can coexist in many patients and may interact.

- In the prospective clinicopathological Nun Study in the USA, in which cognitive testing was performed in life and then compared with pathology at post-mortem, a lesser degree of Alzheimer's (tangle) pathology was needed to produce the same degree of cognitive impairment during life if one or more infarcts was present
- In most autopsy studies on selected older people, mixed Alzheimer's and vascular pathology was the most common cause of cognitive impairment. Many studies have shown it is at least as common, if not more common, than 'pure' vascular dementia
- Several risk factors for vascular disease are also risk factors for Alzheimer's, including hypertension, smoking, and diabetes
- Commonly used definitions of dementia have been designed for Alzheimer's and these are not sensitive to subcortical dementias. The requirement of memory impairment may lead to overrepresentation of Alzheimer's pathology in patients with dementia
- White matter hyperintensities on MRI in up to 50% of AD patients.

How do vascular and Alzheimer's pathologies interact?

- It is uncertain if the two pathologies both cause damage independently or whether they interact. If one pathology, say cerebrovascular disease causes brain damage, this will reduce the capacity of the brain to cope with a second pathology, say Alzheimer's disease (i.e. reduce 'brain reserve'), and therefore exacerbate the effect of the Alzheimer's pathology worsening the cognitive consequences. However increasing evidence suggest the two pathologies may interact, rather than having purely additive effects.
- It has been suggested that vascular changes may exacerbate the formation of Alzheimer's-type pathology. For example, by contributing to vessel wall thickening and reducing the efficiency of the perivascular glymphatic drainage system, this could lead to reduced elimination of amyloid. Secondary to this, increased accumulation of amyloid and a greater likelihood of plaque formation could occur.
- Vascular pathology can lead to hypoxia and hypoperfusion. In animal models both have been shown to increase Alzheimer's pathology. Ischaemia has been shown to accelerate hyperphosphorylation of tau, a crucial step in tangle formation, and increase cleavage of amyloid precursor protein, leading to increased plaque accumulation.

Therapeutic implications

- Considerable epidemiological evidence has associated vascular risk factors with risk of Alzheimer's disease. This raises the possibility that treating risk factors delays onset or progression of Alzheimer's.
- The SPRINT-MIND study supported this. Intensive blood pressure lowering in hypertensive individuals to 120mmHg systolic compared with 140 mm reduced the combined endpoint of dementia and mild cognitive impairment over follow-up up to 8 years.

Investigation of the vascular dementia patient

History
- Details of cognitive decline:
  - Timescale
  - Relationship to stroke.
- Social setting:
  - Effect on patient and carer.

Examination
- Full neurological examination including gait

Cognitive assessment
- MOCA or similar cognitive assessment
- BMET or similar test focused on executive function and processing speed for patients with subcortical vascular disease
- Simple tests of higher cortical function, e.g. parietal function
- Assessment of executive function, e.g. trail making test.

Investigations
- CT
- MRI:
  - Better than CT, particularly for small-vessel disease
  - Gradient echo will show old microbleeds—these occur in small-vessel disease and amyloid angiopathy
- Bloods:
  - Routine stroke screen
  - Rare tests (e.g. CADASIL genetic analysis) when indicated.

Apart from vascular causes, one should also screen for common or reversible causes of dementia:
- Full blood count (anaemia)
- ESR/CRP (vasculitis)
- Renal function—renal failure can cause cognitive impairment
- Liver function—hepatic encephalopathy, when chronic, may masquerade as dementia
- Thyroid function is very common in older people
- Vitamin B_{12}
- Antinuclear antibodies (ANA) and antineutrophil cytoplasmic antibodies (ANCA)—ANA for lupus and ANCA for vasculitis
- Anticardiolipin antibodies
- VDRL (venereal disease research laboratory) test
- In young people with vascular disease, don't forget HIV.

Important differential diagnosis
- Dementia resulting from vascular disease must be distinguished from:
  - Confusion and delirium—an acute and reversible disturbance of cognitive function

- focal disturbances affecting single cognitive domains, e.g. amnesia or aphasia.
- Not uncommonly a patient presenting with acute aphasia is misdiagnosed as confused or demented in the emergency room

Management

One should follow the following plan:
- History, examination, and investigation as described earlier in this topic
- Classification of type of dementia
- Treat rare/reversible causes
- Look for intercurrent depression and treat
- Secondary prevention:
  - Antithrombotic therapy
  - Identify and treat vascular risk factors
- Identify and treat complications
- Provide family and social support.

Therapy of dementia

This can be divided into:
- prevention and treatment of risk factors
- symptomatic treatments
- treatment of complications, including depression
- general supportive care of patient and carers.

Secondary prevention and treatment of risk factors

Few studies have specifically investigated treatment of risk factors in preventing cognitive decline as opposed to stroke. Nevertheless, it seems sensible to treat risk factors as one would for stroke and this is our practice. These include:
- hypertension
- diabetes mellitus
- raised cholesterol
- smoking.

Preventing recurrent stroke is important because this can lead to worsening of the cognitive state and progression from VCI to dementia. This is covered in more detail in Chapter 10 on secondary stroke prevention

Treating hypertension is particularly important in prevention of small-vessel disease and was shown to reduce the progression of MRI white matter hyperintensities, which represent early cerebral small-vessel disease.

In the SPS3 trial, there was a suggestion that more intensive blood pressure therapy aiming for a systolic blood pressure of <130 mmHg was associated with a lower recurrent stroke risk in patients with lacunar stroke.

The SPRINT-MIND trial in hypertensive individuals without stroke reported intensive blood pressure lowering to a target of 120mmHg systolic compared with 140 mm reduced the combined endpoint of dementia and mild cognitive impairment. It also showed this was associated with reduced progression of MRI white matter hyperintensities

In patients with advanced subcortical dementia, it has been suggested that excessive blood pressure lowering in the presence of impaired cerebral autoregulation may reduce cerebral perfusion and therefore worsen cognitive function. However, the PRESERVE trial found that in patients with lacunar stroke and confluent white matter hyperintensities, reducing blood pressure to 125 mmHg systolic, compared with 140 systolic, did not reduce cerebral blood or worsen cognition.

Antiplatelet therapy
- There are little data specifically assessing antiplatelet therapy in preventing dementia. Nevertheless, most authorities recommend single antiplatelet treatment with clopidogrel or aspirin
- Warfarin is contraindicated in patients with small-vessel disease unless there is a specific reason (e.g. cardioembolic source). Leukoaraiosis is associated with an increased risk of cerebral haemorrhage in anticoagulated patients, as shown in the SPIRIT trial
- The SPS3 trial showed aspirin plus clopidogrel is associated with a higher rate of increased risk of intracerebral and systemic haemorrhage in patients with MRI-confirmed cerebral small-vessel disease;

therefore, single-agent antiplatelet therapy with aspirin or clopidogrel is recommended. There was no difference between dual and single antiplatelet therapy on cognition in a secondary analysis of the SPS3 data.

Symptomatic pharmacological treatments

Symptomatic treatments for vascular dementia have been explored:
- Cholinesterase inhibitors:
  - Donepezil
  - Galantamine
- Memantine—an NMDA antagonist.

Trials in vascular and mixed dementia have suggested modest benefits in some outcomes but no major benefit.

Interpretation of the data is difficult due to the following:
- Many patients may have coexistent Alzheimer's disease, which could account for the benefit seen
- The outcome scores are more suited to assessing cognitive deficits in cortical or Alzheimer's-type dementia rather than subcortical vascular dementia (which comprised the majority of patients in some studies)
- To determine whether the cholinesterase inhibitor donepezil was effective in pure VCI, a randomized double-blind study was performed in CADASIL. This autosomal dominant form of small-vessel disease causes a similar cognitive impairment to that seen in sporadic small-vessel disease. However, it occurs at an earlier age when coexistent Alzheimer's pathology is very rare. No effect was found on a traditional trial endpoint, the VADASCog, but a significant (but small) improvement occurred in executive function, although there was no improvement in quality of life. This has two implications:
  - Cholinesterase inhibitors appear to result in improvement in some cognitive features in subcortical dementia, although the effect is small and of little clinical benefit
  - Treatment effects will be detected best using tests targeted to the deficits seen in this group of patients, i.e. executive dysfunction and speed of information processing.

Currently, most bodies (e.g. NICE in the UK) do not recommend the widespread use of cholinesterase inhibitors or memantine for vascular dementia, although they can be considered in cases of mixed dementia (e.g. vascular and Alzheimer's).

Treatment of complications

If there is a sudden or unexpected deterioration in cognitive state, a thorough assessment should be made of treatable comorbid states or complications, including:
- intercurrent infection
- medication side effects
- cardiovascular compromise leading to hypoperfusion
- seizures and post-ictal worsening
- depression.

Recent studies have shown both intercurrent dementia and delirium can lead to a permanent worsening of cognitive function in VCI and therefore avoidance, and prompt treatment are important. Simple measures include avoiding aspiration in patients with dysphagia secondary to stroke, and vaccinations (e.g. flu and COVID-19)

Non-pharmacological therapy

This is an important part of dementia care, and suggested patterns of care are well described in the UK NICE guidelines for dementia ℘ https://www.nice.org.uk/guidance/ng97

Dementia is associated with complex needs and, especially in the later stages, high levels of dependency and morbidity. As the condition progresses, people with dementia can present carers and healthcare staff with complex problems, including aggressive behaviour, restlessness and wandering, eating problems, incontinence, delusions and hallucinations, and mobility difficulties that can lead to falls and fractures. The impact of dementia on an individual may be compounded by personal circumstances such as changes in financial status and accommodation, or bereavement.

Wherever possible and appropriate, agencies should work in an integrated way to maximize the benefit for people with dementia and their carers.

Promoting independence of people with dementia

Healthcare and social care staff should aim to promote and maintain the independence, including mobility, of people with dementia. Care plans should address activities of daily living (ADLs) that maximize independent activity, enhance function, adapt and develop skills, and minimize the need for support. Important considerations in helping maintain independence include:

- consistent and stable staffing
- retaining a familiar environment
- minimizing relocations
- flexibility to accommodate fluctuating abilities
- assessment and care planning advice regarding ADLs, and ADL skill training from an occupational therapist
- assessment and care planning advice about independent toileting skills; if incontinence occurs, all possible causes should be assessed and relevant treatments tried before concluding that it is permanent
- environmental modifications to aid independent functioning, including assistive technology, with advice from an occupational therapist and/or clinical psychologist
- physical exercise, with assessment and advice from a physiotherapist when needed
- support for people to go at their own pace and participate in activities they enjoy.

Capacity and dementia

People with dementia should have the opportunity to make informed decisions about their care in partnership with their health and social care professionals. If they do not have the capacity to make decisions, health professionals should follow national guidelines. Since April 2007, healthcare professionals in the UK need to follow the Mental Capacity Act 2005. It has five key principles:

- Adults must be assumed to have capacity to make decisions for themselves unless proven otherwise
- Individuals must be given all available support before it is concluded that they cannot make decisions for themselves
- Individuals must retain the right to make what might be seen as eccentric or unwise decisions
- Anything done for, or on behalf of, individuals without capacity must be in their best interests
- Anything done for, or on behalf of, individuals without capacity must be the least restrictive alternative in terms of their rights and basic freedoms.

Good communication between care providers and people with dementia and their families and carers is essential.

Depression in VCI

- Depression is common in VCI. This is due not only to the physical and emotional stress caused by the disease and its diagnosis and effects but also (for small-vessel dementia) because of a direct effect of white matter damage on cortical–subcortical circuits
- Depression-complicating dementia can be difficult to detect and is frequently missed
- A high index of suspicion is essential because good treatment responses can be obtained
- Dementia patients with depression do not necessarily present with biological symptoms, but it may result in a global deterioration, which may be taken as a progression of their underlying disease instead of depression
- It can be difficult to diagnose. Multidisciplinary team assessment and carer opinion are important. Sometimes, a carefully monitored trial of therapy is required
- Treatment should consider both pharmacological and non-pharmacological approaches.

Psychological interventions

- Care packages for people with dementia should include assessment and monitoring for depression and/or anxiety
- For people with dementia who have depression and/or anxiety, cognitive behavioural therapy, which may involve the active participation of their carers, may be considered as part of treatment
- A range of tailored interventions, such as reminiscence therapy, music therapy, multisensory stimulation, animal-assisted therapy, and exercise, should be available for people with dementia who have depression and/or anxiety.

Pharmacological treatment

- People with dementia who also have major depressive disorder should be offered antidepressant medication
- Antidepressant drugs with anticholinergic effects should be avoided because they may adversely affect cognition, particularly in patients with coexistent Alzheimer's pathology or a mixed dementia picture.

Apathy in VCI

- Apathy is a behavioural syndrome characterized by a loss of motivation that occurs in about 1 in 3 patients after stroke.
- It is clinically under-recognized and poorly understood.
- It can be defined as a reduction in goal-directed behaviours occurring in the cognitive/behavioural, emotional, or social domains of an individual's life.
- It is particularly common in cerebral small-vessel disease, in which it can occur without clinical stroke.

Diagnosis of apathy

- Apathy can be suspected in routine clinical practice during the history taking and examination from an observed loss of motivation.
- Informant histories are particularly useful. They may reveal symptoms of apathy, such as loss of interest in previous activities and hobbies or doing little when left alone. It is important to ask the informant as the patient may underplay symptoms, due to their apathy.
- There are a number of apathy scales. The most commonly used is the Apathy Evaluation Scale. Other scales, such as the Dimensional Apathy Index, allow detailed evaluation of different components of apathy (Behavioural/Cognitive Initiation, Executive, and Emotional).
- Apathy needs to be differentiated from depression. The two share a number of symptoms but can be differentiated (see Fig. 15.2). This

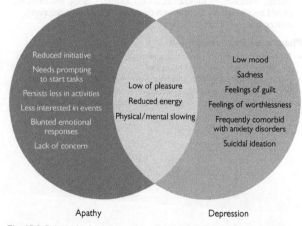

Fig. 15.2 Relationship between apathy and depression. The Venn diagrams show symptoms which are distinct, and which overlap, the two. From Tay J, Morris RG, Markus HS (2012). Apathy after stroke: Diagnosis, mechanisms, consequences, and treatment. *Int J Stroke* 16:510–518.

is important as it has major implications for choosing the appropriate therapy

- Core symptoms of a depressive episode include low mood and diminished pleasure (anhedonia).
- Negative emotionality is a key characteristic of depression that distinguishes it from apathy. Depressed patients present with pessimism and hopelessness, while those with apathy show a lack of emotional distress. Depressed patients can actively engage in avoidant behaviour, resisting socializing and treatment attempts, while apathetic patients are passive and indifferent to these activities.
- Apathy and depression can coexist but both can also occur without the other.

Mechanisms of post-stroke apathy

- Post-stroke apathy occurs as a consequence of neurobiological changes triggered by a stroke
- Apathy is traditionally described as the result of damage to specific brain structures related to goal-directed behaviour, such as the basal ganglia and prefrontal cortex.
- However there is no clear relationship between lesion location and apathy.
- This has led to the recent hypothesis that apathy in cerebrovascular disease occurs due to disruption of to brain networks underlying goal-directed behaviour.
- This network-based theory suggests that apathy follows secondary to focal lesions in key network regions, or from diffuse cerebrovascular pathology disrupting connections within networks.
- Acute infarcts to core brain regions underlying goal-directed behaviour can result in apathy, recapitulating the lesion-deficit view. Alternatively, diffuse white matter damage due to cerebral small-vessel disease can lead to network disruption, explaining associations between MRI markers of small-vessel disease and apathy.

Treatment of apathy in VCI and post-stroke

- There is a lack of trials and, therefore, high-quality evidence to guide management of post-stroke apathy.
- No drug therapies have been shown to improve apathy.
- There is no evidence that antidepressants improve apathy. However, they can improve depressive symptoms, hence the importance of differentiating apathy from depression.
- A number of behavioural approaches have been suggested, many of which involve focusing on goal setting with an emphasis on planning future goals and evaluating success to help re-establish GDB.
- Simple measures may be helpful, including timetabling activities with reminders, to increase the chance the patient engages in activities. Often, they may lose the motivation to engage in activities but when they do, they may enjoy them.

- The symptoms of apathy can be distressing for the partner. It is important to explain to them that the apathetic symptoms are part of the brain damage and not because the patient is 'not trying'. We find a neuropsychologist appointment to advise both the patient and the partner on strategies can be helpful.

Further reading

Epidemiology

Pendlebury ST, Rothwell PM (2009). Prevalence, incidence, and factors associated with pre-stroke and post-stroke dementia: a systematic review and meta-analysis. *Lancet Neurol* **8**, 1006–18.

El Husseini N, Katzan IL, Rost NS *et al*. American Heart Association Stroke Council; Council on Cardiovascular and Stroke Nursing; Council on Cardiovascular Radiology and Intervention; Council on Hypertension; and Council on Lifestyle and Cardiometabolic Health. (2023) Cognitive Impairment After Ischemic and Hemorrhagic Stroke: A Scientific Statement From the American Heart Association/American Stroke Association. *Stroke*. 54:e272-e291.

Definitions of vascular dementia

Folloso MC, Villaraza SG, Yi-Wen, et al. (2024). The AHA/ASA and DSM-V diagnostic criteria for vascular cognitive impairment identify cases with predominant vascular pathology. *Int J Stroke* **19**, 925–934.

Post-stroke dementia and VCI

El Husseini N, Katzan IL, Rost NS, et al. American Heart Association Stroke Council; Council on Cardiovascular and Stroke Nursing; Council on Cardiovascular Radiology and Intervention; Council on Hypertension; and Council on Lifestyle and Cardiometabolic Health (2023). Cognitive impairment after ischemic and hemorrhagic stroke: a scientific statement from the American Heart Association/American Stroke Association. *Stroke* **54**, e272–e291.

Small-vessel disease dementia (subcortical vascular dementia)

Brookes RL, Hollocks MJ, Khan U, Morris RG, Markus HS (2015). The Brief Memory and Executive Test (BMET) for detecting vascular cognitive impairment in small vessel disease: a validation study. *BMC Med* **13**, 51.

Elahi FM, Wang MM, Meschia JF (2023). Cerebral small vessel disease-related dementia: more questions than answers. *Stroke* **54**, 648–660.

Overlap with Alzheimer's disease

Jellinger KA, Attems J (2014). The overlap between vascular disease and Alzheimer's disease—lessons from pathology. *BMC Med* **12**, 206.

Snowdon DA, Greiner LH, Mortimer JA, et al. (1997). Brain infarction and the clinical expression of Alzheimer's disease. The Nun Study. *JAMA* **277**, 813–817.

Sweeney MD, Montagne A, Sagare AP, et al. (2019). Vascular dysfunction—the disregarded partner of Alzheimer's disease. *Alzheimers Dement* 15(1), 158–167.

Therapy of dementia

Battle CE, Abdul-Rahim AH, Shenkin SD, Hewitt J, Quinn TJ (2021). Cholinesterase inhibitors for vascular dementia and other vascular cognitive impairments: a network meta-analysis. *Cochrane Database Syst Rev* **2**(2), CD013306.

Dichgans M, Markus HS, Salloway S, et al. (2008). Donepezil in patients with subcortical vascular cognitive impairment: a randomised double-blind trial in CADASIL. *Lancet Neurol* **7**, 310–318.

Markus HS, Egle M, Croall ID, et al. (2021). PRESERVE: randomized trial of intensive versus standard blood pressure control in small vessel disease. *Stroke* **52**, 2484–2493.

Mok VCT, Cai Y, Markus HS (2024). Vascular cognitive impairment and dementia: mechanisms, treatment, and future directions. *Int J Stroke* **19**, 838–856.

Pearce RL, McClure LA, Anderson DC, et al. (2014). Effects of long-term blood pressure lowering and dual antiplatelet treatment on cognitive function in patients with recent lacunar stroke: a secondary analysis from the SPS3 randomised trial. *Lancet Neurol* **13**, 1177–1185.

Quinn TJ, Richard E, Teuschl Y, et al. (2021). European Stroke Organisation and European Academy of Neurology joint guidelines on post-stroke cognitive impairment. *Eur J Neurol* **28**(12), 3883–3920.

SPRINT MIND Investigators for the SPRINT Research Group; Williamson JD, Pajewski NM, et al. (2019). Effect of intensive vs standard blood pressure control on probable dementia: a randomized clinical trial. *JAMA* **321**, 553–561.

Depression in VCI

Brookes RL, Willis TA, Patel B, et al. (2013). Depressive symptoms as a predictor of quality of life in cerebral small vessel disease, acting independently of disability; a study in both sporadic small vessel disease and CADASIL. *Int J Stroke* **8**, 510–517.

Hackett ML, Köhler S, O'Brien JT, Mead GE (2014). Neuropsychiatric outcomes of stroke. *Lancet Neurol* **13**, 525–534.

Apathy in VCI

Tay J, Morris RG, Markus HS (2012). Apathy after stroke: diagnosis, mechanisms, consequences, and treatment. *Int J Stroke* **16**, 510–518.

Organization
of stroke services

Introduction

- Stroke has been recognized in medicine for more than 3000 years but only recently has stroke medicine been considered a specialty in its own right
- As a disease of ageing, stroke has been susceptible to age-related prejudice, which has hindered the development of services and investment in research
- In the context of a worldwide ageing population and advances in evidence-based interventions, stroke care has changed all over the world with the recognition that stroke is now a treatable condition
- Since the landmark work of the Stroke Unit Trialists' Collaboration in the 1990s, stroke units now feature in hospitals worldwide, although large geographical disparities remain
- There is still much to be done and an organizational (evidence-based) framework is the cornerstone of delivering effective stroke care
- In England and Wales, this was first set out for the first time since the creation of the NHS in The National Stroke Strategy (2007). The process of continual improvement has continued with the publication of The NHS Long Term Plan (2019), Get It Right First Time—Stroke (GIRFT-Stroke 2021), National Sentinel Audit of Stroke (2021) and National Clinical Guideline for Stroke (2023)
- Stroke services should be organized to fit within the structure of the existing healthcare system but require a systematic approach to provide a 'pathway' along which a patient with stroke may 'journey'. Such a pathway should have five components:
  - Effective primary prevention and public awareness of stroke symptoms
  - Direct access to specialist acute stroke services for diagnosis, treatment, and secondary prevention
  - Stroke unit care in hospital
  - Specialist stroke rehabilitation
  - Re-integration into community life after stroke.

The pathway will involve primary and secondary healthcare as well as social care providers and voluntary sector bodies.

For the purpose of this chapter, the stroke pathway will be divided into three phases:

- Pre-hospital care
- Acute hospital care
- Post-hospital care.

Pre-hospital care

- Acute stroke care begins with the timely recognition of the symptoms of stroke and treating stroke as a 'medical emergency'. This involves both public education and education of the wider healthcare community
- With the advent of reperfusion therapy for acute ischaemic stroke and time-critical intervention for intracerebral haemorrhage, the need for an acute stroke 'pathway' and early symptom recognition is paramount
- Rapid transportation to an acute stroke centre (alerting the hospital in advance to the patient's imminent arrival) is a prerequisite for delivering reperfusion treatment for threatened ischaemic stroke as outcomes are time-dependent
- A key concept when planning pre-hospital care is that 'Time is brain'
- Simple tools have been developed to help with stroke symptom recognition by paramedics. Pre-hospital stroke recognition instruments were first introduced in the mid-1990s in the USA (Los Angeles Paramedic Stroke Scale [LAPSS] and Cincinnati Prehospital Stroke Scale [CPSS]) and in the late 1990s in the UK (Face Arm Speech Test [FAST], a modification of the Cincinnati scale)
- The FAST was designed to be an integral part of a training package for UK ambulance personnel. As with the CPSS, the FAST consists of three items (facial weakness, arm weakness, and speech disturbance) but avoids the need for the patient to repeat a sentence as a measure of speech. Instead, language fluency and clarity are assessed by the paramedic during conversation with the patient (see Fig. 16.1)
- The FAST is being increasingly used as a method for the public to be alerted to the symptoms of stroke
- The FAST is particularly good at detecting large hemispheric stroke (e.g. MCA stroke syndromes) but is less good at detecting posterior circulation stroke syndromes
- The FAST has approximately a 20–25% false-positive rate and is not a substitute for taking a proper history and carrying out a complete clinical examination to determine a likely diagnosis of stroke in a hospital emergency department
- Other pre-hospital screens have been introduced (e.g. paramedic crews using ROSIER pre-hospital) but have not proven to be significantly superior to the FAST in terms of sensitivity and specificity, although some screening tests, such as ACT-FAST and RACE (Rapid Arterial ocClusion Evaluation) may be better at identifying patients with a large intracranial vessel occlusion (potentially suitable for thrombectomy)
- Recently, the concept of the Mobile Stroke Unit (MSU) has been tested in a number of different trials. MSUs are specialist ambulances, equipped with onboard brain imaging capability (currently limited to CT), point-of-care testing, and stroke expertise with a specialist nurse and/or stroke neurologist. The latter may be available by a telehealth link. Although trialled only in large metropolitan areas, MSUs have been associated with increased odds of excellent outcomes (both in reducing onset to reperfusion times and proportion of patients receiving

reperfusion therapy and also, importantly, in reducing the chances of severe disability) when compared to usual care

• Pre-hospital specialist stroke care has been delivered further away from stroke centres using stroke-capable helicopters and light aircraft to enable patients in rural and remote areas to access timely stroke care. Equipping aircraft with new lightweight CT scanners or alternative brain imaging modalities (e.g. using microwave technology) is key and at the time of the third edition, this is a topic for research rather than clinical practice.

The FAST test

• F = FACE: Ask the person to smile. Does one side of the mouth or face droop?
• A = ARMS: Ask the person to raise both arms. Does one arm drift downward or can't be raised?
• S = SPEECH: Ask the person to repeat a sentence. Can they repeat it correctly? Do they slur the words?
• T = TIME: If the person exhibits any problems with these, call for emergency help.

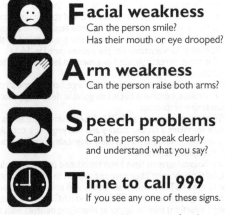

Facial weakness
Can the person smile?
Has their mouth or eye drooped?

Arm weakness
Can the person raise both arms?

Speech problems
Can the person speak clearly
and understand what you say?

Time to call 999
If you see any one of these signs.

Fig. 16.1 A poster designed to promote public awareness of stroke using the FAST test.
© Stroke Association. Reproduced with permission.

Acute hospital care

This starts with fast and accurate stroke diagnosis.

Initial emergency room diagnosis

In hospital, a stroke diagnosis can be assisted speedily, relatively accurately, and reliably by non-specialist healthcare professionals using the ROSIER scoring system (Fig. 16.2). The aim of this assessment tool is to enable medical and nursing staff to differentiate patients with stroke from stroke mimics.

Other aspects of acute stroke care organization

- Brain imaging is always required to confirm the diagnosis of stroke
- In all cases, especially in cases potentially suitable for thrombolysis, imaging is an emergency. Emergency CTA with or without CT perfusion to confirm the presence of intracranial occlusion or hypoperfusion is now often used as an adjunct to anatomical brain imaging to help select cases for endovascular reperfusion therapy
- A formal thrombolysis and thrombectomy protocol with appropriate training for staff is essential
- Acute stroke should be managed in an organized acute stroke unit
- If the stroke diagnosis is subarachnoid haemorrhage, the patient is best managed in a centre with neuroradiology and neurosurgical expertise as well as a specialist intensive care unit
- The use of documented protocols for major aspects of management (such as for thrombolysis and intracerebral haemorrhage 'care bundle') and of proformas for data collection are important
- Continuous audit of processes of care and clinical outcome is an essential part of a good stroke service
- Transfer of care from acute hospital should involve a comprehensive multidisciplinary discharge summary. Appropriate follow-up is needed if there are outstanding matters involving diagnosis, secondary prevention, or other issues around stroke recovery.

Thrombolysis as a driver for change

Thrombolysis treatment for acute stroke, offering the possibility for the first time of cure for stroke, was the one thing more than any other that changed how stroke services were organized. It was this treatment that predominantly led to stroke now being considered a 'medical emergency'.

Potential barriers to stroke thrombolysis occur in both the pre-hospital and acute hospital care pathway and include the following:

- Failure to recognise symptoms of stroke by patient or family and/or failure to seek urgent help
- Failing to go directly to the hospital (i.e. calling the general practitioner/ family doctor rather than an ambulance first)
- Paramedics and emergency department staff triaging stroke as non-urgent or failing to diagnose stroke
- Delays in neuroimaging
- Inefficient process of in-hospital emergency stroke care
- Physicians' uncertainty about administering thrombolysis

- Evidence from acute stroke services in England also suggests a significant effect of the volume of cases on the effective process of care in terms of door-to-needle time. In units that thrombolyse more than 50 cases per year, the median door-to-needle time was around 30 minutes shorter than those who treated fewer cases. The effect was even more marked in centres thrombolysing more than 100 cases/year
- All of these issues and more apply to delivering thrombectomy for acute ischaemic stroke, including a volume/outcome effect
- With thrombectomy being delivered in specialist centres, coordinated care and transfer between a receiving hospital and the thrombectomy centre is required to safely facilitate a process known as 'drip and ship' transfer. The time it takes for a hospital to assess, diagnose a large vessel occlusion, treat with thrombolysis, refer to a thrombectomy centre and then transfer out is called the Door In Door Out (DIDO) time.

Exclude BM <3.5 mmol/L, treat urgently, and reassess once blood glucose normal

Has there been loss of consciousness or syncope?	Y (−1)✍	N (0)✍
Has there been seizure activity?	Y (−1)✍	N (0)✍
Is there a *new acute* onset (or on awakening from sleep)?		
I. Asymmetric facial weakness	Y (+1)✍	N (0)✍
II. Asymmetric arm weakness	Y (+1)✍	N (0)✍
III. Asymmetric leg weakness	Y (+1)✍	N (0)✍
IV. Speech disturbance	Y (+1)✍	N (0)✍
V. Visual field effect	Y (+1)✍	N (0)✍

*Total score____ (−2 to +5)
Provisional diagnosis: ✍ Stroke
✍ Non-stroke (specify) ________

*Stroke is likely if total scores are >0. Scores of </=0 have a low possibility of stroke but it is not completely excluded

Fig. 16.2 The ROSIER scale designed to aid in emergency room diagnosis of stroke patients.

Reproduced from *Lancet Neurology*, 4(11), Nor AM, Davis J, Sen B, *et al.*, The Recognition of Stroke in the Emergency Room (ROSIER) scale: development and validation of a stroke recognition instrument, pp. 727–734, Copyright (2005), with permission from Elsevier.

Stroke units

The evidence from over 30 trials, in 7000 stroke patients, is that organized care on a specialized stroke unit reduces death, disability, and the number of stroke patients needing discharge into institutionalized long-term care.

Although the evidence is based on a number of different models of stroke unit care, the best results come from those which are based in a dedicated ward.

What is a stroke unit?

There are a number of models of stroke unit—acute, rehabilitation, mixed—all of which have the same core features of:
• geographically defined area in a hospital
• evidence-based protocols for treating stroke and its complications
• τηε ethos of promoting stroke recovery and rehabilitation
• coordinated multidisciplinary care
• programmes of education in stroke.

Acute stroke units must have:
• access to urgent brain imaging
• rapid assessment protocols for thrombolysis
• proactive/anticipatory management of common complications of stroke
• non-invasive physiological monitoring for:
  • heart rate (arrhythmia)
  • blood pressure
  • respiratory rate
  • O_2 saturation
  • temperature
  • glucose
• protocols and guidelines in all areas of acute stroke management.

Why do stroke units succeed?

Although evidence shows that stroke units reduce mortality there is no definite information on what aspects of care result in this improvement. It is likely that many aspects of care result in this improvement, such as the following:
• Interested and motivated staff
• Evidence-based, protocol-driven management
• Reduction of complications (e.g. DVT, pneumonia)
• More intensive medical intervention: observational studies have shown interventions such as IV fluids in the first 24 hours, insulin therapy, antibiotic therapy, and O_2 are more common in stroke units
• More organized and intensive therapy: e.g. observational studies have shown that early mobilization is more common in stroke units
• What is clear is that thrombolysis does not account for the difference in mortality or other outcomes in the historical stroke unit trials. Only a small minority of patients received it in the trials.

Staffing a stroke unit

- There is no single correct answer to how many staff are required on a stroke unit, although there are some interesting proposals
- Most of the time, the issue is limited resources
- Stroke units should have an establishment of medical, nursing, physiotherapy, and occupational therapy, speech and language therapy, dietician, and clinical psychology healthcare staff
- In England, the Department of Health suggested a workforce establishment based on consensus views and compared it to an actual survey. A survey of recommendations is shown in Table 16.1
- Within the table, the estimated number of whole working-time equivalent members of each profession per ten beds of stroke unit are shown
- Sources of data and guidance include the Stroke Unit Trialists' Collaboration (SUTC), the National Sentinel Stroke Audit, the British and Irish Association of Stroke Physicians (BIASP), and the National Clinical Guideline for Stroke (2023)
- Evidence from National Audit data from England, Wales, and Northern Ireland has shown that nursing staff numbers over a 24-hour period at weekends on a stroke unit directly correlate with mortality. This has given weight to the call for the minimum number of acute stroke unit nurses on duty at any time to be three per ten beds 24/7
- Staffing in stroke units inevitably varies. In another western European country, Austria, an acute stroke unit of four to eight beds would typically have:
  - One neurologist
  - One nurse per bed
  - One physiotherapist, one occupational therapist, and one speech and language therapist per four beds.

This is similar to the aspirational levels of staffing proposed by the English Department of Health.

Stroke unit certification and accreditation

- Stroke Unit Certification allows units to benchmark themselves against recognized standards and can be useful in driving up standards of care.
- There are many different accreditation processes worldwide.
- In the United States the Get with the Guidelines Certification process ℬ https://www.heart.org/en/professional/quality-improvement/get-with-the-guidelines/get-with-the-guidelines-stroke/get-with-the-guidelines-stroke-recognition-criteria).
- A similar awards-based recognition system is promoted by the World and European Stroke Organization called the 'Angels' awards (ℬ https://www.world-stroke.org/what-we-do/education-and-research/improving-access-to-quality-stroke-care/wso-awards).
- Obtaining an award can be highly motivating for the local stroke team

Table 16.1 Recommended levels of staffing for hyperacute, acute, and rehabilitation units.

Empty cell	PT WTE/ Five beds	OT WTE/ Five beds	SLT WTE/ Five beds	Psy WTE/ Five beds	Dietn WTE/ Five beds	Nurse WTE/ One bed	Consultant Physician
HASU	1.02	0.95	0.48	0.28	0.21	2.9	24/7 availability: minimum six thrombolysis trained physicians on rota
ASU and SRU	1.18	1.13	0.56	0.28	0.21	1.35	ASU: daily ward round with 7 day cover SRU: twice weekly ward round*

Reproduced from Ajay Bhalla, Louise Clark, Rebecca Fisher, Martin James. The new national clinical guideline for stroke: an opportunity to transform stroke care. *Clin Med* 2024, 24(2). https://doi.org/10.1016/j.clinme.2024.100025

ASU = acute stroke unit, HASU = hyperacute stroke unit, SRU = stroke rehabilitation unit.

PT = physiotherapy, OT = occupational therapy, SLT = speech and language therapy, Psy = psychology.

Dietn = dietician, WTE = whole time equivalent.* can be provided by a non-medical stroke consultant.

Telehealth in stroke care

- Telehealth utilization in stroke care has increased enormously since the COVID-19 pandemic
- Video-enabled remote consultation, either pre-hospital or in emergency departments, has been shown to be safe and increase access to reperfusion therapies to patients in rural or remote non-specialist hospitals
- Telehealth has now been used to conduct stroke unit ward rounds and outpatient clinics as well as administer rehabilitation intervention ('telerehab') and is an important aspect of delivering equitable, organized, and specialist care

In-hospital stroke

- 2–17% of all strokes occur in patients already in hospital.
- Outcomes are historically much worse for this cohort of patients—many of whom suffer stroke related to a procedure (e.g. cardiac surgery) or because their usual stroke prevention medication is stopped during the admission (e.g. cessation of anticoagulation for AF).
- Cohort studies have demonstrated delays in symptom recognition and imaging—which seems paradoxical given the events that happen in a hospital.
- While many in-hospital strokes have a contraindication to thrombolysis, the advent of thrombectomy has meant many are still potentially eligible for reperfusion therapy as large intracranial vessel occlusion strokes are overrepresented in this group.
- Outcomes from thrombectomy are more uncertain than stroke occurring in the community and often depend upon the underlying comorbidity responsible for hospitalization.
- Local pathways of care (and staff education) to manage in-hospital strokes are important in 'high-risk' areas such as cardiac wards.

Post-hospital care

Early supported discharge (ESD)

- For patients with mild to moderate disability after stroke, 'early supported discharge' by a specialist multidisciplinary (rehabilitation) team reduces death and disability (as well as length of hospital stay)
- Such models of stroke care have, however, been associated with a suspicion of increased carer burden.

Bed-based stroke rehabilitation

- This is likely to be the most appropriate post-acute stroke care for patients with severe and complex neurological disability from stroke
- Coordinated multidisciplinary care with a 'goal planning' approach is usual in a bed-based setting, which would have 24-hour nursing supervision and a geographical setting removed from the acute hospital (see ➲ Chapter 14).

Community stroke services

- Unidisciplinary or multidisciplinary community-based rehabilitation services are an important part of post-acute stroke care
- Ideally, patients should move seamlessly into a bespoke programme of community-based neurorehabilitation according to their needs, as early intervention is likely to have the greatest impact on functional outcome
- This may be either administered at home or in a community-based rehabilitation centre
- Such a service is also essential for the management of ongoing symptoms for those left with chronic long-term neurological conditions as a result of stroke (e.g. wheelchair services, spasticity clinics, and orthotics).

Role of the voluntary sector

Voluntary sector organizations and peer groups of patients and carers can help with rebuilding confidence after stroke and provide valuable social, emotional, and practical support, enabling integration back into a community setting.

Further reading

Pre-hospital care

Turc G, Hadziahmetovic M, Walter S, et al. (2022). Comparison of mobile stroke unit with usual care for acute ischemic stroke management: a systematic review and meta-analysis. *JAMA Neurol* **79**, 281–290.

Acute hospital care

Bray B, Campbell J, Cloud GC, et al. (2013). Bigger, faster? Associations between hospital thrombolysis volume and speed of thrombolysis administration in acute ischemic stroke. *Stroke* **44**, 3129–3135.

Kleinig TJ, McMullan P, Cloud GC, et al. (2024). Hyper-acute stroke systems of care and workflow. *Curr Neurol Neurosci Rep* **24**, 495–505.

Stroke units

Bray BD, Ayis S, Campbell J, et al. (2014). Associations between stroke mortality and weekend working by stroke specialist physicians and registered nurses: prospective multicentre cohort study. *PLoS Med* **11**, e1001705.

Bhalla A, Clark L, Fisher R, James M (2024). The new national clinical guideline for stroke: an opportunity to transform stroke care. *Clin Med (Lond)* **24**, 100025.

Langhorne P (2021). The stroke unit story: where have we been and where are we going? *Cerebrovasc Dis* **50**, 636–643.

Langhorne P, Ramachandra S 2020. Organised inpatient (stroke unit) care for stroke: network meta-analysis. *Cochrane Database Syst Rev* **4**, CD000197.

Post-hospital care

Early supported discharge

NICE (2023). *Evidence Reviews for Early Supported Discharge: Stroke Rehabilitation In Adults* (update): evidence review A2. London: National Institute for Health and Care Excellence (NICE. NICE Guideline, No. 236.). Available online from: https://www.ncbi.nlm.nih.gov/books/NBK600621/

Clinical pathways in stroke rehabilitation

Platz T, Owolabi M (2021). Clinical pathways in stroke rehabilitation: background, scope, and methods. In: Platz, T. (ed.). *Clinical Pathways in Stroke Rehabilitation*. Cham: Springer. https://doi.org/10.1007/978-3-030-58505-1_2

Telehealth in Stroke care

Kasab S, Martini SR, Meyer BC, Demaerschalk BM, Wozniak MA, Southerland AM (2021). Telestroke across the continuum of care: lessons from the COVID-19 pandemic. *J Stroke Cerebrovasc Dis* **30**, 105802.

Bonita A, Clarke T, Roy A, James R (2024). The new national clinical guideline for stroke: an expert consensus from the new and future One Medicine in 14. *IJSO V3*.

Eco Enterprise P (2021). The future ten: One medicine hierarchy and what's great. *Journal of Common Care.* 1: 58, 615–665.

Lippmann R R, matthews Koy v 2020. Cognitive assessment forms drug cues to a surgical recovery care. *medline Science. Dataframe hot hot v 6. CL3000191*

Post-hospital care

Early supported discharge

NICE (2023). Stroke in over 16s: Early supported Recovery. Stroke Rehabilitation in adults, the social evidence review A1: London national institute for health and Care Excellence. (NICE Guideline L and C43.) [online]. Available online from: https://www.nice.org.uk/guidance/ng236

Dietary behaviour in stroke rehabilitation

Park T, Edwards M (2021). Dietary patterns in stroke rehabilitation overview: scope and outcomes in older. T Reg J Clinical review a b multidisciplinary. Online Sciences M 92. *Viral Medical 10.1001/1916.2020-61201.*

Telehealth in Stroke care

Appel S, Peter M, McGary GC, Buts and e de. Webber MA, Schmidt and MA (2021). Telemedicine in the treatment of acute stroke T J online. J Clinical Technology Science handbook 68. 80.100002.

Ethical issues
in stroke care

Background and legal framework

When making any clinical decision, a healthcare professional needs to be sure that they are firmly on the 'playing field of medical ethics' which has as its boundaries the four cornerstones of:

• *Autonomy* (what the patient wants/patient choice)
• *Beneficence* (to do good by the patient)
• *Non-maleficence* (to do no harm to the patient)
• *Justice/equity* (to be 'fair').

The final consideration is *legality*. Healthcare professionals cannot act outside the law. Considerations of legality differ between countries. For example, physician-assisted suicide is a criminal offence in the UK and the USA, but is legal within strictly regulated guidelines in some other countries such as Switzerland, the Netherlands, and Australia.

While much of what is outlined in this chapter is based on UK and European legislation, the principles discussed are generally applicable to all those working with stroke patients.

European Law of Human Rights—The Human Rights Act 1998

This came into force in the UK at the beginning of October 2000.
The articles of the act most relevant to clinical care are:

• Article 2: right to life
• Article 3: prohibition of torture and inhuman and degrading treatment. This was termed as an 'absolute human right'
• Article 5: right to liberty
• Article 8: right to respect for private and family life, home, and correspondence
• Article 10: freedom of expression and right to information
• Article 14: right not to be discriminated against on grounds of, for example, race, sex, etc.

Details of the act can be found at the following web address: ℘ http://www.opsi.gov.uk/ACTS/acts1998/ukpga_19980042_en_1

Confidentiality

Confidentiality is essential to respect a patient's confidentiality. The following points are taken from guidance issued by the General Medical Council (GMC)—the regulatory body of the medical profession in the UK. They are, however, widely applicable and represent a good standard of practice.

- Patients have a right to expect that a doctor will not disclose any personal information which they learn during the course of their professional duties, unless the patient gives permission
- Disclosure of medical information between medical teams in hospital and between the hospital and general practitioner (family doctor) is clearly required for treatment to which a patient has agreed and, as such, the patient's explicit consent is not needed. The same goes in cases of medical emergency
- Disclosure to employers and insurance companies should only be undertaken with the patient's written consent
- The following are circumstances where disclosure without the patient's consent may be appropriate:
  - 'In the patient's medical interests'
  - 'In the best interests of others', i.e. in the public interest.

Capacity

- The terms competence and capacity are often used interchangeably:
  - Competence is a legal concept
  - Capacity is a more pragmatic concept related to a clinical setting where a clinician determines the patient's ability to make an informed decision about his or her healthcare.
- The law presumes all adults to have capacity until proven otherwise
- Capacity is specific to the task being considered, not global. For example, in the first few days after a stroke, a patient who has the capacity to decide whether they prefer tea or coffee may not have the capacity to decide whether they wish to enter a research trial of a novel pharmacological agent
- Owing to the high incidence of communication problems following stroke, capacity decisions are often difficult. The common issues that need assessment of capacity involve treatment decisions (e.g. insertion of a feeding gastrostomy tube), discharge planning (e.g. a patient with high-level care needs who refuses help or adaptations but insists on returning home), and finances
- Many patients with aphasia still have capacity provided the assessment is conducted using supported communication techniques, such as 'total communication' which utilizes verbal, written, and gestured communication. In trying to assess capacity in a patient with aphasia, a joint review with a speech and language therapist (and a clinical neuropsychologist if available) is helpful. Where there is doubt (either way), provided there is no life-threatening urgency to the decision, it is always better to wait and return at a different time or day to form a final opinion
- Next are several examples of guidance showing how the concept of assessing capacity has developed—all of which have a similar theme.

Applebaum and Grisso (1988): *Standards for Determining Capacity*

(*The New England Journal of Medicine* **319**, 1635–1638.)
- The ability to maintain and communicate stable choices
- The comprehension of the information presented
- The appreciation of the likely consequences
- The ability to manipulate the information rationally.

Case Law (UK): Legal Capacity and Consent to Treatment: Re C [Adult Refusal of Medical treatment 1994, 1 A11 ER 819]

An adult has the legal capacity to give consent or refuse consent to medical treatment if he or she can:
- understand and retain the information relevant to the decision in question
- believe that information
- weigh that information in the balance to arrive at a choice.

British Medical Association and Law Society (1995):
Assessment of Mental Capacity Guidance for Doctors and Lawyers
(London: BMA, p. 66.)

To be considered to have the capacity to undergo a medical treatment, a patient should:
• understand, in simple language, what the medical treatment is, its purpose, and why it is being proposed
• understand its principal benefits, risks, and alternatives
• understand in broad terms what the consequences would be of not receiving the proposed treatment
• retain the information long enough to make an effective decision
• make a free choice.

Mental Capacity Act (MCA) 2005 (England and Wales)
This came into effect in October 2007 and is a new framework for decision-making on behalf of adults aged 16 and over.

Basic principles include:
• a presumption of capacity in all
• maximizing decision-making capacity (e.g. using 'total communication strategies' with a speech and language therapist to determine capacity in an aphasic patient)
• the freedom to make unwise decisions
• best interests—incorporating the person's past and present wishes (including any advance life directives) and their beliefs or values
• the least restrictive alternative.

The test of capacity should include a patient's ability to demonstrate four things:
• To understand information relevant to the decision
• To retain information relevant to the decision
• To use or weigh the information
• To communicate the decision (by any means).

In practice, it is this test that we routinely use when assessing capacity in the English NHS.
• The Act also changed the role of the holder of 'Power of Attorney', formerly known as Enduring Power of Attorney (EPA) and now known as Lasting Power of Attorney (LPA). Power of Attorney is drawn up by an adult with capacity in anticipation of a future point in time when they may be unable to make decisions for themselves (i.e. lack capacity). The person making the Power of Attorney (the donor) appoints another to act on their behalf (the receiver) and registers this with the Office of the Public Guardian. The Power of Attorney only becomes activated when the donor is deemed to have lost capacity
• Prior to 2007, the holder of Power of Attorney only had control over the donor's financial affairs and estate. Now, the receiver in England, Wales, and Scotland is also the voice of the donor with regard to medical decision-making
• The Act introduced a new process for adults who lack capacity, have neither an appointed Power of Attorney, nor appropriate next of kin. In such a scenario, an Independent Mental Capacity Advocate (IMCA) is

legally required to ensure the patient's best interests are being followed. IMCAs are trained advocates, independent of Health and Social Services
- Where an adult lacks both capacity and an appointed Power of Attorney, but has an appropriate next of kin, the next of kin can still apply for receivership to manage the person's affairs via the Court of Protection. Like LPAs, deputies appointed by the Court of Protection will be able to make decisions on welfare, healthcare, and financial matters but will not be able to refuse consent to life-sustaining treatment
- Finally, the Act introduced a new criminal offence of ill-treatment or neglect of a person who lacks capacity—punishable by imprisonment for up to 5 years
- Full details of the Act are at: ℠ http://www.opsi.gov.uk/ACTS/acts2 005/ukpga_20050009_en_1

Deprivation of Liberty Safeguards (DoLS)

- An amendment to the Mental Capacity Act (MCA) of 2005 and applies in England and Wales in the setting of hospitals and care homes only
- On stroke (rehabilitation) units, this usually only applies to patients who lack capacity around issues of discharge and need to be kept on the unit against their wishes. The least restrictive restraint should be applied in accordance with the MCA. Where restraints are used frequently or for a prolonged period of time, they may in effect deprive a person of their liberty and then DoLS needs to be activated
- The two questions to be considered are:
  - Is the patient subject to continuous supervision and control?
  - Is the patient free to leave permanently?
- Where possible, interventions involving family, friends, and carers should be tried before using the DoLS. The deprivation of a person's liberty is a very serious matter and should only occur when it is absolutely necessary and clearly in their best interests
- In the context of stroke units, hospitals as the 'managing authority' may have to apply for an *urgent* DoLS, which can authorize for 7 days. This can only be extended after applying for DoLS to a 'supervisory body' (Local Authority in England), for an assessment for standard of authorization. This is ideally performed by two trained independent assessors—one a mental health assessor and one a 'best interests' assessor. The former is to ensure that the Mental Health Act should not be applied and in practice seldom happens in the absence of psychiatric diagnosis. In the absence of close family, carers or friends, an IMCA may be appointed during the assessment process
- In applying for a standard of authorization for deprivation of liberty, the managing authority must specify its duration, which should not exceed 12 months. The authorization should be reviewed and possibly revoked if there is a significant change in the person's condition in the meantime
- DoLS cannot be applied for if there is a valid LPA who has objected to the proposed restraints, which in effect cause deprivation of liberty
- The chief coroner issued guidance in 2015 that an inquest should be held after the death of a patient who is under a deprivation of liberty order.

Liberty Protection Safeguards

- The Liberty Protection Safeguards were introduced in the Mental Capacity (Amendment) Act 2019 and are on the horizon to replace the Deprivation of Liberty Safeguards (DoLS) system.
- ℘ https://www.legislation.gov.uk/ukpga/2019/18/notes/division/2/index.htm
- will apply to 16- and 17-year-olds in addition to over 18s.
- will also apply to people in the community and their own homes.
- will affect wider arrangements for a patient's care, so it will incorporate several settings (not just a hospital or care home).
- A responsible body (NHS hospital, integrated care board, local health board, or local authority) will replace the supervisory body.

Consent

Informed consent for clinical procedures

- Without valid consent, a healthcare professional may not lawfully examine or treat a competent adult
- Proceeding to physical examination without consent (or valid refusal) risks committing battery (unconsented touching) or assault
- The principle of respect for autonomy grants patients a right to decline investigations or treatment, even if in doing so they risk ill health or death.

Some key points on consent: the law in England

- The consent process has two possible outcomes—acceptance or refusal
- Issues of consent are principally about acceptance of medical treatment and social care
- Consent can be written, verbal, or implied by actions
- A signature on a consent form is *evidence* that a patient has given consent, but is not *proof* of valid consent
- For consent to be valid, the patient must:
  - have capacity to take the particular decision
  - have received adequate information to take it
  - not be acting under duress (voluntary).

The last point is interesting in the context of gaining informed consent for stroke thrombolysis. In our experience, while in the midst of an acute ischaemic brain injury patients are often incapable of giving informed consent. In such cases it is our practice to gain only *assent* while informing the next of kin about the treatment decision.

What is adequate information?

In 1985, the House of Lords adopted the Bolam test (named after a patient who claimed he had not been given adequate information before receiving electroconvulsant therapy in 1954).

This legal standard when deciding whether adequate information has been given to a patient should be the same as that used when judging whether a doctor has been negligent in their treatment or care of a patient (i.e. they would not be considered negligent if their practice conformed to that of a responsible body of medical opinion).

This can still be open to the courts to decide.

Consent for research trials and other studies

Consenting to enter a research trial involves knowing about:

- the research purpose, questions, aims, and methods
- relevant terms like 'randomize'
- the treatment, if any, which the research investigates
- benefits, risks, harms, or costs to research subjects
- hoped-for benefits to other groups, such as future patients
- confidentiality, indemnity, sponsors, and ethical approval
- the research team and a named contact.

Example: consenting for carotid endarterectomy
- Patient must be able to demonstrate capacity around the decision to accept or refuse the operation, i.e.:
  - Be able to understand the information relevant to the decision (understand that the cause of the stroke episode is a narrowed carotid artery which, if left untreated, leaves them at higher risk of recurrent stroke than if they accept the operation)
  - To retain the information relevant to the decision
  - To use or weigh the information (risks of surgery against risks of medical treatment)
  - To communicate the decision (verbally, in writing, or by gesture)
- Patient must be given sufficient information around the procedure, including risk of stroke, death, other typical complications of surgery (scar, wound healing issues, possible local cranial nerve damage), and any alternative treatments (e.g. stenting if appropriate)

It is well within a patient's remit to ask an individual surgeon their personal rates of success and complication.

Research in adults who lack capacity
- Sections 30–33 of the Mental Capacity Act (MCA) provide lawful authority for intrusive research to be carried out involving people without capacity, provided the research has been approved by an appropriate body. Intrusive research is any normally requiring a competent adult's consent
- Clinical trials of investigational medicinal products (CTIMPs) are not covered in the MCA as adults lacking capacity in CTIMPs are included in Schedule 1 of the Medicines for Human Use (Clinical Trials) Regulations 2004
- In the UK, GMC guidelines suggest research into conditions with adults with incapacity should only be undertaken if it is related to their incapacity or its treatment and should not be undertaken if it could equally well be done with other adults
- Guidance is available in the UK from the GMC, '*Research: The role and responsibilities of doctors*', which suggests that if research involves subjects with incapacity, you must demonstrate that:
  - it could be of direct benefit to their health, or
  - it is of special benefit to the health of people in the same age group with the same state of health, or
  - that it will significantly improve the scientific understanding of the adult's incapacity, leading to a direct benefit to them or others with the same incapacity (e.g. hyperacute stroke research)
  - the research is ethical and will not cause the participants emotional, physical, or psychological harm
  - the person does not express objections physically or verbally.

Withholding treatment and withdrawing medical treatment

This is an extremely emotive and potentially upsetting scenario in stroke care, but one which not infrequently arises—especially where the stroke is associated with a bleak prognosis.

It always requires careful attention, a multidisciplinary team approach, and sensitive communication with family, carers, and friends.

Withdrawing artificial nutrition and hydration

- There is considerable variation in what constitutes 'basic care' and what constitutes 'medical treatment' across Europe.
- Currently, artificial nutrition and hydration (ANH) is not 'basic care' but medical treatment in English law.
- The intention of withholding or withdrawing life-prolonging treatment is to avoid treatment that is not benefiting the patient. Judgements on the value of a patient's life should not be made.
- The British Medical Association (BMA) recommends clinical review by a second specialist not involved in the care team, respecting advance life directives if available, and, if not, seeking information from family members and close friends as to the patient's wishes.

Advance decisions/advanced life directives (ALDs)

Also known as 'living wills' or 'advanced refusals'.
- Must be drawn up by competent patients
- Three main types:
  1. Instructive (legally binding); e.g. 'If I had a stroke and was unable to walk again, I would not want any life-prolonging treatment, including tube feeding'
  2. Values; e.g. 'If I had a stroke which meant I was no longer able to complete my favourite newspaper cryptic crossword I would not want any life-prolonging treatment'
  3. Proxy; e.g. 'If as a result of a disabling stroke I am unable to make my own decisions regarding medical treatment I would want my son to do so on my behalf'
- Should be respected where appropriate and patient now *lacks* mental capacity (*legally binding*)
- In the UK, a person can make an Advance Decision to Refuse Treatment (ADRT)—e.g. to refuse life-sustaining treatment.
- The British Medical Association has developed a straightforward guidance document around advance decisions as part of their consent 'toolkit': ℘ https://www.bma.org.uk/media/1850/bma-best-interests-toolkit-2019.pdf
- An example of a living will is available from ℘ https://compassionindying.org.uk/how-we-can-help/living-will-advance-decision/#make-a-living-will

Prolonged disorders of consciousness

Prolonged disorders of consciousness (PDOC) is the term used for patients in prolonged coma and includes (persistent) vegetative state (VS) and minimally conscious state (MCS).

These are rare consequences of stroke but present significant ethical and emotional issues for the treating teams.

Precise terminology is important as it may have medicolegal implications (see Table 17.1).

(Persistent) Vegetative state

- First described by Jennett and Plum in 1972 as 'the absence of any adaptive response to the external environment, the absence of any evidence of a functioning mind which is either receiving or projecting information, in a patient who has long periods of wakefulness'
- Clinically, patients are able to breathe without mechanical support and cardiovascular, gastrointestinal, and renal function must be stable. The patient may be aroused by painful stimuli (eye-opening or grimacing). Patients also show spontaneous movements such as chewing, teeth grinding, smiling, crying, grunting, or screaming
- Essential criteria *for* VS is no evidence of:
  1. awareness of self or environment or the ability to interact with others
  2. sustained purposeful or voluntary behaviour, either spontaneously or in response to visual, auditory, tactile, or noxious stimuli
  3. language, comprehension, or meaningful expression
- Features that are *not* compatible with VS include:
  - evidence of discriminative perception
  - purposeful actions
  - anticipatory actions
  - communicative acts, e.g. a smile specifically in response to the arrival of a friend or relative would be incompatible with VS, whereas a spontaneous smile would be compatible
  - VS due to stroke is rare and is most often seen where stroke is complicated by a prolonged hypoxic brain injury caused by a secondary complication
  - VS in stroke (i.e. atraumatic) is considered to be permanent after 3 months in the USA, with UK guidance suggesting a more conservative 6-month period needs to be seen
- Prognosis—recovery to a state of severe disability is seen in up to 1.6% of patients with persistent VS at 1 year.

Minimally conscious state

- Defined as 'A state of severely altered consciousness in which minimal but clearly discernible behavioural evidence of self- or environmental awareness is demonstrated'
- A state of unconsciousness in which eyes are closed and sleep–wake cycles are absent. After 4 weeks of fulfilling the definition, a patient can be considered in a state of continuing MCS (CMCS). After 6 months of MCS is the patient said to be in permanent MCS (PMCS).

Table 17.1 Comparison of clinical features associated with coma, vegetative state, minimally conscious state, and locked-in syndrome

Condition	Consciousness	Sleep/wake	Motor function	Auditory function	Visual function	Communication	Emotion
Coma	None	Absent	Reflex and postural responses only	None	None	None	None
Vegetative state	None	Present	Postures or withdraws to noxious stimuli	Startle	Startle	None	None
			Occasional nonpurposeful movement	Brief orienting to sound	Brief visual fixation	None	Reflexive crying or smiling
Minimally conscious state	Partial	Present	Localizes noxious stimuli	Localizes sound location	Sustained visual fixation	Contingent vocalization	Contingent smiling or crying
			Reaches for objects	Inconsistent command following	Sustained visual pursuit	Inconsistent but intelligible verbalization or gesture	
			Holds or touches objects in a manner that accommodates size and shape				
			Automatic movements (e.g. scratching)				

Locked-in syndrome	Full	Present	Quadriplegic	Preserved	Preserved	Aphonic/Anarthric	Preserved
						Vertical eye movement and blinking usually intact	

Reproduced from Neurology 58(3), Giacino JT, Ashwal S, Childs N, et al. The minimally conscious state: Definition and diagnostic criteria, pp. 49–353. https://doi.org/10.1212/WNL.58.3.349. Copyright (2002), with permission from Wolters Kluwer Health, Inc.

Locked-in syndrome
- A differential of persistent VS and MCS in which consciousness is preserved
- Results from brainstem lesions which disrupt voluntary control of movement without abolishing either arousal or content of awareness, e.g. extensive pontine infarction due to basilar artery thrombosis. Patients can typically communicate via eye movements
- For a graphic description of the condition, read Jean-Dominique Bauby's personal account entitled *The Diving Bell and the Butterfly*—or watch the film.

Brainstem death

- Must be independently confirmed by two medically qualified doctors
- Must wait at least 6 hours after onset of coma or, if anoxia or cardiac arrest was the cause of coma, until 24 hours after circulation has been restored
- The two tests must be performed at least 2 hours apart
- No legal requirements for special tests to confirm diagnosis in the UK.

Criteria of brainstem death

- Patient is comatose and apnoeic
- There is irremediable structural brain damage due to head injury or intracranial haemorrhage (and be >6 hours after onset of coma), or prolonged anoxia or cardiac arrest (and be >24 hours after circulation restored)
- The following have been excluded:
  - hypothermia
  - drug or alcohol intoxication
  - metabolic or endocrine derangement
  - neuromuscular blockade (no such drugs for 12 hours)
- There are no brainstem reflexes
- The patient remains apnoeic on disconnection from the ventilator.

Ancillary test for brainstem death

- CT angiography. The scan is performed and reported according to the UK consensus protocol for the use of CT angiography as an Ancillary investigation to support a clinical diagnosis of death using neurological criteria. CT angiography demonstrates a lack of a cerebral circulation.

Resuscitation (CPR) decisions

- Cardiopulmonary resuscitation (CPR) was first described in 1960 and devised to treat cardiorespiratory arrest consequent upon anaesthesia or surgery.
- Cardiac arrest always renders a patient legally incompetent. In England and Wales, up until recently families have had no rights in law over CPR decisions of adults, and doctors have acted as the patient's advocate 'in partnership with those people close to the patient'. Excluding relatives of an incompetent patient from participating in making decisions may be seen as a breach of the Human Rights Act Article 8 (*right to respect private and family life*). However, recent changes outlined in the Mental Capacity Act have now given those with LPA the right to make decisions over medical treatment issues, including CPR.
- Recent changes in the UK have seen that, as well as doctors, nurses with appropriate training can also make valid resuscitation orders (including 'do not attempt resuscitation' or DNAR).
- 'Futility' as a rationale for making CPR decisions has now been rejected, although in practice it is still often cited. Instead 'consideration of the prospect for restoration of pulse and respiration initially and then to consider if this will benefit the patient' should be the guide.
- Outcome from in-hospital CPR is poor; studies have shown 14–66% (mean 39%) immediate recovery, 0–28% (mean 15%) discharged, and 5–17% alive at 6 months.
- Competent patients' attitudes and participation should always be taken into account (unless they indicate they do not want to), especially with decisions regarding DNAR orders. Valid advanced refusals of CPR must be respected.
- Knowledge of the likely individualized prognosis after stroke is key in discussing CPR decisions with patients, LPAs, and family.
- If a competent patient does not want a DNAR order, then one cannot be written—but at the same time, 'doctors cannot be required to give treatment contrary to their clinical judgement, but should, whenever possible, respect patients' wishes to receive treatment which carries only a very small chance of success or benefit'.
- Published guidelines regarding good practice are available here: ✍ https://www.resus.org.uk/library/additional-guidance/guidance-dnacpr-and-cpr-decisions.

Palliative care

- Stroke is a common cause of death, and most stroke deaths occur in hospital
- Mortality is greatest in the first 30 days of admission
- Where the diagnosis is one of 'end of life' or 'dying', palliation or symptom control will be the most appropriate form of medical and multidisciplinary treatment
- Equally, advance decisions may determine palliative management
- Palliation is alleviating without curing
- Predictors of mortality in stroke include:
  - deep coma
  - stroke severity, e.g. NIHSS >25
  - brain imaging evidence of diffuse intracerebral bleeding, including intraventricular blood, massive hemispheric infarction with mass effect, brainstem stroke
  - multiorgan failure
  - older age
  - depression
- In principle, all interventions should be aimed at relieving symptoms of suffering, distress, and pain. This includes psychological symptoms such as severe anxiety
- There needs to be clear communication between the members of the treating team and family/carers/friends
- Good palliative care in stroke needs to be individualized but may include interventions such 'at risk' oral intake, which require a multidisciplinary team (MDT) approach
- The religious and cultural needs of the patient should be addressed
- Involvement of a palliative care specialist is appropriate, as well as access to grief or bereavement counselling for family and carers
- Further useful information is available from ℛ https://www.nice.org.uk/guidance/ng31

Deaths reportable to the UK Coroner

This is only applicable to the UK. Under regulation 51 of Registration of Births, Deaths and Marriages Regulations 1968, the following deaths should be reported:

• Element of suspicious death or history of violence
• Death linked to an accident
• Death due to occupation or industrial disease
• Death linked to abortion
• Death during operation or before full anaesthetic recovery
• Death related to medical procedure or treatment
• Actions of deceased may have contributed to their own death (self-neglect, drug, or solvent abuse)
• Death occurred in police custody or prison
• Death within 24 hours of admission
• Deceased was detained under the Mental Health Act
• Deceased was under a Deprivation of Liberty Order

🔊 https://www.legislation.gov.uk/uksi/2019/1112/made

Further reading

Death
Kondziella D (2020). The neurology of death and the dying brain: a pictorial essay. *Front Neurol* **11**, 736.
UK Government (2024). *Guidance for Registered Medical Practitioners on the Notification of Deaths Regulations.* Available online at: https://assets.publishing.service.gov.uk/media/66d044a059b0e c2e151f847e/Guidance_for_registered_medical_practitioners_on_the_Notification_of_Deaths_ Regulations__web_.pdf

Capacity
The Social Care Institute for Excellence (SCIE) (2022). *Deprivation of Liberty Safeguards (DoLS) at a Glance.* Available online at: https://www.scie.org.uk/mca/dols/at-a-glance/

Best interests
British Medical Association (2019). *Best Interests Decision-Making for Adults Who Lack Capacity.* A toolkit for doctors working in England and Wales. Available online at:
https://www.bma.org.uk/media/1850/bma-best-interests-toolkit-2019.pdf

Prolonged disorders of consciousness
Jennett B, Plum F (1972). Persistent vegetative state after brain damage. A syndrome in search of a name. *Lancet* **1**, 734–737.
Royal College of Physicians (2020). *Prolonged Disorders of Consciousness Following Sudden Onset Brain Injury: National Clinical Guidelines.* Available online at: https://www.rcp.ac.uk/improving-care/ resources/prolonged-disorders-of-consciousness-following-sudden-onset-brain-injury-national-clinical-guidelines/

Glossary

Term	Description
Activities of daily living (ADLs)	Tasks performed in the daily routine (e.g. washing, dressing)
Advocate	Someone who acts on the patient's behalf
Agnosia	Impairment of ability to understand the meaning of various sensory stimuli
Agraphia	Inability to write
Alexia	Inability to read
Aneurysm	Weak section of an artery wall that balloons out and may rupture
Angiography	Contrast-enhanced X-ray of the blood vessels
Angioplasty	Insertion of a catheter into a narrow artery and dilatation of the artery; inflation of a balloon on the end of the catheter
Anosognosia	Lack of awareness or denial of disease (e.g. the patient denies anything being wrong with the stroke side)
Anticoagulant	A drug (e.g. warfarin) used to prevent blood clots by inhibiting the blood coagulation protein thrombin
Anticonvulsants	Antiepileptic drugs
Antihypertensives	Blood pressure-lowering drugs
Antiphospholipid syndrome	A condition that results from antibodies that form against the body's phospholipids, producing thrombosis
Antiplatelet therapy	Drugs used to stop platelets in the blood sticking to one another and forming clots. Aspirin is the most widely used. Others include clopidogrel and dipyridamole
Antithrombotics	Drugs that are used to prevent blood clots
Aphasia	The inability to use language. It can either be a problem understanding language (receptive) or speaking it (expressive)
Apoptosis	Programmed, genetically triggered cell death
Apraxia	Loss of ability to do well-practised tasks (e.g. dressing)
Arrhythmia	Irregular heartbeat
Arteriography	X-ray of arteries after the injection of a radio-opaque contrast material
Arteriovenous malformation (AVM)	Disorder characterized by a complex tangle of arteries and veins
Aspiration pneumonia	Chest infection (pneumonia) resulting from the inhalation of foreign material
Asteriognosis	Inability to identify an object by touch

Term	Description
Ataxia	Lack of coordination, unsteadiness
Atheroma	Fatty cholesterol deposits inside of artery walls (*synonym*: plaque)
Atherosclerosis	A disease of arteries characterized by deposits of lipid material which make the artery hard, thick (narrow) and brittle
Atrial fibrillation	Where the heart is beating irregularly. There is an increased risk of a blood clot forming inside the heart, which can break off, travel to the brain, and cause a stroke
Blood pressure	The pressure inside the arteries, pushing blood through the circulation. Pressure is highest when the ventricles in the heart contract (systole) and lowest when they relax (diastole). The normal BP is about 120/80 mmHg
Blood–brain barrier	The walls of blood vessels and capillaries in the brain regulate which elements of the blood can pass through to the neurons
Brainstem	The stem-like, lower part of the brain that connects the brain's right and left hemispheres to the spinal cord
Bruit	The noise that can be heard when listening over a narrowed artery
Capillaries	Tiny blood vessels whose wall consists of endothelium and basement membrane
Cardiac	Relating to the heart
Cardioembolic stroke	Stroke due to a clot that formed in the heart and travelled to the brain
Cardiovascular	Relating to the heart and blood vessels
Carotid artery	There are two carotid arteries located on either side of the neck that supply the front half of the brain with blood. Disease of a carotid artery is a common cause of stroke
Carotid endarterectomy	The operation to remove atheroma from the narrowed internal carotid artery
Carotid stenosis	Narrowing of the carotid artery
Catheter (urine)	A medical device (tube) passed into the bladder to drain urine
Catheterization	The insertion of a tube inside the body—most commonly this is into the bladder to drain the urine directly into a bag
Central pain	Pain caused by damage and altered pain perception in the brain (often the thalamus)

Term	Description
Cerebellum	The part of the brain at the back which is responsible for coordinating voluntary muscle movements
Cerebral	Relating to the brain
Cerebral blood flow (CBF)	The flow of blood through the arteries in the brain
Cerebral cortex	The outer layer of the brain consisting of grey matter
Cerebral haemorrhage	Bleeding into the brain tissue (intracerebral haemorrhage) or into surrounding areas (subarachnoid haemorrhage)
Cerebral hemisphere	One of the two halves of the brain
Cerebral infarct	An area where brain cells have died
Cerebral oedema	Swelling of the brain
Cerebrovascular accident (CVA)	An old term used for stroke (the term is falling into disuse because stroke is no longer viewed as an accident)
Cerebrovascular disease (CVD)	Encompasses all abnormalities in the brain resulting from pathologies of its blood vessels (narrowing, blockage)
Cerebrum	The largest part of the brain, made up of the left and right hemispheres (sides)
Cholesterol	A fatty substance that, if present in excess, can be deposited in the wall of the artery to produce atherosclerosis
Cognition	Higher intellectual (mental) functioning associated with thinking, learning, perception, and memory
Cognitive impairment	A deficiency in a person's short- or long-term memory; orientation as to place, person, and time; thinking; and judgement
Coma	A state of deep unconsciousness when the person is not responsive or able to be aroused
Computed tomography (CT) scan	A series of cross-sectional X-rays of the brain and head; also called computerized axial tomography (CAT)
Confabulation	Filling gaps in memory with imagined events
Continence	The ability to control urinary bladder and bowel functions
Contracture	Static muscle shortening so that the muscle cannot be lengthened and loss of motion of the adjacent joint occurs
Contralateral	The opposite side of the body

Term	Description
Coordination	The control of several muscle groups in the execution of complex movements
CVA	The abbreviation for cerebrovascular accident. Not recommended as the concept of stroke being an accident is not helpful
Deep venous thrombosis (DVT)	A clot of blood usually in the leg veins
Delirium	A temporary state of confusion, often linked with other illnesses such as infection (taken from the Latin de lire, meaning 'out of furrow')
Dementia	Progressive and irreversible loss of intellectual ability (speech, abstract thinking, judgement, memory loss, physical coordination) that interfere with daily activities (e.g. Alzheimer's disease)
Depression	A reversible psychiatric disorder characterized by an inability to concentrate, difficulty sleeping, feeling of hopelessness, fatigue, the 'blues', and guilt
Diplopia	Double vision
District nurse	A nurse who provides skilled, flexible nursing care to people within the community and at home
Diuretics	Drugs given to make you pass more urine. They are used to control heart failure and high blood pressure
Duplex carotid scan (also termed carotid Doppler)	An ultrasound scan of the carotid arteries in the neck
Dysarthria	A motor disorder of the tongue, mouth, jaw, or voice box resulting in slurred speech
Dyslexia	Difficulty reading
Dyslipidaemia	Abnormality in blood lipids
Dysphagia	Difficulty swallowing
Dysphasia or aphasia	Difficulty in using language owing to problems understanding language (receptive) and speaking it (expressive)
Dysphonia	Impairment of the voice
Dyspraxia	Difficulty with performing skilled or purposeful voluntary movement even though the person is physically able to do it
Echocardiogram	Ultrasound scan of the heart
Electrocardiogram (ECG)	A test that measures electrical activity and rhythm of the heart

Term	Description
Electroencephalogram (EEG)	A test used to record electrical activity in the brain by placing electrodes on the scalp
Embolic stroke	A stroke caused by an embolus
Embolism	Blockage of a blood vessel by an embolus
Embolus	A clot or piece of other material which travels distally in the bloodstream, eventually lodging in the blood vessels at a distant site
Emotional lability	A condition in which the mood of the person swings rapidly (unreasonably) from one state to another (such as laughing, crying, or anger)
Endarterectomy	Surgical operation to remove obstructions (usually fatty tissue or blood clot) from inside an artery
Enteral feeding	Feeding using a tube connecting with the stomach
Epidemiology	The study of factors that influence the frequency and distribution of a disease in a population
Epilepsy	Seizures or fits
Extracranial–intracranial (EC–IC) bypass	A type of surgery that restores blood flow to a blood-deprived area of brain tissue by rerouting a healthy artery in the scalp to the area of brain tissue affected by a blocked/narrowed artery
Field of vision	The area that you can see without moving your eyes (or head)
Flaccid	Absence of muscle tone, producing floppy muscles
Gait	Manner of walking
Geriatrician	A doctor who specializes in the care of older people, primarily those who are frail and have complex medical and social problems
Glia	Supportive cells of the nervous system that also play an important role in brain functioning; also called neuroglia
Goal setting	The process whereby the professionals and the patient decide on the main objectives for rehabilitation
Haematoma	A collection of blood forming a definite swelling which compresses and damages the brain around it
Haemorrhagic infarct	An infarct that has had secondary bleeding in it
Haemorrhagic stroke	Bleeding into the brain (intracerebral haemorrhage) or into surrounding areas (subarachnoid haemorrhage)
Handicap	The social consequence of disability for the patient
Hemianaesthesia	Loss of sensation down one side of the body
Hemianopia	Loss of the half field of vision in each eye

Term	Description
Hemi-inattention	Ignoring space on the side of the body; sometimes called unilateral neglect
Hemiparesis	Weakness of one-half of the body
Hemiplegia	Complete paralysis of half of the body
Hemisphere	One-half of the brain
Heparin	A type of anticoagulant
High-density lipoprotein cholesterol (HDL-C)	A compound consisting of a lipid and a protein that carries cholesterol in the blood and deposits it in the liver; also known as 'good' cholesterol
Homeostasis	A state of equilibrium or balance in the body with respect to various functions and to the chemical compositions of the fluids and tissues
Homonymous hemianopia	Loss of the same half field of vision in each eye
Hughes' syndrome	See antiphospholipid syndrome
Hydrocephalus	Raised pressure within the skull caused by excess fluid on the brain
Hypercholesterolaemia	A high level of cholesterol in the blood
Hyperlipidaemia	A high level of fats in the blood
Hypertension	High blood pressure
Hypotension	Low blood pressure
Impairment	Loss of function (e.g. weakness, loss of sensation, loss of speech)
Impotence	Inability to obtain or maintain penile erection
Incidence	Frequency with which cases of a disease occur during a certain period of time in a population
Incontinence	Inability to control urinary bladder (urinary incontinence) or bowel functions (bowel incontinence), or both
Infarct or infarction	Area of dead or dying brain tissue
Intermediate care	Services working together to help people recover from illness and stop them going into hospital if it is not necessary or staying in hospital longer than they need to
Intracerebral haemorrhage	Bleeding into the brain substance
Involuntary	Without being willed or intended

Term	Description
Ischaemia	A loss or reduction of blood flow to tissue resulting in reduce nutrients, oxygen, and removal of waste products (such as lactic acid)
Ischaemic penumbra	Area of damaged, but still living, brain cells arranged in a patchwork pattern around areas of dead brain cells
Ischaemic stroke	An area where brain cells have died (*synonyms*: cerebral infarct, cerebral infarction)
Key worker	The member of the team who is responsible for making sure that health and social care professionals involved in patient treatment and care know what plans and decisions are being made. The key worker is also responsible for keeping the patient and family informed
Lacunar stroke/infarct	A small stroke less than 1.5 cm in diameter when measured on the brain scan (from the French word 'lacune' meaning a lake)
Large artery disease	Stenosis or occlusion of the carotid arteries, often due to atherosclerosis
Lipoprotein	Small globules of cholesterol covered by a layer of protein
Long-term care	This is provided for people who are unable to live independently and who move into residential or nursing homes
Low-density lipoprotein cholesterol (LDL-C)	A compound consisting of a lipid and a protein that carries cholesterol in the blood and deposits the excess along the inside of arterial walls; also known as 'bad' cholesterol
Lumbar puncture	A procedure whereby some of the spinal fluid is removed by the insertion of a needle into the spine
Magnetic resonance angiography (MRA)	An imaging technique involving injection of radio-opaque contrast material into a blood vessel and using magnetic resonance techniques to create an image of brain arteries and veins
Magnetic resonance imaging (MRI)	A type of scan that, instead of X-rays, uses a large, powerful magnet to create an image (picture) of part of the body
Middle cerebral artery	The artery that most frequently becomes blocked, to cause stroke
Monoparesis, monoplegia	Weakness, paralysis of one limb only
Mortality	Describes the number of persons who die during a certain period of time
Nasogastric tube	Tube put down the nose into the stomach

Term	Description
Neglect, one-sided	A term sometimes used for lack of awareness of one side of the body
Neurologist	A doctor specializing in diseases of the nervous system
Neurology	The study of the structure, functioning, and diseases of the nervous system
Neuron	The main functional cell of the brain and nervous system, consisting of a cell body, an axon, and dendrites
Neuroplasticity	After stroke, dead brain cannot regrow. Unaffected brain tissue that surrounds the dead area takes over part of the lost function. This process is called neuroplasticity
Neuroprotective agents	Medications that protect the brain from secondary injury
Nursing home	A generic term for a skilled nursing facility
Nystagmus	Involuntary jerking of the eyes normally caused by damage to the cerebellum or brainstem
Obesity	Being more than 20% over your recommended weight
Occupational therapist (OT)	A therapist who specializes in helping people to reach their maximum level of function and independence in all aspects of daily life
Oedema	Swelling owing to excess water in the tissue
Ophthalmologist	A doctor who specializes in the investigation and treatment of diseases of the eyes
Orthosis	An external orthopaedic appliance, as a brace or splint, that prevents or assists movement of the spine or the limbs
Papilloedema	Swelling of the optic discs in the eyes
Paraesthesia	An abnormal sensation, such as of burning, pricking, tickling, or tingling
Paralysis	Complete weakness and loss of movement
Paraparesis, paraplegia	Weakness, paralysis of both legs (can happen with bilateral strokes or spinal cord problems)
Paraphrasia	Producing unintended phrases, words, or syllables during speech
Paresis	Muscle weakness
Patent foramen ovale (PFO)	A small 'hole' in the heart that may allow blood clots to travel from the right side to the left side without going through the lungs

Term	Description
Peer support	Getting support from people in the same situation as you
PEG tube	Percutaneous endoscopic gastrostomy feeding tube inserted through the abdominal wall into the stomach
Perception	The ability to receive, interpret, and use information
Percutaneous endoscopic gastrostomy (PEG)	Insertion of a tube through the wall of the abdomen into the stomach for the purposes of feeding with a fibreoptic instrument called a gastroscope
Pharmacist	A person who is qualified in pharmacy and authorized to dispense drugs
Phlebotomist	Someone who is trained to take blood specimens from people's veins
Physician	A qualified doctor who specializes in the diagnosis and treatment of disease by other than surgical means
Physiotherapist	A therapist who specializes in physical methods of treatment to promote functional recovery of movement
Plaque	A mixture of fatty substances, including cholesterol and other lipids, deposited inside of artery walls
Plasticity of the brain	See neuroplasticity
Platelets	Blood cells that are known for their role in blood coagulation
Positron emission tomography (PET)	A nuclear medicine scanning technique that uses radioactive isotopes to assess the metabolic function of the brain
Power of Attorney	The legal right to manage financial and other affairs on behalf of another
Prevalence	The number of cases of a disease in a population at any given point in time
Primary care	Care delivered by the GP or healthcare professionals within the community
Prognosis	Expected outcome
Psychiatrist	A specialist in the study and treatment of mental disorders
Psychologist	A person qualified in the scientific study of the mind. A clinical psychologist is trained in the assessment and treatment of people with illness
Pulmonary embolism	A blood clot in the lungs
Randomized controlled trial	A clinical study in which persons are assigned to the experimental or control group by a random selection procedure

Term	Description
Recombinant tissue plasminogen activator (rtPA)	A genetically engineered form of t-PA, a thrombolytic anticlotting substance made naturally by the body [generic name alteplase]
Rehabilitation	The process of regaining function through active treatment
Rehabilitation unit	A place where skilled and experienced staff work to help the stroke patient adjust to the effects of stroke
Respite care	Care given to someone for a short period, usually away from their own home so their family can have a rest from the burdens of caring for them
Rest home	A generic term for a group home, specialized apartment complex, or other institution which provides care services where individuals live; sometimes referred to as a private hospital, residential care facility, or a care home
Risk factors	The possible underlying causes (for the stroke) such as smoking, high blood pressure, ethnic group, and family history of stroke
Small-vessel disease	A disease of small arteries in the brain, often due to hypertension
Social security	A state department which works through the Department of Work and Pensions (DWP) to organize financial aid and assistance in the form of state benefits
Social services	The body run by the local authority or council which provides a number of services for those living at home, including personal care, day centres, equipment, and adaptations
Social worker	Someone from the social services department who gives advice and practical help with social problems
Spasm	Involuntary contraction of a muscle
Spastic paralysis	Paralysis with increased muscle tone and spasmodic contraction of the muscles
Spasticity	Abnormally increased tone in a muscle
Speech and language therapist (SALT)	A therapist who specializes in the rehabilitation of people with speech and language difficulties, helping them to improve their speech and language, and/or to find alternative ways of communicating. They also help with problems with swallowing
Spinal cord	The long elliptical part of the central nervous system joining the brain to the peripheral nerves. It runs in the vertebral canal
Stenosis	A narrowing, normally in an artery
Stroke	An acute focal vascular injury of the brain

Term	Description
Stroke unit	The ward for multidisciplinary team management of patients with acute stroke
Subarachnoid haemorrhage	Bleeding between the brain pial surface and the covering membranes, often caused by a ruptured aneurysm
Thalamus (thalamic)	A part of the brain where the nerves carrying information about sensation from the body join with other nerves
Thrombectomy	The mechanical removal of a clot blocking an artery in the brain
Thromboembolic	A blood clot which has embolized
Thrombolysis	The use of drugs to break up a blood clot
Thrombosis	The formation of a blood clot
Thrombotic stroke	A stroke caused by thrombosis
Thrombus	A blood clot
Tone	A slight constant tension in muscles at rest
Total serum cholesterol	A combined measurement of high-density lipoprotein cholesterol (HDL-C) and low-density lipoprotein cholesterol (LDL-C)
Transcranial magnetic stimulation (TMS)	A small magnetic current delivered to stimulate an area of the brain
Transient ischaemic attack (TIA)	A short-lived mini stroke that lasts from a few minutes up to 24 hours
Vascular	Relating to the blood vessels
Vasospasm	Spasm of a blood vessel
Vein	A blood vessel that carries blood back to the heart
Vertebral arteries	The two arteries on either side of the back of the neck that travel to the brain. They supply the posterior part of the brain
Vertigo	An abnormal sensation of movement
Videofluoroscopy	A video X-ray of the swallowing mechanism
Visuospatial disorder	Inability to interpret special problems correctly
Warfarin	An oral anticoagulant

Useful stroke scales

NIH Stroke Scale

Available at ℗ lohttps://www.ninds.nih.gov/health-information/stroke/assess-and-treat/nih-stroke-scale

Instructions

- Administer stroke scale items in the order listed.
- Record performance in each category after each subscale exam.
- Do not go back and change scores.
- Follow directions provided for each exam technique.
- Scores should reflect what the patient does, not what the clinician thinks the patient can do.
- The clinician should record answers while administering the exam and work quickly.
- Except where indicated, the patient should not be coached (i.e. repeated requests to patient to make a special effort).

Level of consciousness 1

Instructions—Level of consciousness (LOC): The investigator must choose a response if a full evaluation is prevented by such obstacles as an endotracheal tube, language barrier, orotracheal trauma/bandages. A 3 is scored only if the patient makes no movement (other than reflexive posturing) in response to noxious stimulation.

Scale Definition	
0	Alert; keenly responsive.
1	Not Alert; but arousable by minor stimulation to obey, answer, or respond.
2	Not Alert; requires repeated stimulation to attend, or is obtunded and requires strong or painful stimulation to make movements (not stereotyped).
3	Responds only with reflex motor or autonomic effects, or totally unresponsive, flaccid, and areflexic.
	Score

Level of consciousness 2

Instructions—LOC questions: The patient is asked the month and his/her age. The answer must be correct — there is no partial credit for being close. Aphasic and stuporous patients who do not comprehend the questions will score 2. Patients unable to speak because of endotracheal intubation, orotracheal trauma, severe dysarthria from any cause, language barrier, or any other problem not secondary to aphasia are given a 1. It is important that only the initial answer be graded and that the examiner not 'help' the patient with verbal or non-verbal cues.

Scale definition	
0	**Answers** both questions correctly.
1	**Answers** one question correctly.
2	**Answers** neither question correctly.
	Score

Level of consciousness 3

Instructions—LOC commands: The patient is asked to open and close the eyes and then to grip and release the nonparetic hand. Substitute another one-step command if the hands cannot be used. Credit is given if an unequivocal attempt is made but not completed due to weakness. If the patient does not respond to command, the task should be demonstrated to him or her (pantomime), and the result scored (i.e. follows none, one, or two commands). Patients with trauma, amputation, or other physical impediments should be given suitable one-step commands. Only the first attempt is scored.

Scale definition	
0	**Performs** both tasks correctly.
1	**Performs** one task correctly.
2	**Performs** neither task correctly.
	Score

Best gaze

Instructions: Only horizontal eye movements will be tested. Voluntary or reflexive (oculocephalic) eye movements will be scored, but caloric testing is not done. If the patient has a conjugate deviation of the eyes that can be overcome by voluntary or reflexive activity, the score will be 1. If a patient has an isolated peripheral nerve paresis (CN III, IV, or VI), score a 1. Gaze is testable in all aphasic patients. Patients with ocular trauma, bandages, pre-existing blindness, or other disorder of visual acuity or fields should be tested with reflexive movements, and a choice made by the investigator. Establishing eye contact and then moving about the patient from side to side will occasionally clarify the presence of a partial gaze palsy.

Scale definition	
0	**Normal.**
1	**Partial** gaze palsy; gaze is abnormal in one or both eyes, but forced deviation or total gaze paresis is not present.
2	**Forced** deviation, or total gaze paresis is not overcome by the oculocephalic manoeuvre.
	Score

Visual

Instructions: Visual fields (upper and lower quadrants) are tested by confrontation, using finger counting or visual threat, as appropriate. Patients may be encouraged, but if they look at the side of the moving fingers appropriately, this can be scored as normal. If there is unilateral blindness or enucleation, visual fields in the remaining eye are scored. Score 1 only if a clear-cut asymmetry, including quadrantanopia, is found. If the patient is blind from any cause, score 3. Double simultaneous stimulation is performed at this point. If there is extinction, patient receives a 1, and the results are used to respond to item 11.

Scale definition	
0	**No visual loss.**
1	**Partial hemianopia.**
2	**Complete hemianopia.**
3	**Bilateral hemianopia** (blind including cortical blindness).
	Score

Facial palsy

Instructions: Ask—or use pantomime to encourage—the patient to show teeth or raise eyebrows and close eyes. Score symmetry of grimace in response to noxious stimuli in the poorly responsive or non-comprehending patient. If facial trauma/ bandages, orotracheal tube, tape, or other physical barriers obscure the face, these should be removed to the extent possible.

Scale definition	
0	**Normal** symmetrical movements.
1	**Minor paralysis** (flattened nasolabial fold, asymmetry on smiling).
2	**Partial paralysis** (total or near-total paralysis of lower face).
3	**Complete paralysis** of one or both sides (absence of facial movement in the upper and lower face).
	Score

Motor arm

Instructions: The limb is placed in the appropriate position: extend the arms (palms down) 90 degrees (if sitting) or 45 degrees (if supine). Drift is scored if the arm falls before 10 seconds. The aphasic patient is encouraged by using urgency in the voice and pantomime, but not noxious stimulation. Each limb is tested in turn, beginning with the non-paretic arm. Only in the case of amputation or joint fusion at the shoulder, the examiner should record the score as untestable (UN) and clearly write the explanation for this choice.

Scale definition	
0	**No drift**; limb holds 90 (or 45) degrees for full 10 seconds.
1	**Drift; limb holds 90** (or 45) degrees, but drifts down before full 10 seconds; does not hit bed or other support.
2	**Some effort against gravity**; limb cannot get to or maintain (if cued) 90 (or 45) degrees, drifts down to bed, but has some effort against gravity.
3	**No effort against gravity**; limb falls.
4	**No movement.**
UN	**Amputation or joint fusion**, explain:
	Score 5a: Left arm 5b: Right arm

Motor leg

Instructions: The limb is placed in the appropriate position: hold the leg at 30 degrees (always tested supine). Drift is scored if the leg falls before 5 seconds. The aphasic patient is encouraged by using urgency in the voice and pantomime but not noxious stimulation. Each limb is tested in turn, beginning with the non-paretic leg. Only in the case of amputation or joint fusion at the hip, the examiner should record the score as untestable (UN) and clearly write the explanation for this choice.

Scale Definition	
0	**No drift**; leg holds 30-degree position for full 5 seconds.
1	**Drift;** leg falls by the end of the 5-second period but does not hit the bed.
2	**Some effort against gravity;** leg falls to bed by 5 seconds but has some effort against gravity.
3	**No effort against gravity;** leg falls to bed immediately.
4	**No movement.**
UN	**Amputation** or joint fusion, explain:
	Score 6a: Left Leg 6b: Right Leg

Limb ataxia

Instructions: This item is aimed at finding evidence of a unilateral cerebellar lesion. Test with eyes open. In case of visual defect, ensure testing is done in an intact visual field. The finger-nose-finger and heel-shin tests are performed on both sides, and ataxia is scored only if present out of proportion to weakness. Ataxia is absent in the patient who cannot understand or is paralysed. Only in the case of amputation or joint fusion, the examiner should record the score as untestable (UN) and clearly write the explanation for this choice. In case of blindness, test by having the patient touch nose from the extended arm position.

Scale definition	
0	**Absent**
1	**Present in one limb**
2	**Present in two limbs**
UN	**Amputation** or joint fusion, explain:
	Score

Sensory

Instructions: Sensation or grimace to pinprick when tested, or withdrawal from noxious stimulus in the obtunded or aphasic patient. Only sensory loss attributed to stroke is scored as abnormal and the examiner should test as many body areas (arms [not hands], legs, trunk, face) as needed to accurately check for hemisensory loss. A score of 2, 'severe or total sensory loss', should only be given when a severe or total loss of sensation can be clearly demonstrated. Stuporous and aphasic patients will, therefore, probably score 1 or 0. The patient with brainstem stroke who has bilateral loss of sensation is scored 2. If the patient does not respond and is quadriplegic, score 2. Patients in a coma (item 1a = 3) are automatically given a 2 on this item.

Scale definition	
0	**Normal;** no sensory loss.
1	**Mild-to-moderate sensory loss;** patient feels pinprick is less sharp or is dull on the affected side; or there is a loss of superficial pain with pinprick, but patient is aware of being touched.
2	**Severe or total sensory loss;** patient is not aware of being touched in the face, arm, and leg.
	Score

Best language

Instructions: A great deal of information about comprehension will be obtained during the preceding sections of the examination. For this scale item, the patient is asked to describe what is happening in the attached picture (p. 554), to name items on the naming sheet (p. 553), and to read from the list of sentences (p. 556). Comprehension is judged from responses here, as well as to all of the commands in the preceding general neurological exam. If visual loss interferes with the tests, ask the patient to identify objects placed in the hand, repeat, and produce speech. The intubated patient should be asked to write. The patient in a coma (item 1a=3) will automatically score 3 on this item. The examiner must choose a score for the patient with stupor or limited cooperation, but a score of 3 should be used only if the patient is mute and follows no one-step commands.

Scale definition	
0	**No aphasia;** normal.
1	**Mild-to-moderate aphasia;** some obvious loss of fluency or facility of comprehension, without significant limitation on ideas expressed or form of expression. Reduction of speech and/or comprehension, however, makes conversation about provided materials difficult or impossible. For example, in conversation about provided materials, the examiner can identify picture or naming card content from patient's response.
2	**Severe aphasia;** all communication is through fragmentary expression; great need for inference, questioning, and guessing by the listener. Range of information that can be exchanged is limited; listener carries burden of communication. Examiner cannot identify materials provided from patient response.
3	**Mute, global aphasia;** no usable speech or auditory comprehension.
	Score

Dysarthria

Instructions: If patient is thought to be normal, an adequate sample of speech must be obtained by asking patient to read or repeat words from the attached list (p. 555). If the patient has severe aphasia, the clarity of articulation of spontaneous speech can be rated. Only if the patient is intubated or has other physical barriers to producing speech, the examiner should record the score as untestable (UN) and clearly write the explanation for this choice. Do not tell the patient why he or she is being tested.

Scale definition	
0	**Normal.**
1	**Mild-to-moderate dysarthria;** patient slurs at least some words and, at worst, can be understood with some difficulty.
2	**Severe dysarthria;** patient's speech is so slurred as to be unintelligible in the absence of or out of proportion to any dysphasia, or is mute/anarthric.
UN	**Intubated** or other physical barrier, explain:
	Score

Extinction and inattention

Instructions—extinction and inattention (formerly Neglect): Sufficient information to identify neglect may be obtained during the prior testing. If the patient has a severe visual loss preventing visual double simultaneous stimulation, and the cutaneous stimuli are normal, the score is normal. If the patient has aphasia but does appear to attend to both sides, the score is normal. The presence of visual–spatial neglect or anosagnosia may also be taken as evidence of abnormality. Since the abnormality is scored only if present, the item is never untestable.

Scale definition	
0	**No abnormality.**
1	**Visual, tactile, auditory, spatial, or personal inattention,** or extinction to bilateral simultaneous stimulation in one of the sensory modalities.
2	**Profound hemi-inattention or extinction to more than one modality;** does not recognize own hand or orients to only one side of space.
	Score

Total score of patient

ITEM	SCORE
1a	
1b	
1c	
2	
3	
4	
5	
6	
7	
8	
9	
10	
11	
TOTAL SCORE	

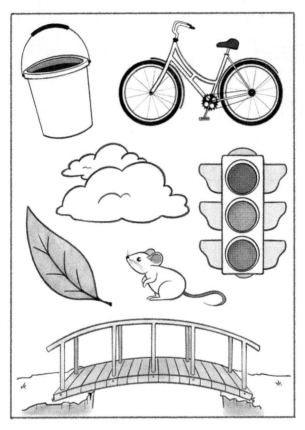

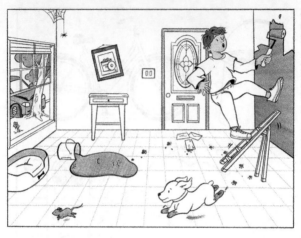

MAMA

TIP-TOP

FIFTY-FIFTY

THANKS

HUCKLEBERRY

BASEBALL PLAYER

CATERPILLAR

You know how.

Down to earth.

I got home from work.

Near the table in the dining room.

They heard him speak on the radio last night.

Reproduced with permission from the National Institute of Neurological Disorders and Stroke and Apex Innovations.

The Rivermead Mobility Index

Name: _____

	Day							
	Month							
	Year							
Topic and Question:								
Turning over in bed: Do you turn over from your back to your side without help?								
Lying to sitting: From lying in bed, do you get up to sit on the edge of the bed on your own?								
Sitting balance: Do you sit on the edge of the bed without holding on for 10 seconds?								
Sitting to standing: Do you stand up from any chair in less than 15 seconds and stand there for 15 seconds, using hands and/or an aid if necessary?								
Standing unsupported: (Ask to stand) Observe standing for 10 seconds without any aid								
Transfer: Do you manage to move from bed to chair and back without any help?								
Walking inside: (with an aid if necessary): Do you walk 10 meters, with an aid if necessary, but with no standby help?								
Stairs: Do you manage a flight of stairs without help?								
Walking outside: (even ground): Do you walk around outside, on pavements, without help?								
Walking inside: (with no aid): Do you walk 10 meters inside, with no caliper, splint, or other aid (including furniture or walls) without help?								
Picking up off floor: Do you manage to walk five meters, pick something up from the floor, and then walk back without help?								
Walking outside: (uneven ground): Do you walk over uneven ground (grass, gravel, snow, ice etc) without help?								
Bathing: Do you get into/out of a bath or shower and to wash yourself unsupervised and without help?								
Up and down four steps: Do you manage to go up and down four steps with no rail, but using an aid if necessary?								
Running: Do you run 10 meters without limping in four seconds (fast walk, not limping, is acceptable)?								
	Total							

The Rivermead Mobility Index is provided courtesy of Dr. Derick Wade and the Oxford Centre for Enablement.

Modified Ashworth Spasticity Scale

0	No increase in tone
1	Slight increase in muscle tone, manifested by a catch and release or minimal resistance at the end of the ROM when the affected part(s) is moved in flexion or extension
1+	Slight increase in muscle tone, manifested by a catch, followed by minimal resistance throughout the remainder (less than half) of the ROM
2	More marked increase in muscle tone through most of the ROM, but affected part(s) easily moved
3	Considerable increase in muscle tone, passive movement difficult
4	Affected part(s) rigid in flexion or extension

Reproduced from Katz RT, Spasticity. In: O'Young B, Young MA, Stiens SA (eds), *Physical Medicine & Rehabilitation Secrets*, pp. 487, Copyright (1997), with permission of Elsevier.

Modified Tardieu Scale

The Tardieu Scale was developed in 1954 by Tardieu and colleagues, being subsequently modified in 1999 by Boyd and Graham to the form in current clinical practice. It explicitly compares the occurrence of a catch at low and high speeds and is effective in measuring the velocity-dependent component of hypertonia (this unique test item gives the Tardieu greater validity than either the Ashworth or modified Ashworth). It is an ordinal rating of hypertonicity which measures the intensity of the muscle reaction at specified velocities (slowest to as fast as possible). The angle at which the catch is first felt is also noted as a clinical estimate similar to the threshold angle. The three variables are considered simultaneously when assessing spasticity.

Procedure

- A constant position of the body must be established, and remain constant from one test to another
- Other joints, in particular the neck, must remain in a constant position throughout the assessment
- The quality of muscle reaction and the angle of muscle reaction must be rated at each of the stretch velocities:
  - Step 1—subject seated in a chair, elbow flexed by 90°
  - Step 2—move the wrist as slowly as possible through pain-free available range into extension (slower than the rate of the natural drop of the wrist under gravity). Rate the quality of muscle reaction (see later) and measure angle of muscle reaction (angle of a catch) as appropriate
  - Step 3—move the wrist as fast as possible through pain-free available range into extension (faster than the rate of the natural drop of the wrist under gravity). Rate the quality of muscle reaction (see later) and measure angle of muscle reaction (angle of a catch) as appropriate.

Score

Quality of muscle reaction: (X)
- 0—No resistance throughout the course of the passive movement
- 1—Slight resistance throughout the course of the passive movement with no clear catch at a precise angle
- 2—Clear catch at a precise angle, interrupting the passive movement, followed by a release
- 3—Fatiguable clonus, less than 10 seconds when maintaining the pressure, appearing at a precise angle
- 4—Unfatiguable clonus, more than 10 seconds when maintaining the pressure, at a precise angle.

Reproduced from Boyd, R.N. and Graham, H.K. (1999), Objective measurement of clinical findings in the use of botulinum toxin type A for the management of children with cerebral palsy. *European Journal of Neurology* 6, s23. © 1999 Blackwell Science Ltd.

Modified Rankin Scale

Score	Description
0	No symptoms at all
1	No significant disability despite symptoms; able to carry out all usual duties and activities
2	Slight disability; unable to carry out all previous activities, but able to look after own affairs without assistance
3	Moderate disability; requiring some help, but able to walk without assistance
4	Moderately severe disability; unable to walk without assistance and unable to attend to own bodily needs without assistance
5	Severe disability; bedridden, incontinent, and requiring constant nursing care and attention

TOTAL (0–5): _____

Modified from *Stroke*, 19(5), Van Swieten JC, Koudstaal PJ, Visser MC, Schouten HJ, van Gijn J, Intraobserver agreement for the assessement of handicap in stroke patients, pp. 604–607, Copyright (1998), with permission from Wolters Kluwer Health, Inc.
NOTE: Some researchers have added an additional category of 6 to indicate dead.

Patient Health Questionnaire (PHQ-9)

This easy-to-use patient questionnaire is a self-administered version of the PRIME-MD diagnostic instrument for common mental disorders. The PHQ-9 is the depression module, which scores each of the nine DSM-IV criteria as '0' (not at all) to '3' (nearly every day). It has been validated for use in Primary Care.

PATIENT HEALTH QUESTIONNAIRE-9 (PHQ-9)

Over the <u>last 2 weeks</u>, how often have you been bothered by any of the following problems? *(Use '✓' to indicate your answer)*	Not at all	Several days	More than half the days	Nearly every day
1. Little interest or pleasure in doing things	0	1	2	3
2. Feeling down, depressed, or hopeless	0	1	2	3
3. Trouble falling or staying asleep, or sleeping too much	0	1	2	3
4. Feeling tired or having little energy	0	1	2	3
5. Poor appetite or overeating	0	1	2	3
6. Feeling bad about yourself — or that you are a failure or have let yourself or your family down	0	1	2	3
7. Trouble concentrating on things, such as reading the newspaper or watching television	0	1	2	3
8. Moving or speaking so slowly that other people could have noticed. Or the opposite—being so fidgety or restless that you have been moving around a lot more than usual	0	1	2	3

PATIENT HEALTH QUESTIONNAIRE-9 (PHQ-9)				
Over the <u>last 2 weeks,</u> how often have you been bothered by any of the following problems? *(Use '✓' to indicate your answer)*	Not at all	Several days	More than half the days	Nearly every day
9. Thoughts that you would be better off dead or of hurting yourself in some way	0	1	2	3
FOR OFFICE CODING	___0___ +	___ +	___ +	___
			= Total Score: _____	

If you checked off <u>any</u> problems, how <u>difficult</u> have these problems made it for you to do your work, take care of things at home, or get along with other people?

Not difficult at all	**Somewhat difficult**	**Very difficult**	**Extremely difficult**
☐	☐	☐	☐

Hamilton Rating Scale for Depression (HAMDS)

THE HAMILTON RATING SCALE FOR DEPRESSION

(to be administered by a health care professional)

Patient's Name

Date of Assessment

To rate the severity of depression in patients who are already diagnosed as depressed, administer this questionnaire. The higher the score, the more severe the depression.

For each item, write the correct number on the line next to the item. (Only one response per item)

1. **DEPRESSED MOOD** (Sadness, hopeless, helpless, worthless)

   0= Absent
   1= These feeling states indicated only on questioning
   2= These feeling states spontaneously reported verbally
   3= Communicates feeling states non-verbally—i.e., through facial expression, posture, voice, and tendency to weep
   4= Patient reports VIRTUALLY ONLY these feeling states in his spontaneous verbal and non-verbal communication

2. **FEELINGS OF GUILT**

   0= Absent
   1= Self reproach, feels he has let people down
   2= Ideas of guilt or rumination over past errors or sinful deeds
   3= Present illness is a punishment. Delusions of guilt
   4= Hears accusatory or denunciatory voices and/or experiences threatening visual hallucinations

3. **SUICIDE**

   0= Absent
   1= Feels life is not worth living
   2= Wishes he were dead or any thoughts of possible death to self
   3= Suicidal ideas or gesture
   4= Attempts at suicide (any serious attempt rates 4)

4. **INSOMNIA EARLY**

   0= No difficulty falling asleep
   1= Complains of occasional difficulty falling asleep—i.e., more than 1/2 hour
   2= Complains of nightly difficulty falling asleep

5. **INSOMNIA MIDDLE**

   0= No difficulty
   1= Patient complains of being restless and disturbed during the night
   2= Waking during the night—any getting out of bed rates 2 (except for purposes of voiding)

6. **INSOMNIA LATE**

   0= No difficulty
   1= Waking in early hours of the morning but goes back to sleep
   2= Unable to fall asleep again if he gets out of bed

7. **WORK AND ACTIVITIES**

   0= No difficulty
   1= Thoughts and feelings of incapacity, fatigue or weakness related to activities; work or hobbies
   2= Loss of interest in activity; hobbies or work—either directly reported by patient, or indirect in listlessness, indecision and vacillation (feels he has to push self to work or activities)
   3= Decrease in actual time spent in activities or decrease in productivity
   4= Stopped working because of present illness

8. **RETARDATION: PSYCHOMOTOR** (Slowness of thought and speech; impaired ability to concentrate; decreased motor activity)

   0= Normal speech and thought
   1= Slight retardation at interview
   2= Obvious retardation at interview
   3= Interview difficult
   4= Complete stupor

9. **AGITATION**

   0= None
   1= Fidgetiness
   2= Playing with hands, hair, etc.
   3= Moving about, can't sit still
   4= Hand wringing, nail biting, hair-pulling, biting of lips

10. **ANXIETY (PSYCHOLOGICAL)**

    0= No difficulty
    1= Subjective tension and irritability
    2= Worrying about minor matters
    3= Apprehensive attitude apparent in face or speech
    4= Fears expressed without questioning

11. **ANXIETY SOMATIC:** Physiological concomitants of anxiety, (i.e., effects of autonomic overactivity, "butterflies," indigestion, stomach cramps, belching, diarrhea, palpitations, hyperventilation, paresthesia, sweating, flushing, tremor, headache, urinary frequency). Avoid asking about possible medication side effects (i.e., dry mouth, constipation)

    0= Absent
    1= Mild
    2= Moderate
    3= Severe
    4= Incapacitating

12. **SOMATIC SYMPTOMS (GASTROINTESTINAL)**

    0= None
    1= Loss of appetite but eating without encouragement from others. Food intake about normal
    2= Difficulty eating without urging from others. Marked reduction of appetite and food intake

13. **SOMATIC SYMPTOMS GENERAL**

    0= None
    1= Heaviness in limbs, back or head. Backaches, headache, muscle aches. Loss of energy and fatigability
    2= Any clear-cut symptom rates 2

14. **GENITAL SYMPTOMS** (Symptoms such as: loss of libido; impaired sexual performance; menstrual disturbances)

    0= Absent
    1= Mild
    2= Severe

15. **HYPOCHONDRIASIS**

    0= Not present
    1= Self-absorption (bodily)
    2= Preoccupation with health
    3= Frequent complaints, requests for help, etc.
    4= Hypochondriacal delusions

16. **LOSS OF WEIGHT**

    A. When rating by history:
    0= No weight loss
    1= Probably weight loss associated with present illness
    2= Definite (according to patient) weight loss
    3= Not assessed

17. **INSIGHT**

    0= Acknowledges being depressed and ill
    1= Acknowledges illness but attributes cause to bad food, climate, overwork, virus, need for rest, etc.
    2= Denies being ill at all

18. **DIURNAL VARIATION**

    A. Note whether symptoms are worse in morning or evening. If NO diurnal variation, mark none
    0= No variation
    1= Worse in A.M.
    2= Worse in P.M.
    B. When present, mark the severity of the variation. Mark "None" if NO variation
    0= None
    1= Mild
    2= Severe

19. **DEPERSONALIZATION AND DEREALIZATION** (Such as: Feelings of unreality; Nihilistic ideas)

    0= Absent
    1= Mild
    2= Moderate
    3= Severe
    4= Incapacitating

20. **PARANOID SYMPTOMS**

    0= None
    1= Suspicious
    2= Ideas of reference
    3= Delusions of reference and persecution

21. **OBSESSIONAL AND COMPULSIVE SYMPTOMS**

    0= Absent
    1= Mild
    2= Severe

Total Score _____

Geriatric Depression Scale (GDS): short form

The Geriatric Depression Scale (GDS) is in the public domain and not protected by copyright. It typically takes 5–7 minutes to perform.

Choose the best answer for how you have felt over the past week:

1. Are you basically satisfied with your life?	YES/**NO**
2. Have you dropped many of your activities and interests?	**YES**/NO
3. Do you feel that your life is empty?	**YES**/NO
4. Do you often get bored?	**YES**/NO
5. Are you in good spirits most of the time?	YES/**NO**
6. Are you afraid that something bad is going to happen to you?	**YES**/NO
7. Do you feel happy most of the time?	YES/**NO**
8. Do you often feel helpless?	**YES**/NO
9. Do you prefer to stay at home, rather than going out and doing new things?	**YES**/NO
10. Do you feel you have more problems with memory than most?	**YES**/NO
11. Do you think it is wonderful to be alive now?	YES/**NO**
12. Do you feel pretty worthless the way you are now?	**YES**/NO
13. Do you feel full of energy?	YES/**NO**
14. Do you feel that your situation is hopeless?	**YES**/NO
15. Do you think that most people are better off than you are?	**YES**/NO

Answers in **bold** indicate depression. Although differing sensitivities and specificities have been obtained across studies, for clinical purposes a score >5 points is suggestive of depression and should warrant a follow-up interview. Scores >10 are almost always depression.

    ✍ https://dementiaresearch.org.au/wp-content/uploads/2016/06/geriatric_depression_scale_short.pdf

Montreal Cognitive Assessment (MoCA)

A freely available* cognitive screen, useful for stroke patients.

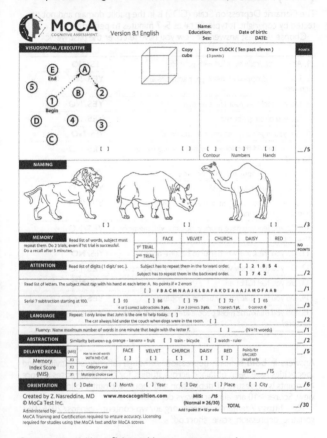

Copies are available at 🔗 https://mocacognition.com/
Copyright © Z. Nasreddine MD. Reproduced with permission.
*Successful completion of the official MoCA training and certification programme is required for healthcare and research professionals administering the MoCA Test. Permission and licensing agreement are required for clinical trials and research studies employing the MoCA Test and/or MoCA Score. The MoCA Test and MoCA Score are copyrighted and protected IP of MoCA Cognition.

The Brief Memory and Executive Test (BMET)

BMET is a freely available short cognitive screen designed to detect the cognitive deficit seen in patients with vascular cognitive impairment (VCI) due to cerebral small vessel disease.

Instructions and further details including scoring as well as downloads are available at ℘ https://www.cambridgestroke.com/bmetcognitivetesting.php

Brief Memory and Executive Test

Name

DOB   Date

Throughout the test, read the black italic text aloud to the patient.

Orientation

What is your full name?	☐	*Which date of the month is it?*	☐
What is your date of birth?	☐	*What year is it?*	☐
How old are you?	☐	*What is the season?*	☐
What day of the week is it?	☐	*What is the name of this place?*	☐
What month are we in now?	☐	*Which floor are we on?*	☐

Score 1 point per correct answer (max score 10) **TOTAL 1** ☐☐

Five Item Repetition Read out the words for all trials, 3 seconds per item.

Instructions: *Listen to the following words and try to remember them. When I have said them all please tell me the ones you remember.*

	Lion	Toe	Book	Light	Three	Trial Total
Trial 1	☐	☐	☐	☐	☐	☐
Trial 2	☐	☐	☐	☐	☐	☐
Trial 3	☐	☐	☐	☐	☐	☐

Score 1 point per correctly recalled word (max score 15) **TOTAL 2** ☐☐

Letter-Number Matching The patient must fill in the boxes in order (left-right) without skipping any boxes. Give sample item (appendix 1a)-explain any errors; Main test (appendix 1b) stopping after 45 seconds.

Instructions: *You see these letters each letter has its own number underneath. Look at the boxes (point); these have the numbers missing. Fill in the correct numbers as quickly as you can, one after the other and do not leave any out.*

Number completed in 45 seconds ☐☐   Errors ☐☐

Score 1 point per correctly filled space (max score 40). **TOTAL 3** ☐☐

Motor Sequencing: Sample test (appendix 2a); Main test (appendix 2b).
Present the sample item (explain any errors); followed by the main test. If errors are made, say *'that is not correct'*, draw a cross at that point and redirect to the previous point (continue timing throughout). Discontinue after 180 seconds.

Instructions: *Start here [point] and draw along the line; keep going until you reach the end [point]. It is okay to cross through the boxes. Don't worry about neatness. Have a go at this sample one. Begin.*

Main test: *This time draw along the line as quickly as you can.*

Score = Time taken to complete the main test (seconds). **TOTAL 4** ☐☐

B-MET

Brief Memory and Executive Test

Letter Sequencing: Sample test (appendix 3a); Main test (appendix 3b). The instructions are as for motor sequencing. Discontinue if the patient has not completed after 180 seconds.

Instructions: *Start here [point] and connect these letters in alphabetical order. Keep going until you reach the end [point].*

Main Test: *This time connect the letters as quickly as you can in alphabetical order, start here [point] and finish here [point]. If you make a mistake, I will correct you as you go along. Begin.*

Score = Time taken to complete the main test (seconds).	TOTAL 5

Letter–Number Sequencing: Sample test (appendix 4a); Main test (appendix 4b).
The instructions as for motor sequencing. Discontinue if the patient has not completed after 300 seconds.

Instructions: *[Demonstrating by pointing at the sample] In this task there are some numbers and letters. You start with number one and draw a line to the first letter in the alphabet [mimic drawing]. Now you draw a line from the A to the next number, which is two [make movement to the box with 2]. You keep going alternating between numbers and letters in order. Remember you have a number, then the first letter, then the next number and then the next letter and so on. Have a go with this practice one*

Main Test: *This time connect the numbers and letters as quickly as you can. Remember you have a number, then the first letter, then the next number and then the next letter. Start here [point] and finish here [point]. If you make a mistake, I will correct you as you go along. Begin.*

Score = Time taken to complete the task (seconds).	TOTAL 6

Five Item Memory (Delayed Recall) Check the boxes for the words remembered and record any additional words as intrusions.

Instructions: *Earlier, I asked you to remember some words. Can you tell me what they were?*

Lion ☐   Toe ☐   Book ☐   Light ☐   Three ☐   Total correct ☐

Additional words: Total Intrusions ☐

Score = Total correct minus total intrusions.	TOTAL 7

Five Item Memory (Delayed Recognition): Word list (appendix 5). Give the patient the word list (appendix 5) and record correct recognition and false positives

Instructions: *Please circle the words that I asked you to repeat earlier.*

Correctly recognized ☐

False Positives ☐

Score = Total correct minus false positives.	TOTAL 8

Brief Memory and Executive Test

Scoring An overall score greater than 7 is indicative of cognitive impairment.

	Impairment (>2SD below the population mean)	Mild impairment (>1.5 SD <2SD below the normal population mean)	Non-impaired	
TOTAL 1	0-5	6-8	9-10	Orientation
TOTAL 2	0-10	11-12	13-15	Working Memory
TOTAL 3	0-14	15-22	23-40	Processing speed
TOTAL 4	25-180	16-24	0-15	Motor speed
TOTAL 5	70-180	50-69	0-49	Executive
TOTAL 6	100-300	70-99	0-69	Executive
TOTAL 7	>0	0-1	1-5	Episodic
TOTAL 8	>1	1-2	2-5	Episodic
	Score 2 points per test falling in this category.	Score 1 point per test falling in this category.		
			TOTAL POINTS =	

Profiling For those patients with overall scores greater than 7 complete the profiling.

Orientation score **x 0.148** =   +

Letter sequencing **x 0.004** =   +

Delayed recall   **x - 0.095** =

TOTAL = [   ] X 100 = [   ]

Transfer to the grid below.

AD											SVD
-6+	-5	-4	-3	-2	-1	0	1	2	3	4	5+

Further reading

National Institutes of Health Stroke Scale (NIHSS)

Goldstein LB, Bertels C, Davis JN (1989). Interrater reliability of the nih stroke scale. *Arch Neuro* **46**, 660–662.

Stockbridge MD, Kelly L, Newman-Norlund S, et al. (2024). New picture stimuli for the NIH stroke scale: a validation study. *Stroke* **55**(2), 443–451.

Rivermead Mobility Index

Collen FM, Wade DT, Robb GF, Bradshaw CM (1991). The Rivermead Mobility Index: a further development of the Rivermead Motor Assessment. *Int Disabil Stud* **13**, 50–54.

Modified Ashworth Scale

Bohannon RW, Smith MB (1987). Interrater reliability of a modified Ashworth scale of muscle spasticity. *Phys Ther* **67**, 206–207.

Modified Tardieu Scale

Boyd RN, Graham HK (1999). Objective measurement of clinical findings in the use of botulinum toxin type A for the management of children with cerebral palsy. *Eur J Neurol* **6**, s23.

Tardieu G, Shentoub S, Delarue R (1954). A la recherche d'une technique de mesure de la spasticite. *Rev Neurol* **91**, 143–144.

Modified Rankin Scale

Bonita R, Beaglehole R (1988). Modification of Rankin Scale: recovery of motor function after stroke. *Stroke* **19**, 1497–1500.

Rankin J (1957). Cerebral vascular accidents in patients over the age of 60. *Scott Med J* **2**, 200–215.

Van Swieten JC, Koudstaal PJ, Visser MC, Schouten HJ, van Gijn J (1988). Interobserver agreement for the assessment of handicap in stroke patients. *Stroke* **19**, 604–607.

Patient Health Questionnaire (PHQ-9)

Kroenke K, Spitzer RL, Williams JB (2001). The PHQ-9: validity of a brief depression severity measure. *J Gen Intern Med* **16**, 606–613.

Hamilton Rating Scale for Depression (HAMDS)

Hamilton M (1967). Development of a rating scale for primary depressive illness. *Br J Soc Clin Psychol* **6**(4), 278–296.

Geriatric Depression Scale (GDS): short version

Marwijk HW, Wallace P, de Bock GH, et al. (1995). Evaluation of the feasibility, reliability and diagnostic value of shortened versions of the Geriatric Depression Scale. *Br J Gen Pract* **45**, 195–199.

Sheikh JI, Yesavage JA (1986). Geriatric Depression Scale (GDS): recent evidence and development of a shorter version. *Clin Gerontol* **5**, 165–173.

Montreal Cognitive Assessment (MoCA)

Chiti G, Pantoni L (2014). Use of Montreal Cognitive Assessment in patients with stroke. *Stroke* **45**(10), 3135–3140.

Nasreddine ZS, Phillips NA, Bédirian V, et al. (2005). The Montreal Cognitive Assessment, MoCA: a brief screening tool for mild cognitive impairment. *J Am Geriatr Soc* **53**, 695–699.

The Brief Memory and Executive Test (BMET)

Brookes RL, Hollocks MJ, Khan U, et al. (2015). The Brief Memory and Executive Test (BMET) for detecting vascular cognitive impairment in small vessel disease: a validation study. *BMC Med* **13**, 51.

Useful websites

Useful websites

Stroke organizations

https://www.ninds.nih.gov/health-information/patient-caregiver-education/brain-attack-coalition

The Brain Attack Coalition is a group of American professional, voluntary, and governmental entities dedicated to reducing the occurrence, disabilities, and death associated with stroke. The site is a good resource of guidelines for stroke treatment.

https://www.stroke.org/en/

Official website of the American Stroke Association.

https://biasp.org/

Official website of the British & Irish Association of Stroke Physicians (BIASP).

https://www.stroke.org.uk/

The Stroke Association is a UK charity for stroke survivors. The site has a lot of useful background facts about stroke and a wealth of patient information.

https://www.world-stroke.org/

The World Stroke Organization (WSO) was established in October 2006 from the merger of the International Stroke Society (ISS) and the World Stroke Federation (WSF), the two lead organizations representing stroke globally. The website has details of presentations from annual meetings and is a window into global stroke care.

https://eso-stroke.org/

European Stroke Organization website with European guidelines and virtual stroke university with compendium of previous European Stroke Conference lectures and symposia.

https://wfnr.co.uk

The World Federation for NeuroRehabilitation (WFNR) is a multidisciplinary organization open to any professional with an interest in neurological rehabilitation. The organization exists to act as a forum of communication between those with an interest in the subject.

Guidelines

https://eso-stroke.org/guidelines/eso-guideline-directory/

European Stroke Organization guidelines

https://www.strokeguideline.org/

The National Clinical Guideline for Stroke for the UK and Ireland provides authoritative, evidence-based practice guidance.

https://www.nice.org.uk/search?q=stroke

Evidence-based resource for stroke. National Institute for Health and Care Excellence (NICE) stroke guidance.

https://www.heart.org/en/professional/quality-improvement/get-with-the-guidelines/get-with-the-guidelines-stroke
Get with the guidelines. Helpful guidance on the implementation of American Stroke Guidelines

Teaching and education resources
https://www.world-stroke-academy.org/
World Stroke Academy: Excellent free resource run by the World Stroke Organization with webinars, e-courses, podcasts, case studies and more.

https://stroke-education.org.uk/
The Stroke-Specific Education Framework (SSEF) describes the knowledge and skills required for those working in stroke health and care services. The framework, based on the 20 quality markers of the National Stroke Strategy (2007), aims to provide a structured and standardized approach to education and training for those working within, and affected by, stroke.

http://www.stroke-in-stoke.info/education-and-training
This provides links to stroke training sites on the internet and to stroke-relevant courses and conferences

https://www.ninds.nih.gov/health-information/stroke/assess-and-treat/nih-stroke-scale
Assess risk by using the NIH Stroke Scale. Developed through research supported by NINDS, the widely used NIH Stroke Scale helps healthcare providers assess the severity of a stroke.

https://clinical-sciences.ed.ac.uk/edinburgh-imaging/education-teaching/short-courses/training-tools/acute-cerebral-ct-evaluation-stroke-study-access
Acute Cerebral CT Evaluation of Stroke Study (ACCESS) helps you to learn about how to read acute stroke CT scans. Participation also helps to increase the amount of data available on observer reliability.

https://clinical-sciences.ed.ac.uk/edinburgh-imaging/education-teaching/short-courses/training-tools/acute-cta-for-thrombectomy-in-stroke-actats
Acute CTA for Thrombectomy in Stroke (ACTATS) teaches about CT & CTA review & interpretation in the context of thrombectomy.

https://radiopaedia.org/?lang=gb
Superb imaging teaching site

Index

For the benefit of digital users, indexed terms that span two pages (e.g., 52–53) may, on occasion, appear on only one of those pages.

Tables, figures, and boxes are indicated by an italic *t*, *f*, and *b* following the page number.